Surgical Procedures for Urology

Surgical Procedures for Urology

Editor: Chris Patterson

AMERICAN
MEDICAL PUBLISHERS
www.americanmedicalpublishers.com

AMERICAN
MEDICAL PUBLISHERS
www.americanmedicalpublishers.com

Cataloging-in-Publication Data

Surgical procedures for urology / edited by Chris Patterson.
p. cm.
Includes bibliographical references and index.
ISBN 979-8-88740-481-3
1. Genitourinary organs--Surgery. 2. Urinary organs--Surgery. 3. Urology.
4. Surgery, Operative. I. Patterson, Chris.
RD571 .S87 2023
61746--dc23

American Medical Publishers,
41 Flatbush Avenue,
1st Floor, New York,
NY 11217, USA

ISBN 979-8-88740-481-3 (Hardback)

Contents

Preface

The scientific, clinical, and surgical aspects related to the study of urine and the genitourinary tract in health and disease is called urology. It involves the management of urinary tract systems and reproductive organs. There are several surgical procedures in urology including cystoscopy, orchiopexy, penile plication, hysterectomy, vasectomy, male circumcision, and penile implants and prosthesis. It also includes surgical procedures to diagnose and treat the conditions of the prostate. Some of the common prostate procedures are transurethral resection of the prostate (TURP), transurethral incision of the prostate (TUIP), and transurethral needle ablation (TUNA). TURP is a surgical procedure that uses minimally invasive technique for treating enlarged prostate. A surgical procedure called penile plication is conducted for treating penis curvature caused by Peyronie's disease. This book provides significant information of this discipline to help develop a good understanding of the surgical procedures used in urology. It presents researches and studies performed by experts across the globe. The extensive content of this book provides the students and professionals of urology with a thorough understanding of the subject.

The researches compiled throughout the book are authentic and of high quality, combining several disciplines and from very diverse regions from around the world. Drawing on the contributions of many researchers from diverse countries, the book's objective is to provide the readers with the latest achievements in the area of research. This book will surely be a source of knowledge to all interested and researching the field.

In the end, I would like to express my deep sense of gratitude to all the authors for meeting the set deadlines in completing and submitting their research chapters. I would also like to thank the publisher for the support offered to us throughout the course of the book. Finally, I extend my sincere thanks to my family for being a constant source of inspiration and encouragement.

Editor

1

Clinical efficacy of enhanced recovery after surgery in percutaneous nephrolithotripsy

Qing Li[2*†], Li Wan[1†], Shucheng Liu[1], Mingyong Li[1], Libo Chen[1], Zhengwu Hou[1] and Wang Zhang[1]

Abstract

Background: To evaluate the feasibility, safety, applied value and efficacy of enhanced recovery after surgery (ERAS) for PCNL for the treatment of renal calculi. Although the ERAS is applied for many urological diseases, its application in percutaneous nephrolithotripsy (PCNL) is still limited.

Methods: This was a prospective study of patients admitted to hospital January and December 2018 and who were only diagnosed with renal calculi and excepted for serious or uncontrollable basic diseases and patients with multiple operation history and medication history. Patients were randomized 1:1 to the ERAS and traditional operation groups starting on the day before operation and end on the day of discharge. Each group was 118 cases. The stone clearance rate, visual analogue scale (VAS) pain score, the occurrence of perirenal hematoma and effusion, the incidence of extravasation of urine, the incidence of fever, bleeding and blood transfusion, and postoperative hospital stay were observed.

Results: The stone clearance rates were similar between the two groups (ERAS: 93.2% (109/117) vs. traditional: 89.8% (106/118), $P=0.800$). The operation time was similar in the two groups (ERAS: 54 ± 12 vs. traditional: 58 ± 11 min, $P=0.656$). VAS pain score that was 0.79 ± 0.76 in the ERAS group at 4 h after surgery and was significantly lower than 2.79 ± 0.98 in the traditional group ($P<0.0001$). The total complication rate was 15 cases in the ERAS group and 22 cases in the traditional group ($P=0.573$). There were no difference in costs ($21{,}348\pm2404$ vs. $21{,}597\pm2293$ RMB, $P=0.529$).

Conclusions: ERAS perioperative management in PCNL was feasible, was without additional complications, and had well economic and social benefits. It is worth of clinical promotion and application.

Keywords: Enhanced recovery after surgery, Perioperative management, Percutaneous nephrolithotripsy, Renal calculi

Background

Renal calculi are one of the most common diseases in urology. The reported lifetime prevalence vary from 1 to 20% [1] and appears to be increasing [2]. A national cross-sectional study suggested that the prevalence of renal calculi in Chinese adults was 6.4% [3]. Percutaneous nephrolithotripsy (PCNL) is one of important surgery methods to treat renal calculi [4].

Enhanced recovery after surgery (ERAS), also called "fast-track surgery" (FTS) can effectively reduce surgical stress and complications, accelerate postoperative rehabilitation, and reduce the physiological, psychological, and economic burden of surgeries [5–7]. ERAS Society in Europe had already popularized the ERAS concept

*Correspondence: liq73@163.com
†Qing Li and Li Wan contributed equally to this work
[2] Department of Urology, The Fifth Affiliated Hospital of Southern Medical University, Guangzhou 510900, China

in multiple fields: gastrointestinal surgery, hepatobiliary surgery, cardiothoracic surgery, and many others [8, 9].

Aim of our study was to examine the safety, feasibility, economic value, and applied value of ERAS perioperative concept in PCNL for the treatment of renal calculi. The urological ERAS in China is still at the trial stage, without clear guidance or support of high-quality evidence-based medicine, while ERAS has been successfully applied for a variety of urological diseases in western countries [10, 11]. Application of ERAS perioperative management in PCNL could help accelerate patients' postoperative rehabilitation and reduce postoperative physiologic and psychological stress response. Considering the economic and social benefits, such a strategy is worthy of clinical trial and application. Therefore, The results should help popularize the application of ERAS in PCNL, which is of clinical importance because of the important numbers of patients undergoing PCNL each year.

Methods

Study design and patients

This was a prospective study of patients (16–85 years of age) admitted to the hospital between January and December 2018 and who were preoperatively diagnosed with renal calculi by abdominal computer tomography (CT) [12]. The study was approved by the ethics committee of the First Affiliated Hospital of University of South China. All patients provided written informed consent prior to any study procedure. For a type 1 error of 0.05 and a power of 0.8, the number of participants needed for each group was 111. Considering that some patients may quit this study, we aimed to recruit 120 participants per group (240 in total).

The indications and contraindications of PCNL were as published [12]. The inclusion criteria were: (1) diagnosed with renal calculus by abdominal CT; (2) scheduled to undergo PCNL; (3) ASA grade I or II; (4) 16–85 years of age; (5) no uncontrolled renal insufficiency (CDK $\leq$ 3), uncontrolled diabetes (postprandial blood glucose $\leq$ 11.1 mmol/L), hypertension (systolic blood pressure $\leq$ 140 mmHg and diastolic blood pressure $\leq$ 100 mmHg), cardiac insufficiency (NYHA $\leq$ 3), and chronic obstructive pulmonary disease (mMRC $\leq$ 3).

The exclusion criteria were: (1) massive intrarenal calculi (stone length > 4 cm); (2) bilateral renal multiple calculi; (3) severe upper urinary tract malformations such as horseshoe kidney malformation, ureteropelvic stenosis (UPJO), giant ureter disease (POM), and other combined calculi that requires complicated surgery, longer operative time, multiple surgeries, or other factors affecting efficacy evaluation; (4) disease considered to affect the process of surgery, postoperative rehabilitation, prognosis and cost; (5) patient with septic shock; (6) requirement for emergency surgery like catheterization or fistula; (7) ipsilateral upper urinary tract surgery history, (8) active severe infection,(as PCT > 0.5, leukocyte + in urine and other patients with UROGENOUS sepsis diagnosis). (9) Patients taking anticoagulant drugs such as aspirin and warfarin in recent 1–2 weeks. The surgery could be performed only when the coagulation function was with normal results.

PCNL was performed by a single surgeon under general anaesthesia in both group. After induction of anaesthesia, with the patient in lithotomy, a 4-F urethral catheter was inserted into the ureter via cystoscopy. Then the patient was repositioned to prone. Then, an 18-G access needle was placed into the preferred calyx under ultrasound guidance. A tiny incision was made in the skin and fascia, and then the 18-F fascial dilator was used to dilate the nephrostomy tract to pass the 18-F semi-rigid plastic sheath. Then, a 9.8-F, 33-cm semi-rigid ureteroscope (Richard Wolf Medical Instruments, Ver- non Hills, IL, USA) was introduced to the sheath. The renal stones were broken into pieces using Holmium laser. Fragmented stones too large for spontaneous passage from the ureter were removed using a grasper. Then a ureter stent was inserted into ureter anterogradely after ureteric catheter removed. Finally, A 16-F nephrostomy tube was placed into calyx through the sheath, then the sheath was removed.

Randomization and blind method

The patients were randomized 1:1 to the ERAS and traditional operation groups using sequential sealed opaque envelopes prepared by a third party biostatistician using a random number table and used double blind method.

Preoperative preparation in all patients

Routine preoperative preparation included blood routine, midcourse urine routine, urine bacterial culture and drug sensitivity test, liver and kidney function, blood coagulation function, intravenous pyelography (IVP), and urinary CT to determine location, size, and number of the stone, split renal function, and anatomical structure. Sensitive antibiotics were used empirically [12] if there were symptoms of urinary tract infection before surgery.

Preoperative preparation in the ERAS group

In the ERAS group, the patients were let to initially accept and cooperate. Education about the ERAS concept was carried out. The patients received detailed preoperative conversation, including PCNL advantages and disadvantages, advantages of compound anesthesia, rough expenses, perioperative complications (such as bleeding, infection, residue, stones recurrence, early manifestations, prognosis, and treatment measures), and the importance of cooperation. Preoperative nervous hypertension was managed by sublingual administration of 0.5 mg of nitroglycerin (or 50 mg of isosorbide mononitrate sustained-release caspsule) and comforting to reduce preoperative anxiety and mental stress. Blood glucose was monitored and controlled to < 6 mmol/L to prevent stress hyperglycemia and insulin resistance.

No routine preoperative bowel preparation was performed, except for patients with long-term constipation and dry stool hardening, who received cleaning enema. Otherwise, all patients were fasted from solid food for 8 h and received 250 mL of 5% glucose solution 2 h before surgery (diabetic patients received xylitol instead of glucose).

For multimodal analgesia, preemptive analgesia was used 30 min before surgery using parecoxib 40 mg or flurbiprofen 50 mg infusion, and dexamethasone 10 mg static infusion for reducing postoperative wound inflammation, improving the antiemetic effect of 5-HT_3 receptor blocker, and reducing postoperative insulin resistance. At 30 min before surgery, third generation cephalosporin was given as prophylaxis.

Preoperative preparation in the ERAS group

The patients were informed of the surgical risks and postoperative complications, and their understanding was obtained. Traditional preoperative intestinal preparation was carried out. The patients fasted overnight and were fasted from all liquids at 4 o'clock in the morning. Parenteral nutrition (glucose and sodium chloride 500 mL iv, vitamins, and potassium chloride) was given to the patients scheduled for surgery late in the day. Third-generation cephalosporin was given as prophylaxis 30 min before surgery.

Intraoperative management in the ERAS group

The patient underwent PCNL under general anesthesia using compound general intravenous anesthesia and epidural anesthesia or paravertebral nerve block anesthesia (ultrasound-guided). Intraoperative temperature was routinely maintained over 36 °C. At the end of the operation, 5 mg of silansetron (or 50 mL of granisetron sodium chloride) were given intravenously to prevent vomiting, and 2 mL of flumacinib were given intravenously to reverse anesthesia.

Intraoperative management in the traditional group

The patients received traditional general anesthesia. At the end of the operation, 2 mL of flumacinib were given to reverse anesthesia.

Postoperative management in the ERAS group

Discharge procedures were completed 1 day after the removal of the nephrostomy tube and when conforming to the discharge criteria. Postoperative visual analog scale (VAS) was pain was used. When coming back to the ward, intramuscular injection of parecoxib 40 mg (or flurbiprofen 50 mg intravenous drip) was done to stop the pain and 15 mL of saline was given orally. One hour later (based on the half-life of 2.5 h for sufentanil), the VAS score was determined again. If VAS was > 4, 2 mL of diclofanac sodium and lidocaine hydrochloride were injected to relieve pain. On the 1st day after surgery, acesodyne was changed to ibuprofen (15 mL orally qd) or celecoxib (200 mg orally qd). At 4 h after surgery, 250 mL of 5% glucose (xylitol for diabetic patients) were given orally, and 5 mg of methoxyclozapine were intramuscularly injected to avoid vomiting. Another dose of 5 mg could be given if nausea still occurred. If there was no serious discomfort, the patients returned to liquid diet 6 h after surgery, and to normal diet the next day. For elderly patients, 0.7 g of Malen capsule orally (bid) or 20 mL of Simo (If it can't be purchased, Macrogol 4000 powder can be used instead) decoction orally (tid) were given when resuming diet to avoid constipation. Postoperative intravenous fluid volume was reduced beyond 1500 mL. If there was no obvious fever, the nephrostomy tube was clamped 2 or 3 days after surgery. After CT, the catheter was removed. Suitable activity on the bed was encouraged on the first day postoperatively. A mild activity out bed was encouraged on the 3 or 4 days after surgery (Additional file 1: Supplementary Table S1).

Postoperative management in the traditional group

If the patient complained of unbearable pain, an intramuscular injection of 2 mL of diclofanac sodium and lidocaine hydrochloride was given to relieve pain. Hyperemesis was broken by an intramuscular injection of 5 mg of methoxyclozapine, and 50 mL of intravenous granisetron were added if there were no improvement. The patient was allowed to drink postoperatively and received liquid diet after the first defecation. Absolute bed rest was prescribed for 3–4 days after surgery. CT was performed on the 3rd or 4th days after surgery. The nephrostomy tube was clipped and bed exercises were encouraged. The urethral catheter was removed 4 or 5 days after surgery, and 5–6 days for nephrostomy tube (Additional file 1: Supplementary Table S1).

Observational indicators

General information, such as sex, age, stone size, stone location, diagnosis, and comorbidities were assessed at baseline. Stone clearance rate [13] and operation time were assessed immediately after operation. Complications, RIRS rate, costs, renal hemorrhage (defined as hematuresis and hemoglobin decrease [14]), indwelling time (nephrostomy tube and catheter), and length of stay were assessed just before discharge. Secondary hemorrhage, urinary fistula, perirenal hematoma, recurrent calculus, and acute renal dysfunction were assessed at 1 month after discharge by follow-up.

Endpoints

The primary endpoints were VAS, blood loss, extubation time, length of hospital stays, costs, and 30-day follow-up that including secondary hemorrhage, urinary fistula, perirenal hematoma, stone recurrence, acute renal insufficiency and other adverse complications. The secondary endpoints were operation time, stone clearance rate, incidence of RIRS, hemorrhage, and blood transfusion.

Discharge criteria

The patients we discharge one day after removing nephrostomy tube, without fever, no chills, no septic shock, no active bleeding, imaging examination showed that D-J tube location was reasonable, defecated, no nausea, no vomiting, no abdominal pain, no ileus after eating, fistula not obviously bleeding and leakage, no obvious hematuria, and ambulation [15]. There was no stone residue (residual stone <5 mm) [9] or residual stone (residual stone >5 mm) that did not cause urinary tract obstruction without will for a second operation.

Statistical analysis

R 3.4.3 (https://www.r-project.org) and R Studio 1.1.385 (https://www.rstudio.com) were used for data analysis, based on a per protocol approach. Continuous data were tested for normal distribution using the Kolmogorov–Smirnov test, are presented as mean ± standard deviation (normal distribution) and median (range) (non-normal distribution), and were analyzed using the Student t test or the Mann–Whitney U test. Categorical data are presented as frequencies and were analyzed using the Pearson chi-square test or the Fisher exact test, as appropriate. P values ≤ 0.05 were considered to be statistically significant.

Results

Characteristics of the patients

Figure 1 presents the patient flowchart. Three hundred patients were assessed for eligibility and 65 were excluded; 235 patients were randomized to the ERAS group (n = 117) and to the traditional group (n = 118).

The average age of the patients in the ERAS group was 51 ± 11 years, and the average stone size was 21.0 ± 9.4 mm. The average age of the patients in the traditional operation group was 54 ± 12 years old, and the average stone size was 19.2 ± 8.2 mm. There were no significant differences between the two groups in sex, age, stone size, and surgical method (all $P > 0.05$) (Table 1).

Surgical outcomes

Table 2 presents the surgical outcomes of the patients. None of the patients had failed puncture and had a conversion to open surgery. The ERAS group had a stone clearance rate of 93.2% (109/117), which is not significantly different from 89.8% in the traditional group (106/118) ($P = 0.800$). The average operation time in the ERAS group was 54 ± 12 min, which was not significantly different from 58 ± 11 min in the traditional group ($P = 0.656$). The immediate VAS pain score in the ERAS group was 0.01 ± 0.09, and was 0.39 ± 0.49 in the traditional group ($P = 0.176$). VAS pain score that was 0.79 ± 0.76 in the ERAS group at 4 h after surgery and was significantly lower than 2.79 ± 0.98 in the traditional group ($P < 0.0001$).

Complications

Table 3 presents the complications. The decrease in hemoglobin was 4.79 ± 5.63 g/L in the ERAS group, which was significantly lower than 8.34 ± 7.23 g/L in the traditional group ($P < 0.01$). In the ERAS group, the urine color was slightly red on postoperative day 1, and normalized with symptomatic treatment including hemostasis, with significantly smaller number of patients with slightly red urine before discharge than in the traditional surgery group (2 vs. 10, $P = 0.04$). None of the patients were observed with impairment of liver, gallbladder, spleen, pancreas, intestines, or other organs. One case of postoperative renal hemorrhage occurred in each of the two groups, and they were relieved after transfusion and selective renal artery embolization ($P > 0.999$).

No obvious perirenal hematoma and urinary extravasation were found at 1-month follow-up. There were no significant difference in postoperative SIRS risk between the ERAS and traditional groups ($P > 0.999$). The total complication rate was 15 cases in the ERAS group and 22 cases in the traditional group ($P = 0.573$). Therefore, ERAS did not increase the incidence of postoperative complications.

Discussion

Surgery is a process of treating and repairing lesions and injury but it also involves significant trauma [9]. The stress response caused by the trauma can directly affect the convalescence [16, 17]. There are many causes of stress during the entire process of an operation, such as mental stress before the operation, hunger, thirst, additional procedures, complications, nausea, etc.

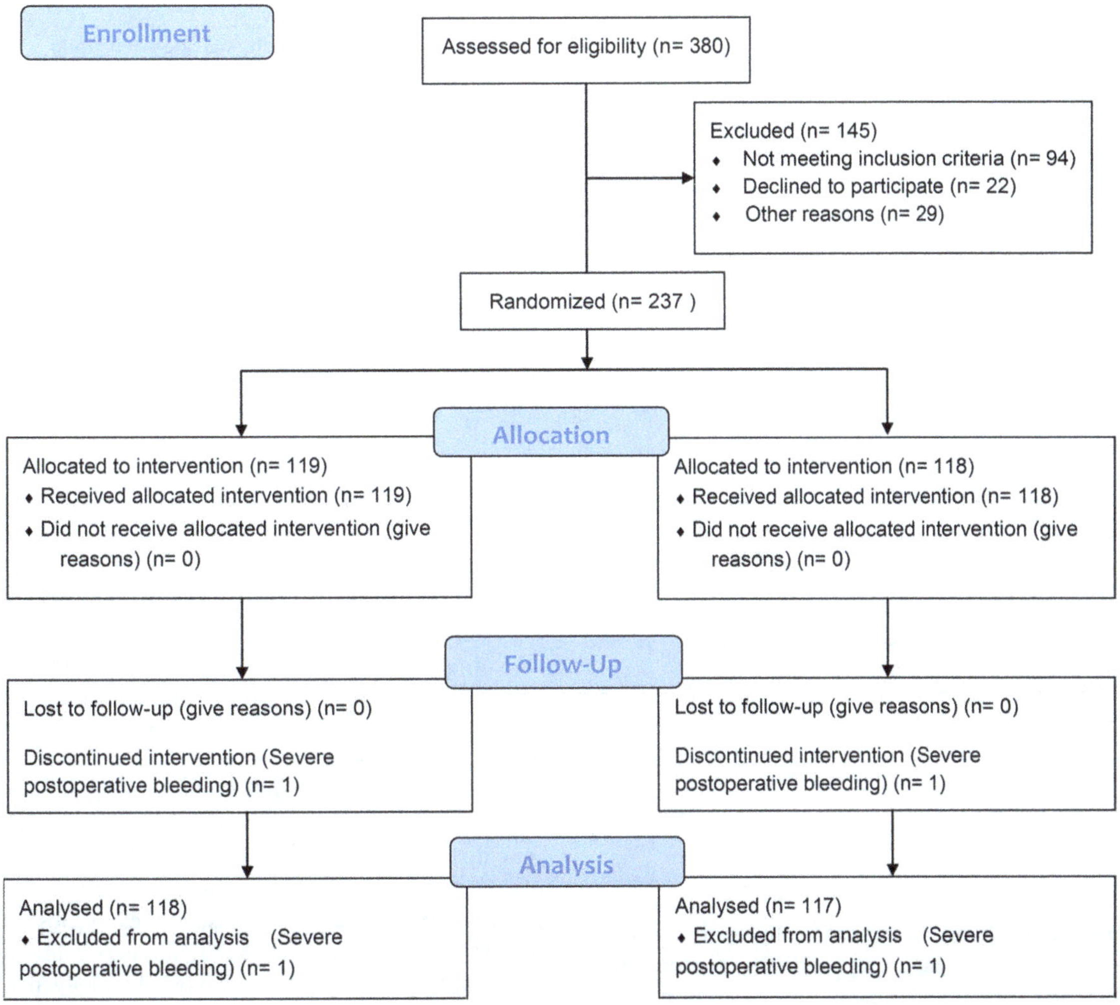

Fig. 1 Patient flowchart

Table 1 Baseline characteristics of the patients

Group	ERAS (117)	Traditional (118)	X^2/t	P
Male/female	72/45	74/44	0.0026	0.9594
Age (years)	51 ± 11	54 ± 12	− 1.4834	0.1393
Stone size (mm)	21.03 ± 9.43	19.19 ± 8.16	1.6653	0.0973
Stone location (ureteropelvic/renal)	51/66	53,564	0.0054	0.9416
Hb	129 ± 18	131 ± 17	0.3942	0.6938

Preoperative education is a key factor for ERAS. Effective preoperative education can help patients better understanding the treatment process, reducing psychological pressure and improving patients' compliance. In advance of analgesia, using anti-inflammatory drugs and long-term fasting was traditionally considered to significantly reduce nausea, vomiting, and aspiration during anesthesia, but this approach increases the burden on the patients. In the ERAS group, shorter preoperative fasting and the preoperative oral administration of sugary liquid can avoid the loss of body fluid and then prevent hypotension and electrolyte disturbance. No intraoperative aspiration occurred in the patients and the incidence of postoperative nausea and vomiting was lower than that in the traditional group, as supported by a previous study [18].

The traditional approach to surgery believes that nephrostomy tube indwelling after PCNL can play a role in pressing the puncture channel, strengthening hemostasis, strengthening drainage, reducing urine extravasation, and reducing the risk of infection. The patients are also more amenable to a second stage surgery in case of residual stones [19]. Nevertheless, the indwelling nephrostomy tube will increase patient discomfort,

Table 2 Surgical characteristics

Observation item	ERAS group	Traditional operation group	P
Operation time (min)	54.2 ± 12	58 ± 11	0.6561
Decrease of hemoglobin (g/L)	4.79 ± 5.63	8.34 ± 7.23	< 0.0001
Stone clearance rate immediately after surgery	93.2%	89.8%	0.7997
Postoperative VAS	0.01 ± 0.09	0.39 ± 0.49	0.176*
VAS 4 h after surgery	0.79 ± 0.76	2.79 ± 0.98	< 0.0001*
Renal bleeding before discharge	2	10	0.0403
Fever > 38 °C	5	6	> 0.999
Postoperative hospitalization (days)	4.6 ± 1.0	6.2 ± 1.1	< 0.0001
Indwelling fistula time (days)	3.6 ± 1.0	5.2 ± 1.1	< 0.0001
Indwelling catheter time (days)	2.6 ± 1.0	4.2 ± 1.1	< 0.0001
Hospitalization costs (RMB)	21,348 ± 2404	21,597 ± 2293	0.5289
Thrombosis of renal artery	0	0	> 0.999
Postoperative shock, death, organ damage and MODS	0	0	> 0.999

* Mann–Whitney U test

Table 3 Complications

Items	ERAS (n = 117)	Traditional (n = 118)	P
Hematuresis	2	10	0.040
SIRS	5	6	> 0.999
Total complications	15	22	0.573
Renal arterial embolization	1	1	> 0.999

with breathing-related pain, hindering early exercise, and increasing the dosage of painkillers, postoperative hospitalization time, and costs [20]. Therefore, some authors believe that early removing or even no nephrostomy tube will not increase the risk of bleeding, infection, and urine extravasation [21]. In the present study, the decrease in postoperative hemoglobin in the ERAS group was significantly lower than in traditional group. In addition, the frequency of hematuria at discharge was also lower for the ERAS group. Mild hematuria was managed using vitamin K_1 30 mg and phenol-sulfoethylamine 1.0 g intravenously, rehydration, and diuresis [22]. It may be hypothesized that the main cause of postoperative bleeding is iatrogenic [23] and contact friction between the tube and the renal pelvis mucosa. ERAS can reduce the indwelling fistula time, lessening pain, and increasing surgery acceptability and compliance with the surgeons' orders, reducing the adverse reactions [7]. Although it cannot reduce the inherent risk of renal bleeding after PCNL at the surgical technique level, it has meaningful effect on reducing the inflammatory response, traumatic stress, fistula friction of oozing blood, pain, and discomfort. Preemptive analgesia and compound anesthesia can effectively reduce the intraoperative anesthesia load and resuscitation time, which are safe and effective during anesthesia resuscitation. Postoperative active analgesia can alleviate pain, so that patients would not refuse to resume exercise because of pain, and also reduce the adverse reactions of the removal of nephrostomy tube and urethral catheter.

It is well known that deficient nutrition is detrimental to postoperative recovery [24]. After major surgery, it may increase hospitalization time and costs [25]. Preoperative nutritional deficiency is an important reason of postoperative metabolic stress, especially postoperative insulin resistance, and it usually appears a few minutes after surgery and continues for weeks or even months. This will lead to weakness and increase mortality by 43% in severe patients and the incidence of postoperative complications such as sepsis and kidney failure by 40–50% [26, 27]. Therefore, shortening perioperative fasting, feeding oral energy mixture preoperatively, reducing the liquid load, and controlling blood glucose during hospitalization are conducive to reducing stress and accelerating recovery, significantly improving immune function, nutritional status, and organ function [5, 6]. In the present study, there were no differences in costs between the two groups, which might be because of using some specific drugs during ERAS perioperative management, and because the postoperative hospitalization time was shorter 1.6 ± 0.1 days.

Although the ERAS had been wildly developed and applied in urology, there are several limitations to the present study. First, the application of ERAS in urology, especially for minimally invasive urology surgeries such as PCNL, is still relatively limited. The sample size was limited and from a single center, and the follow-up was short, leading to bias. Furthermore, the lack of quality of evidence-based medical evidence prevented a formal sample size analysis [28]. Conclusions for safety, efficacy, economy, and feasibility still need to be confirmed and supported by large-scale randomized controlled studies and long-term follow-up. Second, the implementation of ERAS could not be performed by a single clinician. Its success requires the cooperation and support of physicians, surgeons, nurses, and anesthesiologists [29]. Therefore, there are many possible sources of variability and bias. Nevertheless, with the joint efforts of various professional medical staff, ERAS will achieve greater development and benefit more patients.

Conclusions

In conclusion, on the basis of the strict controlled surgical indications and skillful operation, the application of the perioperative ERAS concept in PCNL accelerates rehabilitation and effectively reduces the stress response, and it is a safe and feasible management strategy for PCNL. Furthermore, ERAS has advantages of relieving postoperative pain, shortening hospitalization time and cost, accelerating bed turnover, and improving medical experience, which have socioeconomic value. Therefore, ERAS for PCNL is worth promoting in clinical practice.

Abbreviations

ERAS: enhanced recovery after surgery; PCNL: percutaneous nephrolithotripsy; VAS: visual analogue scale; FTS: fast-track surgery; PCT: procalcitonin; CT: computer tomography; UPJO: ureteropelvic junction obstruction; IVP: intravenous pyelography; VAS: visual analog scale.

Acknowledgements

None.

Authors' contributions

QL and LW carried out the studies, participated in collecting data, and drafted the manuscript. SL and ML and LC performed the statistical analysis and participated in its design. ZH, and WZ helped to draft the manuscript. All authors read and approved the final manuscript.

Competing interests

All authors declare that they have no competing interests.

Author details

[1] Department of Urology, The First Affiliated Hospital of University of South China, Hengyang 421001, China. [2] Department of Urology, The Fifth Affiliated Hospital of Southern Medical University, Guangzhou 510900, China.

References

1. Scales CD Jr, Smith AC, Hanley JM, Saigal CS. Urologic diseases in America P. Prevalence of kidney stones in the United States. Eur Urol. 2012;62:160–5. https://doi.org/10.1016/j.eururo.2012.03.052.
2. Turney BW, Reynard JM, Noble JG, Keoghane SR. Trends in urological stone disease. BJU Int. 2012;109:1082–7. https://doi.org/10.1111/j.1464-410X.2011.10495.x.
3. Zeng G, Mai Z, Xia S, Wang Z, Zhang K, Wang L, et al. Prevalence of kidney stones in China: an ultrasonography based cross-sectional study. BJU Int. 2017;120:109–16. https://doi.org/10.1111/bju.13828
4. Türk C, Petřík A, Sarica K, Seitz C, Skolarikos A, Straub M, Knoll T. EAU guidelines on interventional treatment for urolithiasis. Eur Urol. 2016;69(3):475–82.
5. Surgery EGfERa. Chinese expert consensus on enhanced recovery after surgery in perioperative management. Surg J Chin. 2016;54:413–8.
6. CEgoCCsfpae. Chinese consensus of enhanced recovery after surgery for colorectal surgery. Chin J Gastroenterol Surg. 2015;18:785–7.
7. Jiang ZW, Li N, Li JS. The concept and clinical significance of fast tract surgery. Chin J Surg Pract. 2007;27:131–3.
8. Mortensen K, Nilsson M, Slim K, Schafer M, Mariette C, Braga M, et al. Consensus guidelines for enhanced recovery after gastrectomy: Enhanced Recovery After Surgery (ERAS(R)) Society recommendations. Br J Surg. 2014;101:1209–29. https://doi.org/10.1002/bjs.9582.
9. Wilmore DW, Kehlet H. Management of patients in fast track surgery. BMJ. 2001;322:473–6.
10. Abou-Haidar H, Abourbih S, Braganza D, Qaoud TA, Lee L, Carli F, et al. Enhanced recovery pathway for radical prostatectomy: implementation and evaluation in a universal healthcare system. Can Urol Assoc J. 2014;8:418–23. https://doi.org/10.5489/cuaj.2114.
11. Dutton TJ, Daugherty MO, Mason RG, McGrath JS. Implementation of the Exeter enhanced recovery programme for patients undergoing radical cystectomy. BJU Int. 2014;113:719–25. https://doi.org/10.1111/bju.12533.
12. Yan QB, Ye ZQ, Sun YH. Guidelines for the diagnosis and treatment of urological diseases in China. Urolithiasis. 2014;2014:132–4.
13. Fan D, Song L, Xie D, Hu M, Peng Z, Liao X, et al. A comparison of supracostal and infracostal access approaches in treating renal and upper ureteral stones using MPCNL with the aid of a patented system. BMC Urol. 2015;15:102. https://doi.org/10.1186/s12894-015-0097-3.
14. Gao S. Clinical application of interventional therapy for renal massive hemorrhage after PCNL. Chin Imag J Integr Tradit West Med. 2012;10:559–60.
15. Ping QR, Yan RP, Wang JS. Percutaneous nephrolithotomy combined with flexible ureteroscopy for complex nephrolithiasis. Chin J Minim Invasive Surg. 2017;2017:35–9.
16. Yan Q, Du D. Comparison of percutaneous nephrolithotomy and retrograde intrarenal surgery for residual kidney stones after percutaneous nephrolithotomy. Chin J Endourol. 2017;2017:32–5.
17. Han JM, Zhen ZD. Sodium phosphate Vs castor oil plus manicol in colon preparation. Chin J Dig Surg. 2017;6:346–7.
18. Trudel-Fitzgerald C, Boehm JK, Kivimaki M, Kubzansky LD. Taking the tension out of hypertension: a prospective study of psychological well being and hypertension. J Hypertens. 2014;32:1222–8. https://doi.org/10.1097/HJH.0000000000000175
19. Zhang H. Percutaneous nephrolithotomy surgery and open surgery in the treatment of renal calculi comparative study. Dalian: Dalian Med Univ; 2011.
20. Sac W, Rizkala E, Liu X. Tubeless percutaneous nephrolithotomy: outcomes with expanded indications. Int Braz J Urol. 2014;40:204–11.
21. Etemadian M, Soleimani MJ, Haghighi R, Zeighami MR, Najimi N. Does bleeding during percutaneous nephrolithotomy necessitate keeping the nephrostomy tube? A randomized controlled clinical trial. Urol J. 2011;8:21–6.
22. Chen L, Li JX. Prevention of complications after percutaneous nephrolithotripsy. J Mod Urol. 2013;18:527–31.
23. Zhang J, Wang YB, Wang XL. Risk factors affecting blood loss during and after percutaneous nephrolithotomy. J Mod Urol. 2014;2014:24–7.
24. Durkin MT, Mercer KG, McNulty MF, Phipps L, Upperton J, Giles M, et al. Vascular surgical society of Great Britain and Ireland: contribution of malnutrition to postoperative morbidity in vascular surgical patients. Br J Surg. 1999;86:702. https://doi.org/10.1046/j.1365-2168.1999.0702a.x.
25. Correia MI, Caiaffa WT, da Silva AL, Waitzberg DL. Risk factors for malnutrition in patients undergoing gastroenterological and hernia surgery: an analysis of 374 patients. Nutr Hosp. 2001;16:59–64.
26. Li JS. Nutritional support therapy and accelerated rehabilitation surgery. Chin J Surg. 2015;22:65–7.
27. Fujikuni N, Tanabe K, Tokumoto N, Suzuki T, Hattori M, Misumi T, et al. Enhanced recovery program is safe and improves postoperative insulin resistance in gastrectomy. World J Gastrointest Surg. 2016;8:382–8. https://doi.org/10.4240/wjgs.v8.i5.382

28. Zhang CY, Zhang YH, Cao Y. Clinical analysis of postoperative infection after percutaneous nephrolithotripsy. Chin J Nosocomiol. 2016;26:2550–2.
29. Huang ZY, Zhou WH, Zou P. Effect of TCM comprehensive nursing intervention on pain and occurrence of complications in patients after percutaneous nephrolithotripsy. J Liaoning Univ Tradit Chin Med. 2016;18:254–6.

2

Correlation between body mass index and prostate volume in benign prostatic hyperplasia patients undergoing holmium enucleation of the prostate surgery

Ken Batai[1], Michael Phung[2], Robert Bell[3], Aye Lwin[1], Kieran A. Hynes[4], Elinora Price[5], Karleen M. Meiklejohn[6], Erika R. Bracamonte[6] and Joel T. Funk[1*]

Abstract

Background: Benign prostatic obstruction (BPO) due to benign prostatic hyperplasia (BPH) is a leading cause of morbidity in men over the age of 40. This study examined whether there was an association between body mass index (BMI) and pre-operative prostate volume and whether expression of two genes, alpha-2-macroglobulin (*A2M*) and transforming growth factor beta 3 (*TGFB3*), was correlated with BMI, pre-operative prostate volume, and age at surgery.

Methods: Medical records of patients who underwent holmium enucleation of the prostate surgery for treatment of BPO were retrospectively reviewed. Surgical specimens were obtained from formalin-fixed paraffin-embedded blocks, and expression of the targeted genes was quantified using a real time PCR approach. Linear regression analysis was performed to assess association between BMI and prostate volume adjusting for demographic characteristics and co-morbidity. Spearman's correlation was used to examine whether gene expression was correlated with BMI, prostate volume, and age at surgery.

Results: A total of 278 patients were identified, including 62.9% European Americans ($n = 175$) and 27.7% Hispanic Americans ($n = 77$). BMI was significantly correlated with prostate volume (Spearman's $rho = 0.123$, $P = 0.045$). In linear regression analysis, BMI was positively associated with prostate volume ($\beta = 0.01$, $P = 0.004$), while hyperlipidemia was negatively associated with prostate volume ($\beta = -0.08$, $P = 0.02$). A trend for a positive association was also observed for diabetes ($\beta = 0.07$, $P = 0.099$). In the race/ethnicity stratified analysis, age at surgery showed a trend for significantly positive association with prostate volume in European Americans ($\beta = 0.005$, $P = 0.08$), but not in Hispanic Americans. Expression of the *A2M* gene in the stroma was negatively correlated with age at surgery ($P = 0.006$). *A2M* expression in the gland was positively correlated with prostate volume among older men (Age ≥ 70, $P = 0.01$) and overweight men (BMI 25–30, $P = 0.04$). *TGFB3* expression in the gland was positively correlated with BMI ($P = 0.007$) among older men.

Conclusions: This study demonstrated the positive correlation between BMI and prostate volume. Expression of *TGFB3* and *A2M* was correlated with BMI, prostate volume, and age at surgery.

Keywords: Obesity, Co-morbidity, Health disparities

*Correspondence: jfunk@surgery.arizona.edu
[1] Department of Urology, The University of Arizona, 1501 N Campbell Ave, PO Box 245077, Tucson, AZ 85724-5077, USA

Background

Benign prostatic obstruction (BPO) due to benign prostatic hypertrophy (BPH), enlargement of the prostate gland, is a leading cause of morbidity in men over the age of 40. The prevalence of BPO/BPH increases with advancing age reaching 100% in the ninth decade of life [1]. At present, patients with BPO/BPH are treated with medical therapy consisting of alpha-adrenergic antagonists, 5-alpha-reductase inhibitors or surgery. Medical therapy can lead to considerable side effects including hypotension, erectile dysfunction, gynecomastia, and retrograde ejaculation. Furthermore, surgical treatment can lead to complications such as urinary incontinence, bleeding, urethral stricture disease, or bladder neck contracture [1].

The current guidelines for the management of BPH recommend to treat initially with medical therapy until the disease process progresses to a point at which surgery is a necessity [2]. Unfortunately, BPO/BPH progression is not fully studies [3, 4], and there is a shortage of literature to guide the decisions surrounding when to intervene with definitive surgical therapy in order to avoid adverse outcomes as well as a limited understanding of which patients progress in their disease and why.

Although current BPH and lower urinary tract symptoms (LUTS) studies rarely report racial/ethnic prevalence, it has been reported that men from minority groups, such as Hispanic-Americans (HAs) and African Americans, are at higher risk of developing BPH [5–9]. Additionally, there have been multiple studies reporting the effects of obesity and metabolic syndrome (hypertension, high blood sugar, obesity, waist circumference, and hyperlipidemia) on BPH. Although there is no clear consensus yet, obesity, higher body mass index (BMI), and metabolic diseases were associated risk factors of BPH [7, 9–17]. Despite high prevalence of obesity in HAs and African Americans [18, 19], the relationship between obesity and BPH in these groups and cause for disparities are not fully explored.

It has been hypothesized that pro-inflammatory states due to obesity may be triggers for developing BPH and there may be reactive changes characterized by alterations in the stromal and epithelial microenvironment, reflected in changes in expression of genes involved in inflammatory response and cell growth and development [12, 20]. However, it is still unclear how obesity and metabolic diseases affect BPH pathologic and molecular profiles, especially in medically underserved populations like HAs.

Two main goals of this study were 1) to examine whether there was an association between higher BMI or obesity and prostate volume including HAs who are previously underrepresented in BPH research and 2) to investigate whether expression of three genes, Insulin like growth factor 2 (*IGF2*), alpha-2-macroglobulin (*A2M*), and transforming growth factor beta 3 (*TGFB3*), was correlated with BMI, pre-operative prostate volume, and age at surgery. We also assessed if age and self-identified race/ethnicity modified these relationships.

Methods

BPH patients

Electronic medical record of consecutive patients who underwent (HoLEP) surgery for treatment of BPO/BPH between October 2012 and June 2018 were retrospectively reviewed. Patients who had histologically confirmed BPH were included. Patients with (a) pathology diagnoses other than BPH, (b) a history of prostate cancer, or (c) a prior surgical intervention for BPO/BPH were not included. Chart review was conducted on every eligible patient in the identified timeframe. Clinical (e.g., histology, pre-operative prostate volume, and medication) and demographic (e.g., age and race/ethnicity) characteristics as well as BMI, smoking status, and comorbidities (e.g., diabetes, hypertension, and hypolipidemia) were extracted. The pre-operative prostate volume was estimated using the ellipsoid formula (length x width x height x (π/6) based on either transrectal ultrasound or cross-sectional imaging (MRI or CT). The study protocol was approved by the University of Arizona Institutional Review Board.

Prostate tissue samples

To prepare the surgical specimens for gene expression analysis, hematoxylin and eosin (H&E) slides associated with formalin-fixed paraffin-embedded (FFPE) tissue samples underwent a review by board certified genitourinary pathologists to identify different architectural and cellular components (the stromal-rich and glandular/epithelium-rich areas) on the slides. Then, from the FFPE tissue sample, 1.5 mm^2 punches from each identified area (the stromal-rich or the glandular/epithelium-rich area) were taken.

RNA extraction and gene expression analysis

The Roche high Pure FFPET kit was used to extract RNA, and RNA was quantified using Nanodrop. Three genes, *IGF2*, *A2M*, and *TGFB3*, were selected from Luo et al. [21]. Two genes, *A2M* and *TGFB3*, were successfully amplified, but due to technical issues *IGF2* was not successfully amplified. The samples from 30 patients yielded quantifiable RNA expression data using a real time PCR approach. ΔCt method and a housekeeping gene, 18SrRNA, were used for normalization. ΔCt was log2 transformed for statistical analysis.

Statistical analysis

Chi-square test, independent sample T-test, and Mann–Whitney U-test were performed to characterize eligible patients for this study and patients included for the gene expression study. Linear regression analysis was performed to test the association between BMI and pre-operative prostate volume. Pre-operative prostate volume was log-transformed to normalize. Backward selection approach was used to determine variables to include in the regression mode. Age and race/ethnicity were added to the model to assess if they altered the association between BMI and prostate size. Spearman's correlation was used to examine whether gene expression was correlated with BMI, prostate volume, and age at surgery. Separate analysis was performed for younger men (age < 70) and older men (age ≥ 70) as well as European Americans (EAs) and HAs to assess if associations were different in these groups.

Results

A total of 278 patients who met inclusion criteria were identified. The mean age of patients was 70.6 (SD 8.5). The largest group of patients was EAs (62.9%), and HAs were the second largest group of patients (27.7%). BMI was significantly correlated with pre-operative prostate volume (Spearman's *rho* = 0.123, *P* = 0.045, Fig. 1). Similar correlations were observed when stratified analysis was performed based on age and race/ethnicity (Additional file 1: Supplementary Table 1). Age at surgery was not correlated with prostate volume but was correlated with BMI (Spearman's *rho* = −0.169, *P* = 0.005). The correlation was stronger in EAs than in HAs. Median pre-operative prostate volume was 75 mL (Interquartile Range, 48.8–105.0). Characteristics of patients with smaller prostate volume (≤ 75 mL) and larger prostate (> 75 mL) were compared (Table 1). Patients with larger prostates had significantly higher BMI compared to patients with smaller prostate volume (*P* = 0.03). Urinary retention was more common in men with larger prostate (44.7% and 55.9% in men with small and larger prostate respectively, *P* = 0.04).

The linear regression analysis was performed to assess if BMI was associated with pre-operative prostate volume (Table 2). BMI, hyperlipidemia, and diabetes remained in the model using the backward selection approach. BMI was positively associated with pre-operative prostate volume ($\beta = 0.01$, *P* = 0.004). Hyperlipidemia was negatively associated with prostate volume ($\beta = -0.08$, *P* = 0.02), and a trend for a positive association was observed for diabetes ($\beta = 0.07$, *P* = 0.099). Additionally, including age at surgery and race/ethnicity in the model did not change the association between BMI and prostate volume. In the race/ethnicity stratified analysis, the association between BMI and prostate volume was similar in both groups, but association was no longer significant in HAs, possibly due to small sample size (Additional file 1: Supplementary Table 2). Interestingly, age at surgery showed a trend for significantly positive association with prostate volume in EAs ($\beta = 0.005$, *P* = 0.08), but not in HAs. The analysis

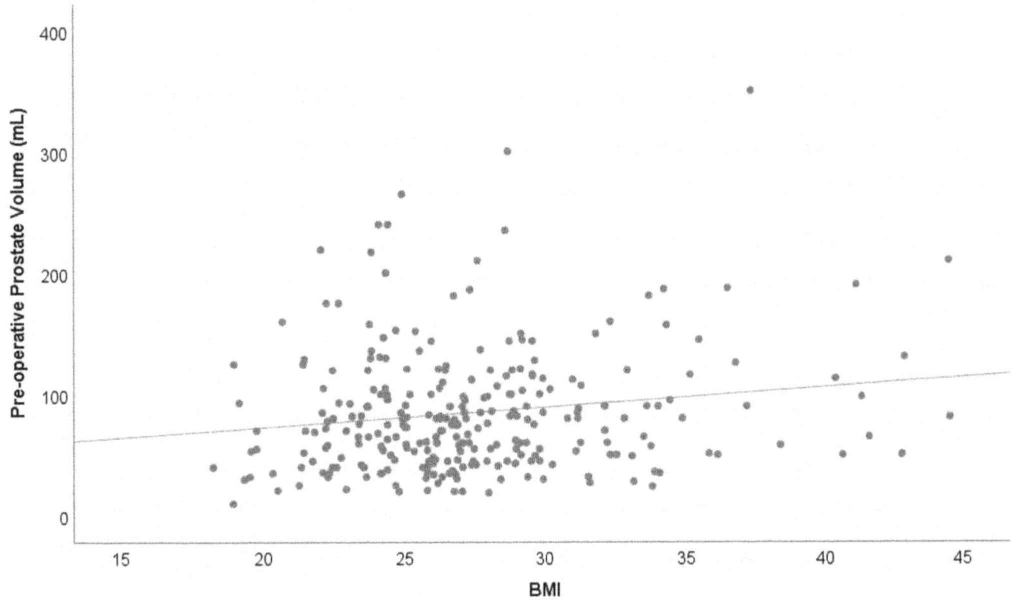

Fig. 1 Correlation between pre-operative prostate volume (mL) and BMI (Spearman's *rho* = 0.123, p = 0.045)

Table 1 BPH patients characteristics stratified by pre-operative prostate volume

	Prostate volume ≤ 75 mL	Prostate volume > 75 mL	P
Age, mean (SD)	70.8 (8.8)	70.5 (8.2)	0.81
Race/ethnicity, n (%)			0.48
European Americans	91 (64.5)	84 (61.3)	
Hispanic/latino	35 (24.8)	42 (30.7)	
Other/unknown	15 (10.6)	11 (8.0)	
BMI, median (IQR)	26.3 (24.1–29.0)	27.2 (24.2–29.9)	**0.03**
Smoking history, n (%)			0.30
Never	79 (60.8)	73 (57.5)	
Former smoker	40 (30.8)	48 (37.8)	
Currently smoker	11 (8.5)	6 (4.7)	
Urinary tract Infection, n (%)			0.39
No	113 (80.1)	111 (82.2)	
Yes	28 (19.9)	24 (17.8)	
Urinary retention, n (%)			**0.04**
No	78 (55.3)	60 (44.1)	
Yes	63 (44.7)	76 (55.9)	
Bladder stone, n (%)			0.19
No	128 (90.8)	117 (86.7)	
Yes	13 (9.2)	18 (13.3)	
Diabetes, n (%)			0.23
No	114 (80.9)	104 (76.5)	
Yes	27 (19.1)	32 (23.5)	
Hyperlipidemia, n (%)			0.21
No	80 (56.7)	84 (62.2)	
Yes	61 (43.3)	51 (37.8)	
Hypertension, n (%)			0.30
No	65 (46.1)	57 (42.2)	
Yes	76 (53.9)	78 (57.8)	

Note: $P < 0.05$ using Independent sample T-test for age and Chi-square tests for other variables. Bold values indicate statistically significant ($P < 0.05$)

BMI body mass index, *BPH* benign prostatic hyperplasia, *IQR interquartile range*, *SD* standard deviation

stratified based on age revealed similar association in younger and older men.

We then assessed the correlation of gene expression with age at surgery, BMI, and pre-operative prostate volume (Table 3). The characteristics of patients selected for gene expression analysis are presented on Additional file 1: Supplementary Table 3. Expression of the *A2M* gene in the stroma was significantly negatively correlated with age at surgery ($P = 0.006$). In the stratified analysis, the correlation was significant in HAs, men with normal BMI (BMI < 25), and obese men (BMI > 30) (Additional file 1: Supplementary Table 4). *A2M* expression in the gland was significantly positively correlated with prostate volume among older men (Age ≥ 70, $P = 0.01$) and overweight men (BMI 25–30, $P = 0.04$). Among older men, *TGFB3* expression in the gland was significantly positively correlated with BMI (Spearman's *rho* = 0.709, $P = 0.007$) and showed a trend for significant correlation with prostate volume ($P = 0.08$).

Discussion

In this study, we demonstrated the positive correlation between BMI and pre-operative prostate volume. We also demonstrated gene expression of *TGFB3* and *A2M* and its associations with BMI, preoperative prostate volume, and age at surgery. We also investigated if age and race/ethnicity modified the patterns of correlations.

Although multiple studies have examined the relationships between obesity, particularly abdominal obesity, and BPH risk [7, 12], there are fewer studies that incorporate pre-operative prostate volume, especially in racial/ethnic groups that are affected by both obesity and BPH. Our findings confirmed findings from previous studies and demonstrated a correlation between BMI

Table 2 Linear regression showing association between body mass index and pre-operative prostate volume

	Unadjusted		Adjusted model 1		Adjusted model 2	P
	β	P	β	P	β	
Age at surgery	0.002	0.19			0.003	0.13
BMI	0.009	**0.006**	0.010	**0.004**	0.010	**0.002**
Race/ethnicity						
HAs versus EAs	0.031	0.38			0.030	0.39
Others versus EAs	– 0.043	0.42			– 0.054	0.16
Smoking						
Non-smokers versus former smokers	0.034	0.32				
Non-smokers versus current smoker	– 0.141	**0.03**				
Diabetes	0.051	0.17	0.066	0.099	0.054	0.16
Hyperlipidemia	– 0.047	0.13	– 0.080	**0.02**	– 0.074	**0.02**
Hypertension	0.001	0.98				
UTI	0.008	0.84				
Bladder stone	0.051	0.29				

Note Adjusted model 1 is based on backward selection, and BMI, diabetes, and hyperlipidemia were retained in the final mode. Additionally adjusted for age at surgery and race/ethnicity in model 2. Bold values indicate statistically significant ($P < 0.05$)

BMI body mass index, *EA* European Americans, *HA* Hispanic Americans, *UTI* urinary tract infection

Table 3 Correlation between clinical/demographic variables and gene expression (Spearman's correlation coefficient and *P*-value)

	Age at surgery	BMI	Pre-operative prostate volume
All (n = 30)			
A2M			
Gland	– 0.068 (0.72)	0.222 (0.16)	0.277 (0.14)
Stroma	**– 0.498 (0.006)**	0.221 (0.27)	– 0.098 (0.61)
TGFB3			
Gland	0.000 (1.00)	0.207 (0.30)	0.326 (0.08)
Stroma	– 0.298 (0.17)	0.321 (0.16)	0.065 (0.77)

Note: Bold values indicates statistically significant ($P < 0.05$)

BMI body mass index

and prostate volume [9–11, 15–17, 20]. Fowke and colleagues showed that prostate volume was significantly positively associated with BMI, waist-hip ratio, waist circumference, percent body fat, total fat mass, and total lean mass [20]. Kim et al. demonstrated positive correlations between BMI and prostate volume and between BMI and International Prostate Symptom Score among Korean men [11]. A study from Japan even developed a validated model to estimate prostate volume (> 40 mL) based on age, PSA, percent free PSA, and body weight [22]. Despite these studies, there are reports that demonstrate no correlation between BMI or body weight and BPH [23, 24]. Contrary to our finding, Yee et al. investigated the relationship between obesity and LUTS, and they found that men with higher BMI had a smaller prostate than men with lower BMI at baseline [25]. Moreover, weight loss did not improve LUTS after intervention.

Previous studies also demonstrated that Hispanic ethnicity was associated with BPH risk with increased rates of reporting LUTS [7, 8]. Obesity is more prevalent among HAs than EAs [26, 27]. The 2014 National Health Interview Survey analysis results also show that HAs have a higher prevalence of diabetes than EAs [28]. Moreover, the prevalence of diabetes is slightly higher in Mexican Americans, especially Mexican American men, than HAs of other origins [26]. We hypothesized that men from minority groups, such as HAs, who were obese and had metabolic diseases were disproportionately affected by BPH. When stratifying by race/ethnicity, both EA and HA had a positive correlation between BMI and preoperative prostate volume, but correlation was significant only for EAs, probably due to small sample size for HAs.

Contrary to our hypothesis, hyperlipidemia was negatively associated with pre-operative prostate volume, and we did not observe significant association for diabetes or hypertension. There have been multiple studies interested in demonstrating the link between metabolic syndrome and BPH, but findings have been inconsistent. Some studies have reported how diabetes [13, 14] and hyperlipidemia [13, 29] were correlated with BPH, while other studies have failed to demonstrate an association [23, 24]. Egan and colleagues investigated the correlation between metabolic diseases and BPH in National Health and Nutrition Examination Surveys [24]. They found that cardiovascular disease, diabetes, or hypertension were not associated with BPH after adjusting for social and behavioral factors. When breaking down the components of metabolic syndrome or looking at metabolic syndrome as a whole, Telli et al. found no evidence to support any association between metabolic syndrome and LUTS [23]. The clinical significance of current and previous studies is uncertain, because of the consistent, but weak association between obesity and prostate volume, and inconsistent associations between metabolic diseases and BPH. Since obesity rates continue to increase in racial/ethnic minority groups, impact of obesity on BPH and its clinical implications need further investigation. The obesity-driven BPH may have a different pathophysiological basis from the hormonally-driven or age related progression of BPH, and understanding of pathophysiological basis of obesity-driven may open up a new avenue for treatment.

To explore the biological basis of obesity-driven BPH, we examined the correlations between obesity and expression of genes that are potentially related to obesity. We demonstrated how expression of two genes, *A2M* and *TGFB3*, were correlated with age at surgery, BMI, or preoperative prostate volume. These two genes along with *IGF2* were selected as genes of interest in BPH because they were over-expressed in BPH compared to normal prostate tissue in a previous study by Luo et al. [21] and these gene may play roles in obesity [30–33]. *A2M* was also over-expressed in BPH compared to normal prostate tissue in another study [34]. *TGFB3* and *IGF2* are both growth factors, and *TGFB3* encodes a ligand of the transforming growth factor-beta (TGF-beta) superfamily. *A2M* encodes a protease inhibitor and cytokine transporter, and the protein encoded by *A2M* can inhibit inflammatory cytokines and interrupt inflammatory cascades. A more recent molecular profiling study using RNA sequencing further demonstrated that *A2M* and *TGFB3* were over-expressed in BPH [35]. However, this study identified *BMP5* and *CXCL13* as the two most significantly over-expressed genes in BPH. *BMP5* (bone morphogenetic protein 5) also encodes a ligand of the TGF-beta superfamily. Ligands of this protein family bind TGF-beta receptors and activate SMAD family transcription factors. Dysregulation of *TGFB3* and *BMP5* may affect expression of downstream genes that are involved in BPH progression. *CXCL13* (C-X-C motif chemokine ligand 13) is an antimicrobial peptide and CXC chemokine, a small cytokine. Both growth factors and immune response are likely to be involved in epithelial and stromal growth in the prostate promoting development and progression of BPH [4, 36–38], but growth factors and inflammatory response gene may not influence prostate volume uniformly in all racial/ethnic and age groups. Moreover, a molecular profiling study identified two distinct subtypes of BPH, subtype A enriched with stromal signatures and subtype B associated with obesity and hypertension [39]. This current study also observed different gene expression correlation patterns for different cell types, race/ethnicity, and age groups. The difference in gene expression patterns between cell types or between patients' demographic backgrounds and co-morbid conditions needs to be further investigated with a larger sample.

The limitations of this study include its retrospective nature and small sample size at a single institution. Only 278 patients met our inclusion criteria, but we provide surgical care for a diverse patient population due to our location in the Southwestern United States. To our knowledge, this is the first study to explore the relationship between obesity and BPH in HA men in the United States. Secondly, the prostate volume was measured using ultrasound, CT, or MR. Different measurement methods may create systematic bias causing false positive or negative associations. Moreover, we explored the correlation between expression of only three genes and BPH characteristics in a small subset of patients, and we failed to amplify one of the genes, *IGF2*. All the patients included were had advanced BPH that required a surgical treatment and they were receiving medical management with alpha blockade and/or 5-alpha reductase inhibitors. Medications may have altered the correction between BMI and prostate volumes or between metabolic diseases and prostate volumes. Inclusion of patients with less severe BPH or BPO who have not undergone surgical or therapeutic treatment and a multi-institutional study with a larger sample size and a more diverse patient population is warranted to further investigate the impact of obesity or obesity related diseases on BPH and BPO characteristics. Finally, there is a paucity of data regarding molecular risk factors in patients with BPH. Further studies are needed to identify genes linked to BPH, so precision medicine can be used to predict disease progression, treatment response, and clinical outcomes.

Conclusions

We demonstrated the positive association between BMI and pre-operative prostate volume. We also demonstrated the association between gene expression of *TGFB3* and *A2M* with BMI, preoperative prostate volume and age at surgery. Further studies are needed to confirm these findings.

Abbreviations

BMI: Body mass index; BPH: Benign prostatic hyperplasia; BPO: Benign prostatic obstruction; CT: Computed tomography; EA: European Americans; FFPE: Formalin-fixed paraffin-embedded; HA: Hispanic Americans; HoLEP: Holmium enucleation of the prostate; LUTS: Lower urinary tract symptoms; MRI: Magnetic resonance imaging; PCR: Polymerase chain reaction; RNA: Ribonucleic acid; SD: Standard deviation.

Acknowledgements

The authors would like to thank everyone who helped prepare clinical data from Banner University Medical Center, particularly Myra Ortega.

Authors' contributions

Study design: KB, MP, ERB, JTF; acquisition of data: KB, MP, RB, AL, KAH, EP, KMM; statistical analysis: KB; Interpretation of data: KB, MP, RB, JTF; manuscript preparation: KB, MP, RB, AL, JTF; project supervision: ERB, JTF. All authors read and approved the final manuscript.

Competing interests

The authors do not have conflict of interest.

Author details

[1]Department of Urology, The University of Arizona, 1501 N Campbell Ave, PO Box 245077, Tucson, AZ 85724-5077, USA. [2]Department of Urology, University of California Los Angeles, 10833 Le Conte Avenue, Box 951738, Los Angeles, CA 90095-1738, USA. [3]Department of Pathology and Immunology, Washington University in St. Louis, 660 S Euclid Ave, Campus, Box 8118, St. Louis, MO 63110, USA. [4]Department of Surgery, University of Mississippi Medical Center, 2500 N State St, Jackson, MS 39216, USA. [5]Department of Surgery, University of Arizona, 1501 N. Campbell Ave., Tucson, AZ 85724, USA. [6]Department of Pathology, University of Arizona, 1501 N. Campbell Ave., Tucson, AZ 85724, USA.

References

1. Wein AJ, Kavoussi LR, Partin AW, Peters CA. Campbell-Walsh urology. Eleventh. Philadelphia: Elsevier; 2016.
2. Foster HE, Dahm P, Kohler TS, Lerner LB, Parsons JK, Wilt TJ, McVary KT. Surgical management of lower urinary tract symptoms attributed to benign prostatic hyperplasia: AUA Guideline Amendment 2019. J Urol. 2019;202(3):592–8.
3. Chughtai B, Forde JC, Thomas DD, Laor L, Hossack T, Woo HH, Te AE, Kaplan SA. Benign prostatic hyperplasia. Nat Rev Dis Primers. 2016;2:16031.
4. De Nunzio C, Presicce F, Tubaro A. Inflammatory mediators in the development and progression of benign prostatic hyperplasia. Nat Rev Urol. 2016;13:613.
5. Egan KB. The epidemiology of benign prostatic hyperplasia associated with lower urinary tract symptoms: prevalence and incident rates. Urol Clin N Am. 2016;43(3):259–97.
6. Platz EA, Kawachi I, Rimm EB, Willett WC, Giovannucci E. Race, ethnicity and benign prostatic hyperplasia in the Health Professinals Follow-up Study. J Urol. 2000;163(2):490–5.
7. Kristal Alan R, Arnold Kathryn B, Schenk Jeannette M, Neuhouser Marian L, Weiss N, Goodman P, Antvelink Colleen M, Penson David F, Thompson Ian M. Race/ethnicity, obesity, health related behaviors and the risk of symptomatic benign prostatic hyperplasia: results from the prostate cancer prevention trial. J Urol. 2007;177(4):1395–400.
8. Van Den Eeden SK, Shan J, Jacobsen SJ, Aaronsen D, Haque R, Quinn VP, Quesenberry CP Jr. Urologic diseases in America P: evaluating racial/ethnic disparities in lower urinary tract symptoms in men. J Urol. 2012;187(1):185–9.
9. Bhindi B, Margel D, Trottier G, Hamilton RJ, Kulkarni GS, Hersey KM, Finelli A, Trachtenberg J, Zlotta A, Toi A, et al. Obesity is associated with larger prostate volume but not with worse urinary symptoms: analysis of a large multiethnic cohort. Urology. 2014;83(1):81–7.
10. Fowke JH, Motley SS, Cookson MS, Concepcion R, Chang SS, Wills ML, Smith JA Jr. The association between body size, prostate volume and prostate-specific antigen. Prostate Cancer Prostatic Dis. 2006;10:137.
11. Kim JM, Song PH, Kim HT, Moon KH. Effect of obesity on prostate-specific antigen, prostate volume, and international prostate symptom score in patients with benign prostatic hyperplasia. Korean J Urol. 2011;52(6):401–5.
12. Wang S, Mao Q, Lin Y, Wu J, Wang X, Zheng X, Xie L. Body mass index and risk of BPH: a meta-analysis. Prostate Cancer Prostatic Dis. 2011;15:265–72.
13. Nandy PR, Saha S. Association between components of metabolic syndrome and prostatic enlargement: An Indian perspective. Med J Armed Forces India. 2016;72(4):350–5.
14. Chen Z, Miao L, Gao X, Wang G, Xu Y. Effect of obesity and hyperglycemia on benign prostatic hyperplasia in elderly patients with newly diagnosed type 2 diabetes. Int J Clin Exp Med. 2015;8(7):11289–94.
15. Gacci M, Sebastianelli A, Salvi M, De Nunzio C, Vignozzi L, Corona G, Jaeger T, Chini T, Russo GI, Maggi M, et al. Benign prostatic enlargement can be influenced by metabolic profile: results of a multicenter prospective study. BMC Urol. 2017;17(1):22.
16. Meng J, Liu Y, Guan SY, Ma H, Zhang X, Fan S, Hu H, Zhang M, Liang C. Age, height, BMI and FBG predict prostate volume in ageing benign prostatic hyperplasia: Evidence from 5285 patients. Int J Clin Pract. 2019;2019:e13438.
17. Li BH, Deng T, Huang Q, Zi H, Weng H, Zeng XT. Body mass index and risk of prostate volume, international prostate symptom score, maximum urinary flow rate, and post-void residual in benign prostatic hyperplasia patients. Am J Mens Health. 2019;13(4):1557988319870382.
18. Hales CM, Carroll MD, Fryar CD, Ogden CL. Prevalence of obesity and severe obesity among adults: United States, 2017–2018. NCHS Data Brief. 2020;360:1–8.
19. Health, United Sates, 2018
20. Fowke JH, Koyama T, Fadare O, Clark PE. Does inflammation mediate the obesity and BPH relationship? an epidemiologic analysis of body composition and inflammatory markers in blood, urine, and prostate tissue, and the relationship with prostate enlargement and lower urinary tract symptoms. PLoS ONE. 2016;11(6):e0156918.
21. Luo J, Dunn T, Ewing C, Sauvageot J, Chen Y, Trent J, Isaacs W. Gene expression signature of benign prostatic hyperplasia revealed by cDNA microarray analysis. Prostate. 2002;51(3):189–200.
22. Nakanishi Y, Masuda H, Kawakami S, Sakura M, Fujii Y, Saito K, Koga F, Ito M, Yonese J, Fukui I, et al. A novel equation and nomogram including body weight for estimating prostate volumes in men with biopsy-proven benign prostatic hyperplasia. Asian J Androl. 2012;14(5):703–7.
23. Telli O, Demirbas A, Kabar M, Karagoz MA, Sarici H, Resorlu B. Does metabolic syndrome or its components correlate With lower urinary tract symptoms in benign prostatic hyperplasia patients? Nephrourol Mon. 2015;7(3):e27253–e27253.
24. Egan KB, Burnett AL, McVary KT, Ni X, Suh M, Wong DG, Rosen RC. The co-occurring syndrome—coexisting erectile dysfunction and benign prostatic hyperplasia and their clinical correlates in aging men: results from the National Health and Nutrition Examination Survey. Urology. 2015;86(3):570–80.
25. Yee CH, So WY, Yip SK, Wu E, Yau P, Ng CF. Effect of weight reduction on the severity of lower urinary tract symptoms in obese male patients with benign prostatic hyperplasia: a randomized controlled trial. Kor J UROL. 2015;56(3):240–6.
26. Flegal KM, Kruszon-Moran D, Carroll MD, Fryar CD, Ogden CL. Trends in obesity among adults in the united states, 2005 to 2014. JAMA. 2016;315(21):2284–91.
27. Story M, Evans M, Fabsitz RR, Clay TE, Rock BH, Broussard B. The epidemic of obesity in American Indian communities and the need for childhood obesity-prevention programs. Am J Clin Nutr. 1999;69(4):747S-754S.
28. Summary Health Statistics: National Health Interview Survey, 2014
29. Shih H-J, Huang C-J, Lin J-A, Kao M-C, Fan Y-C, Tsai P-S. Hyperlipidemia is associated with an increased risk of clinical benign prostatic hyperplasia. Prostate. 2018;78(2):113–20.

30. Petrus P, Mejhert N, Corrales P, Lecoutre S, Li Q, Maldonado E, Kulyté A, Lopez Y, Campbell M, Acosta JR, et al. Transforming growth factor-β3 regulates adipocyte number in subcutaneous white adipose tissue. Cell Rep. 2018;25(3):551-560.e555.
31. Lin E, Kuo P-H, Liu Y-L, Yang AC, Tsai S-J. Transforming growth factor-β signaling pathway-associated genes SMAD2 and TGFBR2 are implicated in metabolic syndrome in a Taiwanese population. Sci Rep. 2017;7(1):13589–13589.
32. Rugsarash W, Tungtrongchitr R, Petmitr S, Phonrat B, Pongpaew P, Harnroongroj T, Tungtrongchitr A. The genetic association between alpha-2-macroglobulin (A2M) gene deletion polymorphism and low serum A2M concentration in overweight/obese Thais. Nutr Neurosci. 2006;9(1–2):93–8.
33. Elam MB, Cowan GS Jr, Rooney RJ, Hiler ML, Yellaturu CR, Deng X, Howell GE, Park EA, Gerling IC, Patel D, et al. Hepatic gene expression in morbidly obese women: implications for disease susceptibility. Obesity (Silver Spring, Md). 2009;17(8):1563–73.
34. Fromont G, Chene L, Latil A, Bieche I, Vidaud M, Vallancien GUY, Mangin P, Fournier G, Validire P, Cussenot O. Molecular profiling of benign prostate hyperplasia using a large scale real-time reverse transcriptase-polymerase chain reaction approach. Urology. 2004;172(4, Part 1):1382–5.
35. Middleton LW, Shen Z, Varma S, Pollack AS, Gong X, Zhu S, Zhu C, Foley JW, Vennam S, Sweeney RT, et al. Genomic analysis of benign prostatic hyperplasia implicates cellular re-landscaping in disease pathogenesis. JCI insight. 2019;5(12):e129749.
36. Lucia MS, Lambert JR. Growth factors in benign prostatic hyperplasia: basic science implications. Curr Urol Rep. 2008;9(4):272–8.
37. Lloyd Granville L, Ricke William A, McVary Kevin T. Inflammation, voiding and benign prostatic hyperplasia progression. J Urol. 2019;201(5):868–70.
38. La Vignera S, Condorelli RA, Russo GI, Morgia G, Calogero AE. Endocrine control of benign prostatic hyperplasia. Andrology. 2016;4(3):404–11.
39. Liu D, Shoag JE, Poliak D, Goueli RS, Ravikumar V, Redmond D, Vosoughi A, Fontugne J, Pan H, Lee D, et al. Integrative multiplatform molecular profiling of benign prostatic hyperplasia identifies distinct subtypes. Nat Commun. 2020;11(1):1987.

3

Association between severity of prenatally diagnosed hydronephrosis and receipt of surgical intervention postnatally among patients seen at a fetal-maternal center

Zoë G. Baker[1*], Arthi Hannallah[1], Melissa Trabold[1], Danielle Estell[2], Cherry Deng[3], Andy Y. Chang[1,2], S. Scott Sparks[1,2], Roger De Filippo[1,2] and Evalynn Vasquez[1,2]

Abstract

Background: Hydronephrosis (HN) is the most common abnormality detected on prenatal ultrasound. This study sought to stratify outcomes of patients by severity of prenatal HN with postnatal outcomes.

Methods: This was a retrospective review of patients referred to a tertiary care fetal-maternal clinic with diagnosis of prenatal HN from 2004 to 2019. HN severity was categorized as mild, moderate, or severe. Data were analyzed to determine the association between HN severity and surgical intervention. Decision for surgery was based on factors including history of multiple urinary tract infections, evidence of renal scarring, and/or reduced renal function. Surgery-free survival time was represented by the Kaplan–Meier method, and hazard ratios were calculated using the log-rank test.

Results: 131 kidneys among 101 infants were prenatally diagnosed with hydronephrosis; 35.9% had mild HN, 29.0% had moderate HN, and 35.1% had severe HN. 8.5% of patients with mild HN, 26.3% of patients with moderate HN, and 65.2% of patients with severe HN required surgery. Patients with severe HN were 12.2 (95% CI 6.1–24.4; $p < 0.001$) times more likely to undergo surgery for HN than patients with mild HN and 2.9 (95% CI 1.5–5.3; $p = 0.003$) times more likely to undergo surgery than patients with moderate HN. Patients with moderate HN were 4.3 times more likely to require surgery than patients with mild HN (95% CI 1.5–12.9; $p = 0.01$). Median age at surgery was 11.8 months among patients with mild HN (IQR 11.7–14.1 months), 6.6 months among patients with moderate HN (IQR 4.2–16.4 months), and 5.4 months among patients with severe HN (3.7–12.4 months).

Conclusion: Among this cohort of referrals from a fetal-maternal clinic, severity of HN correlated with increased likelihood of surgical intervention. Continued assessment of patients with prenatal HN should be evaluated to best determine the role of the pediatric urologist in cases of prenatal HN.

Keywords: Hydronephrosis, Prenatal, Surgery, Fetal, Diagnosis

Background

Hydronephrosis (HN) is a descriptive term for dilation of one or both kidneys. It is the most common prenatal abnormality detected by ultrasound [1] and is diagnosed in one to five percent of pregnancies [2, 3]. Increased prenatal screening has enabled physicians to diagnose

*Correspondence: zobaker@chla.usc.edu
[1] Division of Urology, Children's Hospital Los Angeles, Los Angeles, CA, USA

prenatal HN more readily. Renal ultrasonography (US) and voiding cystourethrogram (VCUG) are often performed postnatally for physicians to assess renal function and consider treatment plans.

The Society for Fetal Urology (SFU) has categorized the severity of HN into grades 1–4. This system takes into consideration the degree of pelvic dilation, presence of calyceal dilation, and thinning of parenchymal tissue in the kidneys. Despite advances in prenatal ultrasound screening for HN, there is still some ambiguity in criteria for diagnosing severity and appropriate management. There is debate about the cutoff values for the SFU grading system, though efforts have been made by various professional groups to consolidate findings into a more comprehensible management guide for practicing urologists [4]. Another highly contested matter is the threshold at which surgical intervention is needed. Gender, age, and the presence of urological comorbidities are factors that must also be considered during the course of treatment.

After HN is detected on prenatal ultrasound, prenatal counseling with pediatric urologists is encouraged in order to form appropriate management plans. Urologists may recommend newborns with prenatal HN to be put on antibiotic prophylaxis in order to reduce the risk of urinary tract infections (UTIs) [5]. This is usually followed by monitoring with ultrasounds to assess the progression and potential resolution of HN. While current literature indicates that a large proportion of cases are stabilized or resolved following conservative management [1, 3, 6], studies have reported differing findings regarding the proportion of patients who go on to require surgery. A recent review found that the rate of complete resolution of prenatally-detected HN in the absence of surgery may range from 33 to 70% [7]. Discrepancies in the rates of patients who require surgery may be largely due to differences in HN severity between populations [8–13]. Variation in the proportion of patients with prenatally diagnosed HN who require surgery after birth may result in difficulty in counseling pregnant women on their child's expected care trajectory. In some patients with HN, surgery may be indicated to prevent or manage recurrent UTIs, kidney dysfunction, ureteropelvic junction obstruction (UPJO) and/or vesicoureteral reflux (VUR) [1, 6–8, 13]. Common surgical interventions for HN, depending on the etiology of hydronephrosis, include pyeloplasties for UPJO, ureteral reimplantations for VUR, and in some cases, nephrectomies for symptomatic, nonfunctional kidneys [7, 9, 13, 14].

The aim of this study is to assess the number and proportion of patients diagnosed with mild (SFU Grade 1 or 2), moderate (SFU Grade 3), and severe (SFU Grade 4) prenatal HN at a fetal-maternal center that progress to surgery, and to assess the correlation between severity of prenatal diagnosis and probability of postnatal surgical intervention. Time to surgery by prenatal severity score will also be assessed. The results of this study may assist providers in delivering more accurate prenatal counseling to parents following identification of HN, illustrate the importance of prenatal visits, and may also aid pediatric urologists in taking appropriate precautions while identifying the etiology among pediatric patients with HN.

Methods

Electronic medical records were reviewed among patients who received prenatal HN diagnoses by neonatologists and referred to pediatric urologists at a fetal-maternal center in a large urban setting between 2004 and 2019. Information on prenatal urologic diagnoses and severity of hydronephrosis was recorded from mothers' pediatric urology notes, radiology reports, and/or radiology images. Patients' demographic, clinical, and surgical information were similarly recorded and linked to their mothers' data.

Patients were included in the study if severity of HN was recorded at the prenatal visit, they attended at least one urology appointment postnatally, and they were at least 12 months old at the time of data analysis. Patients with prenatal anteroposterior (AP) diameters of less than 10 mm were excluded, as this was the cut-off for patients to receive pediatric urology referrals. Patients were also excluded if they did not survive to term or were less than 12 months old at the time of data analysis. Patients were followed until the date of their surgical intervention, until the date their HN resolved, or until the date of their last follow-up with a pediatric urologist, up until age 6 years. Prenatal images were reviewed and hydronephrosis severity was assessed by each patient's pediatric urologist. HN severity was classified as mild (SFU 1–2), moderate (SFU 3), or severe (SFU 4). Classifications were based on the status of the calices, extent of pelvic dilation, and presence of parenchymal atrophy. SFU grades of 1 and 2 were combined as some prenatal notes did not differentiate between the two and instead indicated "SFU grade 1/2." Data on both kidneys were recorded among patients prenatally diagnosed with bilateral HN.

The probability of undergoing surgical intervention for HN was stratified by prenatally diagnosed HN severity. Patients' diagnoses were classified postnatally. If a specific diagnosis was not given due to the transient nature of the patient's HN, it was classified as transient. Decision for surgical intervention was based on the clinical characteristics of the patient including history of multiple recurrent urinary tract infections, evidence of renal scarring, and/or decreased renal function. Surgical interventions of interest included: pyeloplasty, nephrectomy, ureteral reimplantation, ureterostomy, ureterocele incision, and other urologic surgeries related to a diagnosis of HN. Among patients who underwent surgery, age at time of surgery was recorded. Kaplan–Meier curves and estimates with confidence intervals were created to assess the probability of receiving surgery versus proceeding with conservative management over time, stratified by HN severity. Whether patients were discharged from the clinic after resolution of HN without surgery or were receiving continued follow-up and monitoring for HN at the time of data analysis was also noted. Patients who did not undergo surgery and who had persistent HN at the time of data analysis were censored at the time of last clinic follow-up visit. Hazard ratios (HR) were calculated using the log-rank test, to determine differences in probability of surgery between patients with severe versus mild HN, severe versus moderate HN, and moderate versus mild HN. Etiology of HN by prenatal severity was also reported. Pearson X^2 tests were utilized to evaluate whether there were any differences in probability of receiving surgery by patient gender, race/ethnicity, primary language, medical insurance type (public versus private), or vesicoureteral reflux (VUR) presence.

This study was reviewed and approved by the institutional review board at Children's Hospital Los Angeles.

Results

Overall results

This study included 101 infants and 131 kidneys prenatally diagnosed with HN (Table 1). Mean gestational age at first detection of hydronephrosis was 23.5 weeks (IQR 20–31), though mothers were not referred to pediatric urology until AP diameter was at least 10 mm. There were no significant differences in gestational age at HN detection by HN severity. Postnatally, patients were followed for a median of 1.2 years (IQR 0.8–2.3 years). The majority of patients were male (n = 75, 74.3%), and 40% (n = 41) identified as Hispanic. Approximately 70% of patients were diagnosed with unilateral HN (n = 71), and 30% with bilateral HN (n = 30). Overall, 33.6% (n = 44) of hydronephrotic kidneys required surgical intervention, including 8.5% of kidneys diagnosed with mild HN, 26.3% of those diagnosed with moderate HN, and 65.2% of those diagnosed with severe HN (Table 2). Of the remaining kidneys, 30 (22.9%) spontaneously resolved, and 57 (43.5%) did not yet require surgical intervention and were being conservatively managed with serial ultrasound.

The likelihood of requiring surgery varied significantly by prenatal HN severity. Additionally, among those patients who required surgery, age at surgery varied by HN severity; patients with moderate and severe HN generally underwent surgery at younger ages than patients with mild HN (Fig. 1). Patients with severe HN were 12.2 times more likely to require surgery than patients with mild HN (95% CI 6.1–24.4; $p < 0.001$), and 2.9 times more likely to require surgery than patients with moderate HN (95% CI 1.5–5.3; $p = 0.003$). Additionally, patients with moderate HN were 4.3 times more likely to require surgery than patients with mild HN (95% CI 1.5–12.9; $p = 0.01$). There was no significant difference in probability of receiving surgery by patient gender, race/ethnicity, primary language, or medical insurance type. Additionally, there was no significant difference in the probability

Table 1 Demographic and prenatal factors among patients prenatally diagnosed with hydronephrosis at fetal-maternal center and followed post-birth from 2004–2019 (n = 101)

Demographic/prenatal factor	n	%
Gender		
Male	75	74.3
Female	26	25.7
Race/ethnicity		
Hispanic	41	40.6
Non-Hispanic White	19	18.8
Other	28	27.7
Unknown	13	12.9
Parent primary language		
English	64	63.4
Non-English	36	35.6
Unknown	1	1.0
Medical insurance type		
Public	68	67.3
Private	33	32.7
Hydronephrosis side		
Unilateral	71	70.3
Bilateral	30	29.7
Prenatally-diagnosed hydronephrosis severity (among n = 131 kidneys)		
Mild	47	35.9
Moderate	38	29.0
Severe	46	35.1

Table 2 Number and rate of kidneys requiring surgical intervention among 131 kidneys diagnosed prenatally with mild, moderate, and severe hydronephrosis

Hydronephrosis severity	Total (n)	Surgical intervention (n)	Surgical intervention (%)
Mild	47	4	8.5%
Moderate	38	10	26.3%
Severe	46	30	65.2%
Total	131	44	33.6%

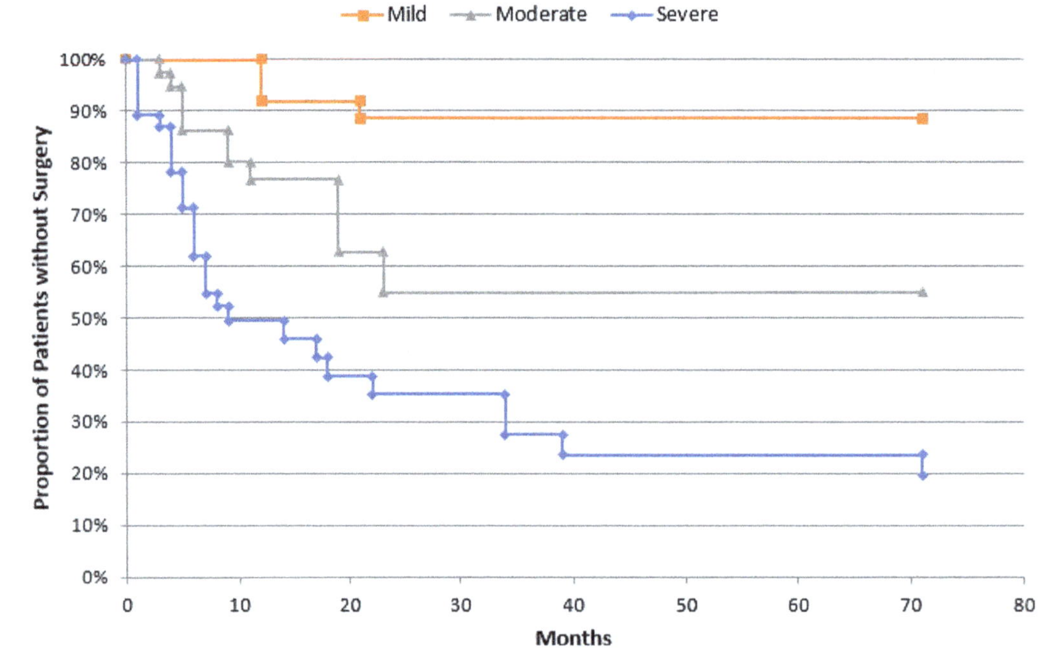

Fig. 1 Kaplan–Meier curves indicating surgery-free survival time in months, by prenatally-diagnosed hydronephrosis severity type

of surgical intervention among patients with evidence of VUR, compared to those with no evidence of VUR (45.5% vs. 43.8%; X^2 $p = 0.72$).

Patients with mild prenatally diagnosed hydronephrosis

Among the 131 kidneys included in the study, 47 (35.9%) were prenatally diagnosed with mild HN. Most patients (74.5%, n = 35) who were diagnosed with mild HN had transient etiologies that self-resolved (Table 3; Fig. 2). Overall, four patients (8.5%) with mild HN required surgery for HN postnatally, which occurred at a median age of 11.8 months (IQR 11.7–14.1 months; Fig. 1). At the time of analysis, 20 kidneys with mild HN had spontaneously resolved, and 23 were still being followed with serial ultrasound. The Kaplan–Meier estimate indicates that 8.1% (95% CI 0.0–16.9%) of patients with mild HN require surgery by one year of age, and 11.4% (95% CI 0.8–22.0%) require surgery by six years of age (Fig. 1). HN-related diagnoses among patients who required surgery included UPJO in three cases, and ureterocele in one case (Table 3; Fig. 2). Three of these patients underwent pyeloplasty, and one patient underwent ureteral reimplantation, ureterocele incision, and bladder neck reconstruction (Table 3). In addition to transient etiologies, other etiologies that did not require surgical intervention among patients with mild HN included partial UPJO that did not meet the requirements for surgical intervention in five kidneys, VUR in three patients, and ureterocele in one patient.

Patients with moderate prenatally diagnosed hydronephrosis

A total of 38 kidneys (29.0%) were diagnosed with moderate prenatal HN, of which 10 (26.3%) required surgery (Table 2). Four kidneys with moderate HN spontaneously resolved, and the majority (n = 24) were still being followed for moderate HN at the time of data analysis. The Kaplan–Meier estimate indicates that 23.4% (95% CI 10.2–36.6%) of patients with moderate HN require surgery by one year of age, and 45.4% (95% CI 22.5–68.3%) may require surgery by six years of age (Fig. 1). Patients with moderate HN who required surgery were a median of 6.6 months old at the time of surgery (IQR 4.2–16.4 months). The majority of patients who required surgery had UPJO (n = 7; 70% of patients who underwent surgery; Table 3; Fig. 2). Additionally, one patient who required surgery had a ureterocele, and two had VUR. Most patients (n = 7) who required surgery underwent pyeloplasty, two patients underwent ureteral reimplantations, and one patient each underwent a ureteroureterostomy and a nephroureterectomy (Table 3). Patients who did not require surgery most frequently had a transient etiology of their HN (n = 19; Table 3; Fig. 2). Additionally, among patients who did not require surgical intervention, six had UPJO not meeting the requirements for surgical intervention, three had VUR, and one had a ureterocele.

Table 3 HN-related diagnoses, number of patients who required surgery, and surgical interventions among patients with mild, moderate, and severe prenatally-diagnosed HN

HN severity	HN-related diagnoses*	Total kidneys n	Kidneys requiring surgery n	Surgical intervention: Surgery type	n
Mild	UPJ obstruction	8	3	Pyeloplasty	3
	Ureterocele	2	1	Ureterocele incision, ureteral reimplantation, bladder neck reconstruction	1
	VUR	3	0	–	–
	Transient	35	–	–	–
	Total	47	4	–	–
Moderate	UPJ obstruction	13	7	Pyeloplasty	7
				Ureteroureterostomy	1
	VUR	5	2	Ureteral reimplantation	2
	Ureterocele	2	1	Nephroureterectomy	1
	Transient	19	–	–	–
	Total	38	10	–	–
Severe	UPJ obstruction	25	21	Pyeloplasty	17
				Partial nephrectomy	3
				Cutaneous ureterostomy	1
				Vesicostomy	1
	PUV	4	4	Valve ablation	4
	Ureterocele	4	2	Ureterocele incision	2
	VUR	3	3	Vesicostomy	2
				Ureteral reimplantation	1
	UVJ obstruction	2	2	Ureteral reimplantation	2
	Megaureter	1	1	Circumcision	1
	Transient	10	–	–	–
	Total	46	30	–	–

*Patients may have more than 1 diagnosis and may have undergone more than 1 type of surgical intervention

Patients with severe prenatally diagnosed hydronephrosis

Kidneys with severe HN accounted for 35.1% of kidneys included in the study (n=46). Postnatal surgical intervention was required among 65.2% (n=30) of kidneys with severe HN, and patients received surgery at a median of 5.4 months of age (3.7–12.4 months; Fig. 1). Of the remaining kidneys, six self-resolved and 10 were being followed conservatively. The Kaplan–Meier estimate indicates that 50.5% (95% CI 36.3–64.8%) of patients with severe HN require surgery by one year of age, and 80.3% (95% CI 66.0–94.7%) may require surgery by six years of age (Fig. 1). UPJO remained the most common HN-related diagnosis among patients with severe HN who underwent surgery, occurring in 70.0% (n=21) of these patients (Table 3; Fig. 2). Other HN-related diagnoses among patients who underwent surgery included posterior urethral valves (PUV), ureterocele, ureterovesical junction obstruction (UVJO), VUR, and megaureter. Among the 30 kidneys requiring surgery, 17 underwent pyeloplasty (Table 3). Additional surgical interventions included valve ablation, partial nephrectomy, cutaneous ureterostomy, vesicostomy, ureterocele incision, ureteral reimplantation, and circumcision for recurrent urinary tract infections (Table 3). Among the 16 patients with severe prenatal HN who did not require surgical intervention, diagnoses included transient etiologies (n=10), UPJO not meeting the requirements for surgical intervention (n=4), and ureterocele (n=2).

Discussion

Prenatal HN is the most common prenatal abnormality detected on ultrasound and is a common referral to pediatric urologists [1]. How this HN can be managed depends on the severity of HN and concurrent findings that are identified in postnatal evaluation, generally by VCUG and renal US [4, 6]. The aim of this study was to stratify the proportion of patients with mild, moderate, and severe HN who eventually require surgical intervention in order to gain greater insight into how to adequately counsel families prenatally on the management of HN. There was a relatively homogenous spread of the severity of HN in this cohort of 101 patients (35.9%

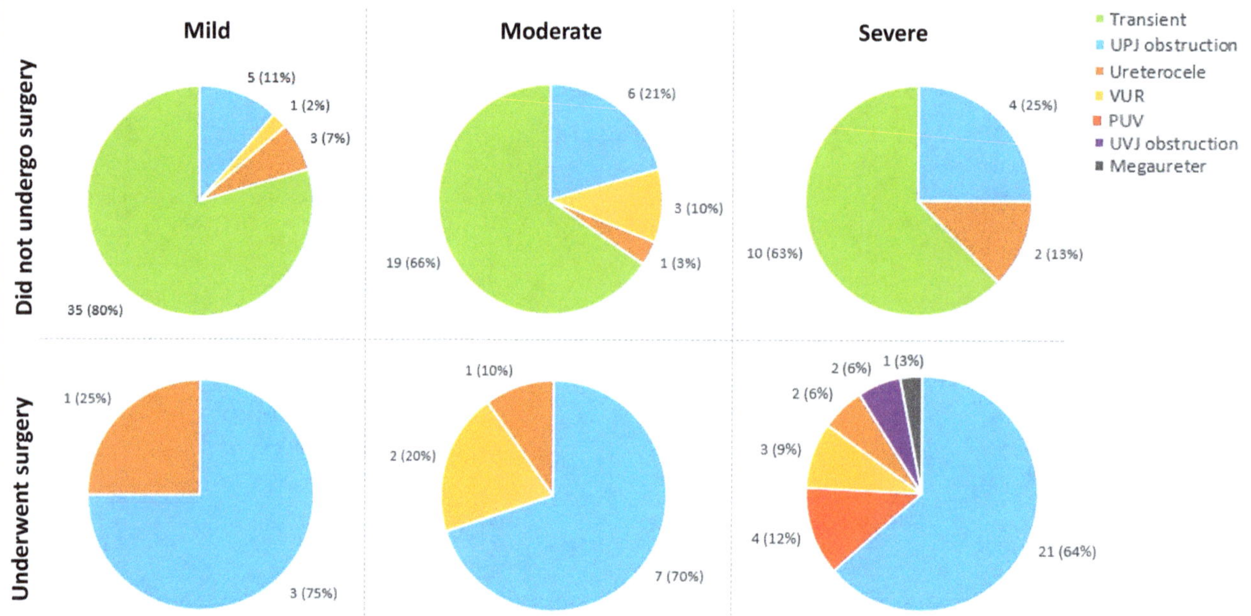

Fig. 2 Number and percentage of hydronephrosis-related diagnoses among 101 patients, by prenatally-diagnosed hydronephrosis severity and receipt of surgical intervention

mild, 29.0% moderate, and 35.1% severe). It has been previously reported that 35–50% of patients with antenatal HN will have no HN on postnatal renal US [6]. The etiology of HN in our cohort also similarly reflected findings from previous studies. The most common pathological finding in our cohort was also UPJO, but the most common cause overall of HN was transient HN [6].

Patients with mild prenatally diagnosed hydronephrosis

Among patients with mild prenatal HN, 74.5% had a transient etiology that resolved postpartum, none of whom had surgical intervention. As with previously reported studies, patients with transient HN determined to no longer be present postnatally may not warrant close urologic follow-up after a negative ultrasound result [4]. However, 8.5% of patients with mild prenatal HN did require surgical intervention, suggesting that postnatal follow-up of patients diagnosed with mild prenatal HN is warranted.

Patients with moderate prenatally diagnosed hydronephrosis

As with the patients with mild HN, those with moderate HN who were determined to have transient HN did not require surgical intervention. While transient HN was less common in patients with moderate versus mild prenatal HN, it still occurred in half of all patients diagnosed with moderate prenatal HN. Approximately one quarter of all kidneys prenatally diagnosed with moderate HN required surgery. Time to surgery in this cohort was notable. The median time to surgery for patients with moderate HN was 6.6 months, compared to 11.8 months in those with mild HN and 5.4 months in those with severe HN. Liu et al. noted that the rate of pathology in those with moderate prenatal HN was 45.1% (25.3–66.6) [15]. This raises the question of why those with moderate HN were likely to undergo intervention around the same as those with more severe findings. While fewer patients with moderate HN underwent surgery overall compared to those with severe HN, one must consider what prompts practitioners to consider intervention particularly in this moderate group.

Patients with severe prenatally diagnosed hydronephrosis

Like those in the mild and moderate cohorts, those patients with severe HN who were determined to have transient HN did not undergo surgical intervention. As one would expect, the patients with severe prenatal HN were significantly more likely to require some form of surgical intervention, which occurred at the earliest median time, as compared to mild and moderate cohorts. Among all kidneys with severe prenatal HN, almost 50% required surgical intervention due to UPJO. Surgical interventions required for HN-related diagnoses were also broader than patients with mild or moderate HN, including valve ablation, vesicostomy, cutaneous ureterostomy, partial nephrectomy, and circumcision for recurrent urinary tract infection in some cases. Data from this study suggest that patients with severe prenatal HN require close postnatal follow-up and may require surgery within the first six months of life.

Limitations

This study is not without its limitations. Due to the retrospective nature of this study, classifications of HN severity were not standardized; while some providers used SFU grades, others used descriptions of "mild," "moderate," or "severe" to diagnose prenatal HN severity. Additionally, with only 101 patients in the cohort, our study is underpowered to be able to adequately stratify the severity of HN with the type of surgical procedure; however, it was possible to assess the association between increased HN severity and increased risk of surgical intervention of any type. The decision to recommend surgery was based on the patients' clinical characteristics and the pediatric urologists' judgements, which may vary depending on the surgeon. Additionally, as the median length of follow-up time in this study was 1.2 years, the Kaplan–Meier estimator for surgery-free survival through six years may be unreliable as it relies on data from few participants. The broad confidence intervals provided reflect the uncertainty of the six-year Kaplan–Meier estimates. For this reason, the six-year surgery-free survival estimate should be considered with caution, and the Kaplan–Meier estimator for surgery-free survival through one year is more reliable. Furthermore, assessment of outcomes among patients with prenatal HN in a multi-institutional setting would hold more impact in being able to determine how to manage the equivocal cases of prenatal HN.

Conclusions

The experience from this maternal fetal health center provides further reassurance that patients with transient HN will not likely require surgical intervention in the future, despite severity. However, regardless of the nature of HN, those with moderate and severe HN do require further urologic work up beyond postnatal renal US to evaluate for potential pathologies and prevent infection or loss of renal function. Additionally, it reiterates the importance of prenatal counseling for close postnatal follow-up no matter the degree of prenatal hydronephrosis as it is difficult to predict the likelihood of surgery or resolution of HN on prenatal ultrasound alone. Even the mild form of prenatal HN may have pathology that requires surgical intervention. However, patients who are diagnosed with prenatal HN are significantly more likely to require surgical intervention and at an early age if they are found to have severe HN. Close follow-up and adequate family counseling in those with more severe HN prenatally are warranted.

Abbreviations

AP: Anteroposterior; CI: Confidence Interval; HN: Hydronephrosis; HR: Hazard Ratio; IQR: Interquartile Range; PUV: Posterior Urethral Valves; SFU: Society for Fetal Urology; UPJO: Ureteropelvic Junction Obstruction; UVJO: Ureterovesical Junction Obstruction; US: Ultrasonography; UTI: Urinary Tract Infection; VCUG: Voiding Cystourethrogram; VUR: Vesicoureteral Reflux.

Acknowledgements

Not applicable.

Authors' contributions

ZB collected and analyzed data and wrote the manuscript. AH assisted with data analysis and writing the manuscript. MT and DE assisted with data collection and analysis. CD assisted with data collection and analysis and writing the manuscript. AC, SS, and RD helped to conceptualize the study design, saw patients, and reviewed and edited the manuscript. EV oversaw the project, conceptualized the study, saw patients, and reviewed and edited the manuscript. All authors have read and approved the final manuscript.

Competing interests

The authors have no financial or non-financial competing interests to be declared.

Author details

[1] Division of Urology, Children's Hospital Los Angeles, Los Angeles, CA, USA. [2] Keck School of Medicine of Medicine of USC, University of Southern California, Los Angeles, CA, USA. [3] Thomas J. Long School of Pharmacy, University of the Pacific, Stockton, CA, USA.

References

1. Yalcinkaya F, Ozcakar ZB. Management of antenatal hydronephrosis. Pediatr Nephrol. 2019. https://doi.org/10.1007/s00467-019-04420-6.
2. Lee RS, Cendron M, Kinnamon DD, Nguyen HT. Antenatal hydronephrosis as a predictor of postnatal outcome: A meta-analysis. Pediatrics. 2006;118(2):586–93. https://doi.org/10.1542/peds.2006-0120.
3. Arnaud A, Hossini SL, de Lara ST, Dobremez E, Chateil J, Harper L. Managing children with hydronephrosis: Common pitfall during ultrasound follow-up to remember. Arch Dis Child. 2019. https://doi.org/10.1136/archdischild-2019-317386.
4. Kohno M, Ogawa T, Kojima Y, Sakoda A, Johnin K, Sugita Y, Nakane A, Noguchi M, Moriya K, Hattori M, Hayashi Y, Kubota M. Pediatric congenital hydronephrosis (ureteropelvic junction obstruction): Medical management guide. Int J Urol. 2020;27:369–76.
5. Braga LH, Mijovic H, Farrokhyar F, Pemberton J, DeMaria J, Lorenzo AJ. Antibiotic prophylaxis for urinary tract infections in antenatal hydronephrosis. Pediatrics. 2013;131(1):e251–61. https://doi.org/10.1542/peds.2012-1870.
6. Woodward M, Frank D. Postnatal management of antenatal hydronephrosis. BJU Int. 2002. https://doi.org/10.1046/j.1464-4096.2001.woodward.2578.x.
7. Passoni NM, Peters CA. Managing ureteropelvic junction obstruction in the young infant. Front Pediatr. 2020;8:242.
8. Chertin B, Pollack A, Koulikov D, Rabinowitz R, Hain D, Hadas-Halpren I, Farkas A. Conservative treatment of ureteropelvic junction obstruction in children with antenatal diagnosis of hydronephrosis: Lessons learned after 16 years of follow-up. Eur Urol. 2006;49(4):734–9. https://doi.org/10.1016/j.eururo.2006.01.046.
9. Sadeghi-Bojd S, Kajbafzadeh A, Ansari-Moghadam A, Rashidi S. Postnatal evaluation and outcome of prenatal hydronephrosis. Iran J Pediatr. 2016;26(2):e3667.
10. Yang Y, Hou Y, Niu ZB, Wang CL. Long-term follow-up and management of prenatally detected, isolated hydronephrosis. J Pediatr Surg. 2010;45(8):P1701-1706.

11. Ulman I, Jayanthi VR, Koff SA. The long-term followup of newborns with severe unilateral hydronephrosis initially treated nonoperatively. J Urol. 2000;164(3):1101–5.
12. Arena S, Chimenz R, Antonelli E, Peri FM, Romeo P, et al. A long-term follow-up in conservative management of unilateral ureteropelvic junction obstruction with poor drainage and good renal function. Eur J Pediatr. 2018;177:1761–5.
13. Leong SY, Afolabi TM, Tsu LV. The management of antenatal hydronephrosis U.S. Pharmacist. 2016;41(5):112–6.
14. Sung J, Skoog S. Surgical management of vesicoureteral reflux in children. Pediatr Nephrol. 2012;27(4):551–61. https://doi.org/10.1007/s00467-011-1933-7.
15. Liu DB, Armstrong WR 3rd, Maizels M. Hydronephrosis: prenatal and postnatal evaluation and management. Clin Perinatol. 2014;41(3):661–78. https://doi.org/10.1016/j.clp.2014.05.013.

4

Infection-related hospitalization following ureteroscopic stone treatment: Results from a surgical collaborative

Adam Cole[1*], Jaya Telang[1], Tae-Kyung Kim[1], Kavya Swarna[1], Ji Qi[1], Casey Dauw[1], Brian Seifman[2], Mazen Abdelhady[3], William Roberts[1], John Hollingsworth[1] and Khurshid R. Ghani[1] on behalf of for the Michigan Urological Surgery Improvement Collaborative

Abstract

Background: Unplanned hospitalization following ureteroscopy (URS) for urinary stone disease is associated with patient morbidity and increased healthcare costs. To this effect, AUA guidelines recommend at least a urinalysis in patients prior to URS. We examined risk factors for infection-related hospitalization following URS for urinary stones in a surgical collaborative.

Methods: Reducing Operative Complications from Kidney Stones (ROCKS) is a quality improvement (QI) initiative from the Michigan Urological Surgery Improvement Collaborative (MUSIC) consisting of academic and community practices in the State of Michigan. Trained abstractors prospectively record standardized data elements from the health record in a web-based registry including patient characteristics, surgical details and complications. Using the ROCKS registry, we identified all patients undergoing primary URS for urinary stones between June 2016 and October 2017, and determined the proportion hospitalized within 30 days with an infection-related complication. These patients underwent chart review to obtain clinical data related to the hospitalization. Multivariable logistic regression analysis was performed to determine risk factors for hospitalization.

Results: 1817 URS procedures from 11 practices were analyzed. 43 (2.4%) patients were hospitalized with an infection-related complication, and the mortality rate was 0.2%. Median time to admission and length of stay was 4 and 3 days, respectively. Nine (20.9%) patients did not have a pre-procedure urinalysis or urine culture, which was not different in the non-hospitalized cohort (20.5%). In hospitalized patients, pathogens included gram-negative (61.5%), gram-positive (19.2%), yeast (15.4%), and mixed (3.8%) organisms. Significant factors associated with infection-related hospitalization included higher Charlson comorbidity index, history of recurrent UTI, stone size, intra-operative complication, and procedures where fragments were left in-situ.

Conclusions: One in 40 patients are hospitalized with an infection-related complication following URS. Awareness of risk factors may allow for individualized counselling and management to reduce these events. Approximately 20% of patients did not have a pre-operative urine analysis or culture, and these findings demonstrate the need for further study to improve urine testing and compliance

Keywords: Ureteroscopy, Infection, Outcomes, Quality improvement, Urolithiasis

*Correspondence: aicole@med.umich.edu
[1] Department of Urology, University of Michigan, Ann Arbor, MI 48103, USA

Background

Ureteroscopy (URS) is now the most common treatment modality for treating upper urinary tract stones in North America [1, 2]. Due to technological advances and widespread availability of equipment, URS is often performed in the outpatient setting [3]. Despite this, morbidity, especially infection-related complications, may occur in up to 5–18% of patients [4–8]. These often result in hospital admission and can have a significant impact on patients, providers, and payers [3, 9–11]. A hospital admission for sepsis can cost approximately $20,000 [12]. Therefore, efforts to mitigate infection-related complications following URS would be beneficial in reducing healthcare expenditures.

Prior studies investigating infection-related complications after URS have provided some insights on risk factors, which include stone, patient, and operative characteristics. However, most are single institution series from tertiary referral or academic medical centers [4–10], which may limit generalizability of the results to the wider swathe of urologic patients commonly treated by diverse practitioners in community or multi-specialty group practices.

In the state of Michigan, we have developed a quality improvement (QI) initiative and a clinical registry—Reducing Operative Complications from Kidney Stones (ROCKS)—to better understand processes of care, outcomes, and quality indicators for patients undergoing URS for urinary stones. A strength of this registry is its diversity of patients and practicing urologists. In our drive to improve outcomes for URS, we sought to better understand risk factors for infection-related hospitalization using data from this surgical collaborative. We also sought to assess care in relation to guideline-based practice. We hypothesize that there are modifiable factors which lead to infection related morbidity. Identifying high-risk patients may allow for individualized counseling, and development of QI interventions that reduce adverse events, and the associated patient morbidity and healthcare costs.

Methods

Data source

The Michigan Urological Surgery Improvement Collaborative (MUSIC) was established in 2011 in partnership with Blue Cross Blue Shield of Michigan. The ROCKS QI initiative within MUSIC comprises diverse community and academic urology practices in the state of Michigan and started in 2016. For patients with urinary stones undergoing URS, trained abstractors prospectively record standardized data elements in a web-based registry including patient and stone characteristics, surgical details and complications. Patient data are entered into the registry 60 days after a URS procedure, and data entry is guided by standard variable definitions and collaborative-wide operating procedures. To ensure data quality, the coordinating center performs on-site data audits on a semi-annual basis.

Patient selection and outcomes

We identified all patients undergoing URS for primary treatment of urinary stones between June 2016 and October 2017. During this period, ROCKS consisted of 11 practices. To be included in the ROCKS registry, a patient had to be at least 18 years of age and undergone unilateral URS for urinary stones. Patients who underwent bilateral URS, had an ipsilateral nephrostomy at the time of URS, or underwent URS after percutaneous renal surgery were ineligible. We identified all patients who were discharged after surgery and then subsequently hospitalized (at any institution) within 30 days of their procedure. An infection-related hospitalization was determined by chart review, based on the presence of SIRS criteria with or without bacteriuria. Patients admitted for other indications (pain, hematuria, etc.) were classified as a non-infectious hospitalization. Stone-free rate (SFR) was defined as absence of any fragment on X-ray, CT or ultrasound reports obtained within 60 days. Chart review was performed on all patients with infection-related hospitalizations, including urine culture pathogen data, length of stay, and timing from surgery.

Statistical analyses

We generated descriptive summary statistics of all patients in the analytic sample. Chi-square tests and student's *t* tests were performed for categorical and continuous variables, respectively, to compare demographic and operative factors between the two groups. Significant pre-operative and operative variables were then used as covariates in a multivariable analysis to determine which factors were associated with higher odds of an infection-related hospitalization. Multivariable analysis was performed using a logistic regression model. The odds ratios and 95% confidence intervals were reported. Significant variables with less than 10 events were not included in the multivariable final model. All analyses were performed with SAS 9.4 (SAS Institute, Cary, NC) at a 5% significance level.

Results

A total of 1817 URS procedures in 1737 patients from 11 practices were analyzed. In total, 80 (4.4%) patients were hospitalized within 30 days of their URS. Forty-three (2.4%) patients were hospitalized with an infection-related complication (Fig. 1). Median time from surgery to admission was 4 days (range 0–30) and median length of stay was 3 days (range 1–33) for the patients admitted with an infection-related complication. The majority of admissions (74.4%) occurred within 7 days of surgery,

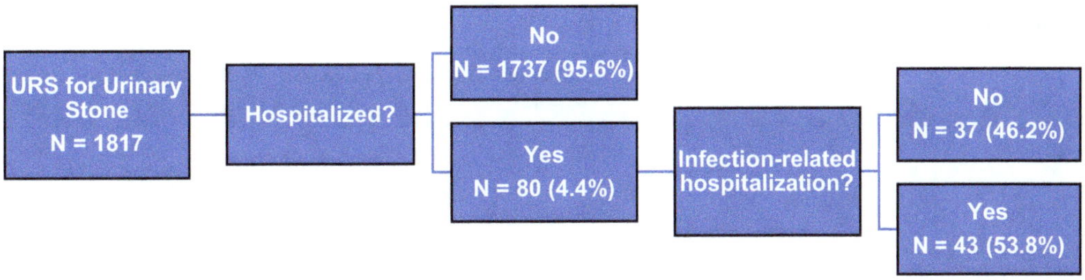

Fig. 1 Post-operative hospitalization events following ureteroscopy for urinary stones in 1817 patients in a statewide surgical collaborative (MUSIC)

and more than half of patients (55.8%) were admitted for longer than 2 days. One (2.3%) patient had a prior ureteroscopy within 1 month of the index surgery. Of patients with a positive urine culture during hospitalization (n = 26), isolated pathogens included 16 (61.5%) gram-negative, 5 (19.2%) gram-positive, 4 (15.4%) yeast, and 1 (3.8%) with gram-positive and -negative cocci. Only 9 of these 26 patients (34.6%) had positive urinalysis (defined by positive nitrite) or urine culture prior to surgery. Three patients died during their hospitalization (mortality rate 0.2%).

Pre-operative, intra-operative, and post-operative characteristics among infection-related hospitalized, and non-hospitalized patients, are provided in Table 1. Significant factors for hospitalization with an infection-related complication on bivariate analysis were public insurance status, older age, higher Charlson Comorbidity Index (CCI), history of recurrent UTI (registry variable based on clinic note by physician indicating history of prior UTIs), spinal cord injury, urinary diversion, intra-operative complication, and larger stone size. Patients that were hospitalized were less likely to be on pre-operative alpha-blockers. There was no statistical difference in the proportion of patients who had an indwelling ureteral stent prior to URS. Of those hospitalized with an infection-related complication, 9 (20.9%) did not have a pre-procedure urinalysis or urine culture, compared to 355 (20.5%) in the non-hospitalized group ($p = 0.95$). 12 (27.9%) patients who were hospitalized with an infectious indication had a positive urinalysis or urine culture prior to surgery, compared to 261 (15.4%) in the non-hospitalized patients ($p = 0.08$). None of the 12 patients with abnormal pre-operative urine studies who were hospitalized were treated with antibiotics prior to surgery.

Patients who were hospitalized for infectious reasons were more likely to have an intra-operative complication (7.0%). Complications included inability to complete procedure due to bleeding or perforation. There was no difference in the rate of ureteral stent placement, ureteral dilation, or use of ureteral access sheath at the time of surgery between the infection-related hospitalization group and the non-admitted group. Those hospitalized with an infection-related complication were more likely to have lithotripsy with fragments left in situ at the conclusion of the operation.

On multivariable analysis (Table 2), significant risks factors associated with hospitalization for infection-related causes included higher CCI, history of recurrent UTI, increasing stone size, history of intra-operative complication, and lithotripsy with fragments left in-situ. The strongest risk factors were the presence of an intra-operative complication (OR 3.7) and history of recurrent UTI (OR 3.74).

Discussion

We found that in 11 diverse urology practices across the state of Michigan, 1 in 40 patients were hospitalized with an infection-related complication following URS for urinary stones. During admission the most commonly identified organisms were gram-negative, however a small proportion of patients had yeast identified. Risk factors for an infection-related admission were higher Charlson comorbidity index, history of recurrent UTI, larger stone size, intra-operative complication and cases where lithotripsy was performed with fragments left in-situ. Overall, 20% of all patients did not have a documented urinalysis or urine culture prior to URS. Collectively, these findings represent an opportunity for the development of QI initiatives to decrease the risk of infection and sepsis after URS, as well as better adherence to American Urological Association (AUA) guidelines.

Previous investigators have examined risk factors for infectious complications following URS. Zhong et al. examined 250 patients that underwent URS for stone treatment, and found an 8.1% incidence of systemic inflammatory response syndrome (SIRS) following the procedure. Risk-factors included stone size, smaller caliber ureteral access sheath, higher irrigation flow rate, and presence of struvite calculi [8]. Other studies have also identified female gender [5, 6, 13], history of

Table 1 Patient characteristics for patients undergoing ureteroscopy for urinary stones in MUSIC ROCKS stratified by post-operative course

Risk factor	Infection-related hospitalization (n = 43)	Non-hospitalized (n = 1737)	*P* value
Pre-operative characteristics			
Public insurance	25 (58.1%)	669 (39.7%)	0.01
Mean age (SD)	60.1 (15.8)	54.4 (15.5)	0.02
Male gender	19 (44.2%)	867 (50.1%)	0.44
BMI > 30	24 (58.5%)	788 (46.8%)	0.13
CCI ≥ 1	26 (60.5%)	495 (28.5%)	< 0.01
CCI ≥ 2	14 (32.6%)	241 (13.9%)	< 0.01
Presence of hydronephrosis on pre-operative imaging	27 (67.5%)	1048 (66.7%)	0.92
Largest stone size (mm), mean (SD)	10.1 (6.5)	7.8 (5.4)	< 0.01
Solitary kidney	2 (4.7%)	25 (1.5%)	0.13
Horseshoe kidney	1 (2.3%)	6 (0.4%)	0.16
History of recurrent UTI	9 (20.9%)	88 (5.1%)	< 0.01
Urinary diversion	2 (4.7%)	7 (0.4%)	0.02
Spinal cord injury	2 (4.7%)	3 (0.2%)	< 0.01
Anti-platelet therapy	13 (30.2%)	345 (20.4%)	0.12
Pre-operative urinalysis/urine culture not performed	9 (20.9%)	355 (20.5%)	0.95
Positive pre-operative urinalysis/urine culture	12 (27.9%)	266 (15.4%)	0.08
Positive pre-operative urinalysis/urine culture treated	0 (0%)	59 (22.2%)	0.07
Urgent/emergent surgery	1 (2.3%)	146 (8.4%)	0.15
Peri-operative antibiotic use	38 (95%)	1513 (96.9%)	0.49
Alpha-blocker therapy prior to URS	11 (26.2%)	755 (45.1%)	0.01
Pre-stenting (ureteral stent in place)	20 (46.5%)	649 (37.5%)	0.23
Stone location			
Renal	17 (45.9%)	502 (31.0%)	0.07
Ureter	14 (37.8%)	906 (56.0%)	
Both	6 (16.2%)	211 (13.0%)	
Intra-operative characteristics			
Intra-operative complication	3 (7.0%)	33 (1.9%)	< 0.01
Complication: bleeding	2 (4.7%)	14 (0.8)	
Complication: perforation	0 (0.0%)	4 (0.2%)	
Complication: other	1 (2.3%)	15 (0.9%)	
Ureteral dilation	6 (13.9%)	340 (19.7%)	0.44
Ureteral access sheath use	18 (41.9%)	626 (36.6%)	0.49
Lithotripsy with fragments left in-situ	30 (69.8%)	716 (42.3%)	< 0.01
Stenting during URS	31 (72.1%)	1248 (72.1%)	0.99
Post-operative characteristics			
Discharged with antibiotics	15 (36.6%)	638 (39.2%)	0.74
Discharged with antibiotics and stent placed	9 (20.9%)	509 (29.3%)	0.23
Discharged with alpha-blocker	27 (65.8%)	911 (55.9%)	0.21
Stone free rate	19 (57.6%)	579 (77.5%)	< 0.01

obstructive pyelonephritis [5, 6], positive pre-operative urine culture [5, 6], and prolonged ureteral stent dwell time [5] as risk factors for SIRS/sepsis, with rates of SIRS/sepsis from 0.30–8% [5–8, 14]. We also found similar risk factors for hospitalization related to infectious complications, including higher Charlson comorbidity index, history of recurrent UTI, intra-operative complication, and stone size. Interestingly, female gender and pre-operative ureteral stenting were not risk factors in this analysis. Female gender has been a reported risk factor in some series [5, 6, 13], however in other studies this was not a risk factor [7, 14] suggesting differences in

Table 2 Multi-variable logistic regression demonstrating association between patient characteristics and risk of infection-related hospitalization

Risk factor	OR	CI	*P* value
Age	1.01	0.98–1.03	0.95
Comorbidity (CCI 0 vs. 1)	3.12	1.37–7.14	<0.01
Comorbidity (CCI 0 vs. 2)	2.72	1.16–6.37	0.02
Stone size	1.04	1.01–1.07	0.02
History of recurrent UTI	3.74	1.55–9.00	<0.01
Insurance (public vs. private)	1.57	0.75–3.25	0.23
Alpha-blocker prior to URS	0.51	0.24–1.06	0.07
Complete fragment removal	0.32	0.16–0.65	<0.01
Intra-operative complication	3.70	1.22–11.25	0.02

study design. Perhaps a prospective study would be helpful. Additionally, public insurance was associated with an increased risk of an infectious-hospitalization on univariate analysis. However, this association was not seen in our multi-variable model, suggesting that the association of insurance and infection may be due to other factors.

Awareness of risk factors can allow for an individualized approach to pre-operative antibiotic selection, adoption of intra-operative technical factors such as considering a ureteral access sheath or limiting the irrigation flow rate, and post-operative antibiotic therapy in patients at risk for developing sepsis. Since there was a strong relationship between an intra-operative complication and subsequent hospitalization, patients who suffer this event could be considered for prolonged observation in the recovery room or even admission and observation. Likewise, patients with a history of recurrent UTI should be considered for pre-operative urine culture (not urinalysis) and be managed with culture-directed pre-operative antibiotics. While almost all patients received peri-operative antibiotics, more patients in the hospitalized group had an abnormal urine study prior to surgery, and none of these patients were treated with antibiotics. There are a very small number of patients in both groups with untreated positive urine cultures prior to ureteroscopy. This represents a focus for subsequent quality improvement initiatives with the goal to improve pre-operative testing and follow-up.

We found that in patients with a positive urine culture during hospitalization, only 34.6% had a positive UA or urine culture prior to surgery. It is possible this discordance lies in our definition of a positive urinalysis (nitrite positivity), which can be altered by medications such as pyridium. Additionally, any positive pre-op culture, regardless of organism or colony count, is deemed positive. These represent limitations of our study, however, previous studies have also reported discordance between pre-operative, intra-operative and post-operative urine cultures in patients undergoing stone surgery. Paonessa et al. examined pre-operative urine cultures and intraoperative stone cultures in patients undergoing percutaneous nephrolithotomy and found that 9.7% of patients with negative pre-operative urine cultures had positive stone cultures. In patients with both positive pre-operative urine and intra-operative stone cultures, the organisms differed in 13.3%, representing an overall discordance in almost a quarter of cases [15]. Marien et al. also demonstrated 27% discordant voided and upper tract urine cultures after decompression for obstructing stones [16].

The AUA Guidelines on Surgical Management of Stones advises clinicians to obtain a urinalysis prior to URS, and in patients with clinical or laboratory signs of infection, a urine culture should be obtained [17]. EAU Guidelines state a urine culture or urinary microscopy are mandatory before treatment [18]. In our cohort, approximately 20% of patients who were admitted with an infectious complication did not have a urinalysis or urine culture prior to surgery. This aspect of care, where patients are not managed in accordance with current guidelines represents an area for improvement. Interestingly, this rate was similar in the group of non-hospitalized patients. It would appear that obtaining a pre-operative urinalysis or urine culture did not alter the risk of hospitalization for an infection-related reason. One major limitation of our work is that we do not differentiate between urine culture or urinalysis in our registry. Additionally, the pre-operative screening requirements vary by center due to institutional protocols, work-flow, staffing, and resources. Some institutions require a urine culture within 30 days of surgery, while others use urinalysis with reflex culture. Despite these difference, pre-operative urine studies were not obtained in approximately 20% of all patients, likely for a variety of reasons: urine studies may not have been ordered, urine studies were ordered but not performed by the patient, or they were performed at outside institutions but not available. Our findings warrant further investigation to address these quality of care gaps.

Lithotripsy with fragments left in-situ was associated with an increased risk of infection-related hospitalization in our cohort. This variable is determined by review of the operative notes by data abstractors based on key phrases, such as "all fragments were removed," or "all remaining fragments were 1 mm of less." The database does not detect specific stone treatment technique, and it is difficult to ascertain if this indicates dusting technique, or a hybrid technique of basketing and dusting. It is possible that our results are confounded by patients with large stone burden. Also, while patients in the non-hospitalized group were more likely to be on pre-operative alpha-blockers, this was not significantly associated with a lower risk of an infection-related hospitalization on multi-variate analysis. In a recent study, 1 week of pre-operative alpha-blocker therapy was associated with lower overall complications after URS [19]. The same mechanism by which alpha-blockers are prescribed to facilitate ureteral stone passage—inhibition of the alpha receptors in the distal ureter and reduced ureteral muscle tone and peristalsis—has been proposed to facilitate ureteroscopy and instrumentation of the ureter [20]. This is an area of interest that will be the subject of future investigation.

Our work has several limitations. First, our patients are located in a single state and it is possible these results are not applicable to all patients in the United States or outside the country. Our registry does not collect information on pre-operative ureteral stent dwell-time, technical intraoperative details such as size of access sheath, irrigation rate, surgical time, and other factors that may place patients at higher risk for developing an infectious complication. In addition, stone cultures are not captured by registry. Additionally, it is possible we are underreporting the number of events based on our study design. From the registry we were able to identify all patients that were hospitalized within 30 days. We then made a determination if the hospitalization was due to infectious or non-infectious etiologies (pain, hematuria, etc.) based on chart review. Along with the admission notes, SIRS criteria were used to determine if the admission was due to infectious-indication, as culture data was not available or obtained after administration of antibiotics. Therefore it is possible that some patients were admitted with infectious-indications without SIRS criteria. Finally, the small number of hospitalization events may alter the fit of our multi-variable model.

Our findings do have several implications. URS is among the most commonly performed urologic surgeries, and unplanned healthcare encounters following URS are not uncommon. We demonstrate suboptimal statewide compliance with guidelines regarding pre-operative urine screening. Efforts should be taken to comply with best practice statements, and this will be the subject of future QI initiatives in MUSIC. In particular we are considering collecting information on which specific pre-operative urine study was performed to determine whether urinalysis is insufficient as a screening tool to mitigate the risk of sepsis after URS.

Conclusion

We found that nearly 1 in 40 patients are hospitalized with an infection-related complication following URS for urinary stones in diverse practices in Michigan. Awareness of risk factors may allow for individualized counselling and management to reduce these events. Approximately 20% of patients did not have a pre-operative urine analysis or culture, and these findings demonstrate the need for further study to improve urine testing and compliance.

Abbreviations

URS: Ureteroscopy; AUA: American Urological Association; ROCKS: Reducing Operative Complications from Kidney Stones; MUSIC: Michigan Urological Surgery Improvement Collaborative; QI: Quality improvement; SFR: Stone-free rate; UTI: Urinary tract infection; CCI: Charlson Comorbidity Index; OR: Odds ratio; SIRS: Systemic inflammatory response syndrome; UA: Urinalysis; EAU: European Association of Urology.

Acknowledgements

We would like to thank the significant contribution of the clinical champions, urologists and data abstractors in each participating MUSIC ROCKS practice. In addition, we would like to acknowledge the support provided by the Value Partnerships program at BCBSM.

Authors' contributions

Made substantial contributions to the conception: AC, KG. Made substantial contributions to design of the work: AC, JT, TK, KS, JQ, Made substantial contributions to the acquisition and analysis of the data: AC, JT, TM, KS, JQ. Made substantial contributions to interpretation of the data: AC, CD, WR, JH, KG. Made substantial contributions to drafting and revising the manuscript: AC, CD, BS, MA, WR, JH, KG. All authors read and approved the final manuscript.

Competing interests

The authors declare that they have no competing interests.

Author details

Department of Urology, University of Michigan, Ann Arbor, MI 48103, USA. [2] Michigan Institute of Urology, West Bloomfield, MI 48322, USA. [3] Detroit Medical Center, Department of Urology, Detroit, MI 48201, USA.

References

1. Oberlin DT, Flum AS, Bachrach L, Matulewicz RS, Flury SC. Contemporary surgical trends in the management of upper tract calculi. J Urol. 2015;193:880–4.
2. Ordon M, et al. The surgical management of kidney stone disease: a population based time series analysis. J Urol. 2014;192:1450–6.
3. San Juan J, Hou H, Ghani KR, Dupree JM, Hollingsworth JM. Variation in spending around surgical episodes of urinary stone disease: findings from Michigan. J Urol. 2018;199:1277–82.
4. Mitsuzuka K, Nakano O, Takahashi N, Satoh M. Identification of factors associated with postoperative febrile urinary tract infection after ureteroscopy for urinary stones. Urolithiasis. 2016;44:257–62.
5. Nevo A, Mano R, Baniel J, Lifshitz DA. Ureteric stent dwelling time: a risk factor for post-ureteroscopy sepsis. BJU Int. 2017;120:117–22.
6. Uchida Y, Takazawa R, Kitayama S, Tsujii T. Predictive risk factors for systemic inflammatory response syndrome following ureteroscopic laser lithotripsy. Urolithiasis. 2018;46:375–81.
7. Blackmur JP, et al. Analysis of factors' association with risk of postoperative urosepsis in patients undergoing ureteroscopy for treatment of stone disease. J Endourol. 2016;30:963–9.
8. Zhong W, Leto G, Wang L, Zeng G. Systemic inflammatory response syndrome after flexible ureteroscopic lithotripsy: a study of risk factors. J Endourol. 2015;29:25–8.
9. Bloom J, Matthews G, Phillips J. Factors influencing readmission after elective ureteroscopy. J Urol. 2016;195:1487–91.
10. Du K, et al. Unplanned 30-day encounters after ureterorenoscopy for urolithiasis. J Endourol. 2018;32:1100–7.
11. Scales CD, et al. The impact of unplanned postprocedure visits in the management of patients with urinary stones. Surgery. 2014;155:769–75.
12. Arefian H, et al. Hospital-related cost of sepsis: a systematic review. J Infect. 2017;74:107–17.

13. Martov A, et al. Postoperative infection rates in patients with a negative baseline urine culture undergoing ureteroscopic stone removal: a matched case–control analysis on antibiotic prophylaxis from the CROES URS global study. J Endourol. 2015;29:171–80.
14. Somani BK, et al. Complications associated with ureterorenoscopy (URS) related to treatment of urolithiasis: the Clinical Research Office of Endourological Society URS Global study. World J Urol. 2017;35:675–81.
15. Paonessa JE, Gnessin E, Bhojani N, Williams JC, Lingeman JE. Preoperative bladder urine culture as a predictor of intraoperative stone culture results: clinical implications and relationship to stone composition. J Urol. 2016;196:769–74.
16. Marien T, Mass AY, Shah O. Antimicrobial resistance patterns in cases of obstructive pyelonephritis secondary to stones. Urology. 2015;85:64–8.
17. Assimos D, et al. Surgical management of stones: American urological association/endourological society guideline, PART I. J Urol. 2016;196:1153–60.
18. Türk C, et al. EAU guidelines on interventional treatment for urolithiasis. Eur Urol. 2016;69:475–82.
19. Sokhal A, et al. Do pre-operative alpha blockers facilitate ureteroscope insertion at the vesico-ureteric junction? An answer from a prostective case–controlled study. Eur Med J. 2017;2:82–6.
20. Alsaikhan B, Koziarz A, Lee J, Pace K. Preoperative alpha-blockers for ureteroscopy for ureteral stones: a systematic review and meta-analysis of randomized controlled trials. J Endourol. 2020;34:33–41.
21. Margel D, et al. Clinical implication of routine stone culture in percutaneous nephrolithotomy—a prospective study. J Urol. 2006;67:26–9.

5

Laparoscopic resection of a large clinically silent paraganglioma at the organ of Zuckerkandl

Xiang Ren[1], Jiwen Shang[1,2*], Ruimin Ren[2], Huajun Zhang[2] and Xue Yao[2]

Abstract

Background: Large paraganglioma of the Zuckerkandl organ (POZ) is extremely rare. The patient can occasionally be paucisymptomatic, further obscuring the diagnosis and carrying high mortality. Recommended treatment for large paraganglioma (PGL) is open surgical removal. We report a case of successful laparoscopic resection of a large POZ with normal blood pressure in a 45-year-old man.

Case presentation: A 45-year-old man was hospitalized because of hyperglycemia. Computed tomography of the abdomen and the serum and urinary catecholamine levels confirmed the diagnosis of large POZ. But his blood pressure was normal and he underwent laparoscopic tumor excision successfully. During 6 months follow-up after laparoscopy, serum and urinary catecholamines were normal but glycaemia remained high level. DNA analysis of the succinate dehydrogenase complex subunits B (SDHB) and SDHD revealed no mutation.

Conclusions: POZ is an unusual mass and preoperative diagnosis can be difficult in clinically silent cases. PGL cannot be excluded in patients with normal blood pressure. Even a large POZ can be excised laparoscopically by following proper techniques.

Keywords: Paraganglioma, Large, Silent, Organ of zuckerkandl, Laparoscopy, Genetic testing

Background

PGLs are catecholamine-producing tumors that may occur anywhere along the sympathetic paraganglionic chain [1]. The treatment of PGL including its diagnosis is difficult, especially when some patients lack typical clinical signs and symptoms (headache, palpitations, sweating, or hypertension) which are due to the direct actions of secreted catecholamines. About 53% of PGLs occur in the organs of Zuckerkandl [2], which are a collection of paraganglia located anterolaterally to the distal abdominal aorta between the origin of the inferior mesenteric artery or renal artery and the aortic bifurcation. The majority of POZs are non-functional [3], so misdiagnosis and missed diagnosis are common. Traditional treatment for large POZ was open surgical resection, and only a few cases of laparoscopic approach to this pathology have been reported (Table 1). We report a case of successful laparoscopic resection of a large POZ with normal blood pressure in a 45-year-old man and review the related literature on POZ.

Case presentation

A 45-year-old man with a half-year history of hyperglycemia presented to endocrinology. The patient denied attacks of headache, hypertension, palpitation and sweating. He was kept for observation with 24-h

*Correspondence: sjw139@126.com
[1] Graduate School, Shanxi Medical University, Taiyuan 030000, China

electrocardiography (ECG) and blood pressure monitoring which was normal. His glycaemia returned to normal level under the action of insulin. Haematological and biochemical investigations were normal except for elevated serum and urinary catecholamines (Table 2). Abdominal-pelvic CT scan with contrast injection had revealed a 7.2 × 6.5 cm inhomogeneous, right para-aortic mass located at the level of the inferior mesenteric artery (Fig. 1). Both the adrenals were normal. With these findings, a diagnosis of POZ was reached. However, due to

Table 1 Cases of laparoscopic resection of a large POZ reported in the literature

Case	References	Misdiagnosis	Age (years)	Size (cm)	Time (min)	Blood loss (mL)	Genetic screening	Gene mutation
1	Kravarusic et al. [4]	No	14	6	NA	NA	Yes	SDHB
2	Thapar et al. [5]	No	20	6.5 × 5	NA	300	No	–
3	Cozzupoli et al. [6]	NA	20	10	NA	NA	NA	NA
4	Salgaonkar et al. [3]	No	22	8 × 7	125	40	No	–
5	Joshi et al. [7]	Yes	28	7.5 × 6.6 × 7.5	NA	NA	No	–
Present		Yes	45	7.2 × 6.5	120	50	Yes	No

NA not available

Table 2 Blood and urinary analysis

	Upon presentation	6 months follow-up	Reference values
Blood pressure (max)	118/76 mmHg	115/75 mmHg	100–120/60–80 mmHg
Fasting blood-glucose (max)	7.5 mmol/L	7.4 mmol/L	3.9–6.1 mmol/L
Blood			
Adrenaline	1050 pg/mL	39.7 pg/mL	0–100 pg/mL
Noradrenaline	650 pg/mL	168.0 pg/mL	0–600 pg/mL
Dopamine	102 pg/mL	59.17 pg/mL	0–100 pg/mL
Urine			
Metanephrines 24 h	2120 mg/24 h	190 mg/24 h	64–350 mg/24 h
Normetanephrines 24 h	4252 mg/24 h	260 mg/24 h	120–490 mg/24 h
Vanillylmandelic acid 24 h	35 mg/24 h	6.0 mg/24 h	2.0–7.1 mg/24 h

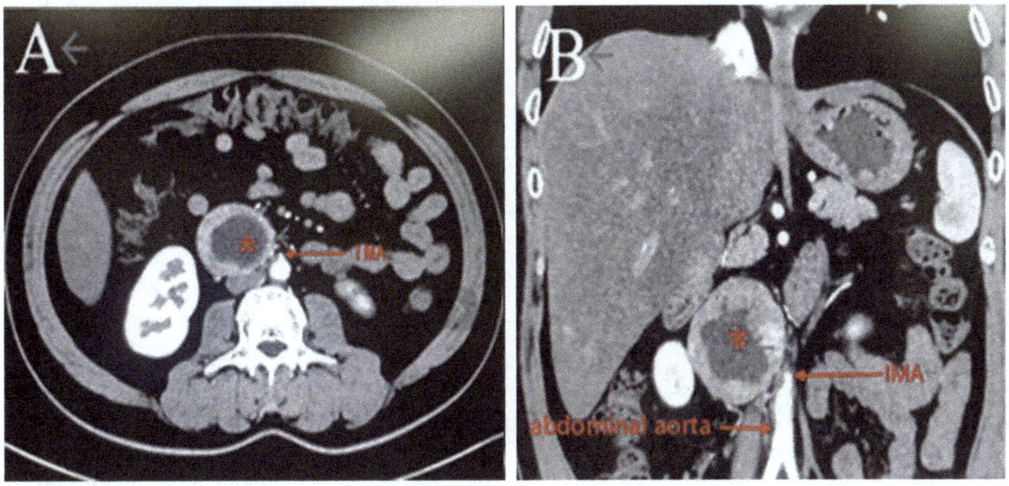

Fig. 1 CT findings: CT shows a 7.2 × 6.5 cm right para-aortic mass (asterisk) located at the level of the inferior mesenteric artery (IMA). Transverse plane (**a**). Coronal plane (**b**)

the patient's family economic reasons and the lack of MIBG scan examination equipment in our hospital, our patient did not undergo further MIBG scan examination. Then he was transferred to our center where attempts to preoperative preparation included expansion of intravascular volume and alpha blockade with phenoxybenzamine for 2 weeks even with the situation of normal blood pressure.

We made full consideration and preparation for possible conversion to open surgery before deciding to adopt laparoscopic surgery. If there were acute bleeding, small operation space, malignant tumor invasion or other parts of the injury that have to be converted to open surgery, we will use a longitudinal incision under the right costal margin for open surgery. In addition, we also communicated with vascular surgeons that if the aorta or the inferior vena cava were damaged, open resection and reconstruction of these vessels might be warranted.

The patient was placed in 70° left lateral decubitus position, and a 10-mm trocar was inserted above the umbilicus for telescope using. Another 10-mm, 10-mm and 5-mm trocar were placed under the right costal margin, right anterior axillary line and subxiphoid, respectively (Fig. 2). A steep Trendelenburg position allowed the small bowel and omentum to be moved away from the mass. First, cut the hepatic triangular ligament and hepatocolicum ligament with an ultrasonic shears, and lift the liver to expose the upper pole of the right kidney. The ascending mesocolon is then longitudinally incised and pushed open to expose the right kidney and the right renal vein, and the descending and horizontal parts of the duodenum are separated and pushed open, showing that the upper pole of the exposed tumor is filled with nourishing vessels. Then the vessels of nutritional tumors were separated and ligated one by one. Uncovering the lower part of the tumor, it can be seen that the inferior vena cava and abdominal aorta, and the abdominal aorta send out a thicker vascular supply tumor, which was ligated by Hem-o-lock. The tumor and its surrounding tissues were then clipped along the tumor capsule and separated gradually. The well-encapsulated mass was excised. The mass was placed in a sample collection bag and removed through a 5-cm right upper abdomen incision that incorporated the incision made for the costal margin 10-mm port. Except for upon contact with the tumor blood pressure rose up to 160 mmHg he remained stable throughout surgery. The total operative time was 120 min and intraoperative blood loss was around 50 mL. The post-operative period was uneventful and he was discharged on post-operative day 5. The histopathology found the tissue was consistent with a benign PGL and DNA analysis of SDHB and SDHD revealed no mutation. During 6 months follow-up after post-operative, urinary and serum catecholamines were within normal range but glycaemia remained high level (Table 2).

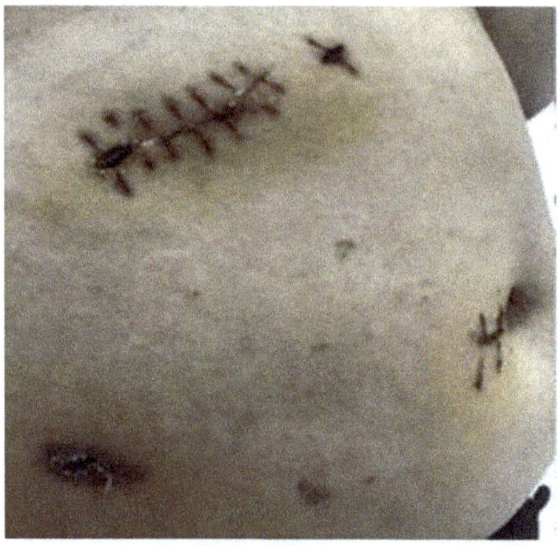

Fig. 2 Positions of the ports. A 10-mm trocar was inserted above the umbilicus, and another 10-mm, 10-mm and 5-mm trocar were placed under the right costal margin, right anterior axillary line and subxiphoid, respectively

Discussion and conclusion

PGLs are rare catecholamine-secreting neuroendocrine tumors that arise from the extra-adrenal paraganglia. Most PGLs occur in the subdiaphragmatic region, most commonly within the organ of Zuckerkandl [8]. The clinical presentation of pheochromocytomas/PGLs can vary remarkably, from dramatic symptoms and signs to minimal or no symptoms whatsoever [9]. This latter situation is often termed "clinically silent" pheochromocytoma/PGL [10, 11]. Even though the patient with a clinically silent PGL experiences no symptoms and shows no signs of a PGL, blood and urine levels of catecholamines are often elevated [10–12]. This situation usually leads to misdiagnosis and missed diagnosis. Therefore, understanding its clinical characteristics is very important for the standardized diagnosis and treatment of clinical diseases. In our case, the patient without characteristic paroxysmal attacks of headache, sweating, palpitation and hypertension only presented with hyperglycemia. Although pheochromocytomas/PGLs can cause hyperglycemia and even induce diabetes type 2 [13], the patient's glycaemia remained high level at 6-month follow-up after post-operative when urinary and serum catecholamines were normal. It confirmed that this hyperglycemia was presumably not related to the POZ, but merely coincided by chance.

A giant PGL/pheochromocytoma usually present with paucity of clinical signs and symptoms [14, 15]. The mechanism of clinically silent PGL/pheochromocytoma remains unclear. The reasons for the same can be due of the presence of tumoral necrosis, high loads of interstitial tissue compared to chromaffin cells or the paucity of the release of the catecholamines due to encapsulation by the connective tissues [15]. These cause normal catecholamine values during their serum and urinary assays [16]. There are also studies that believe that there is a self-metabolism mechanism of catecholamines inside the tumor, which prevents active catecholamines from being released into the blood [17]. These explanations are not consistent with our case. Therefore, the mechanism of this situation needs to be further explored in subsequent studies.

Previously, it was considered that there were no guidelines to ensure adequate preoperative preparation in these clinically silent tumors [10]. The present view holds that patients suspected of clinically silent pheochromocytoma should be given a high sodium diet and adequate fluid intake before surgery, and alpha blockade should be prepared for 7–14 days to avoid possible cardiovascular damage caused by abrupt blood pressure rise and fall and insufficient blood volume during and after surgery [18]. Surgical resection is the treatment of choice for POZ, and laparoscopic resection is suited for small (<7 cm) tumors [3]. Only eight cases of laparoscopic resection of POZ have been described till to 2020. Depending on their location, strategies utilized to approach the tumor included duodenal Kocherisation as well as colonic mobilization [3]. Under the situation of our patients with tumors>7 cm, we chose laparoscopic resection with duodenal Kocherisation, exposed the tumor directly after freeing the kidney, and early controlled the blood vessels from the abdominal aorta to reduce intraoperative bleeding and minimize intraoperative hemodynamic instability.

Most PGLs appear to be sporadic; however, about 30–35% of tumors are associated with hereditary syndromes, mainly multiple endocrine neoplasia type 2 (MEN-2), von Hippel Lindau (VHL) disease, and neurofibromatosis type 1(NF1) [19]. 70% of POZ cases are associated with SDHB or less commonly SDHD gene mutations [20]. In our case, blood calcitonin, serum free T3, free T4, and TSH levels were normal. These results make MEN-2 disease unlikely. Ophthalmological screening showed an absence of retinal hemangioblastoma that makes VHL disease unlikely. The lack of cutaneouscafé-au-lait spots suggested the absence of NF1. DNA analysis of SDHB and SDHD revealed no mutation. In addition, genetic testing should be performed for at-risk family members [21].We once advised his family members to do the related genetic tests, but they refused due to the cost. Nonetheless, a predisposing genetic factor cannot be excluded since current research has revealed several other genes linked to familial and sporadic cases of pheochromocytoma [22]. Thus, we advised the patient to return for regular follow-up.

In conclusion, POZ is an unusual mass and preoperative diagnosis can be difficult in clinically silent cases. PGL cannot be excluded in patients with normal blood pressure. Even a large POZ can be excised laparoscopically by following proper techniques.

Abbreviations

POZ: Paraganglioma of the Zuckerkandl organ; PGL: Paraganglioma; CT: Computed tomography; SDHB: Succinate dehydrogenase complex subunit B; SDHD: Succinate dehydrogenase complex subunit D; ECG: Electrocardiography; Max: Maximum; IMA: Inferior mesenteric artery; MEN-2: Multiple endocrine neoplasia type 2; VHL: Von Hippel Lindau; NF1: Neurofibromatosis type 1; TSH: Thyroid stimulating hormone.

Acknowledgements

Not applicable.

Authors' contributions

XR made contributions to the acquisition of history, image and wrote the manuscript. JS performed the treatment, and reviewed the manuscript to give clinical opinions. RR made supervision and helped reviewing the manuscript. HZ and XY reviewed the manuscript and were involved in its critical revision before submission. All authors read and approved the final manuscript.

Competing interests

The authors declare that they have no competing interests.

Author details

[1] Graduate School, Shanxi Medical University, Taiyuan 030000, China.
[2] Department of Urology, Shanxi Bethune Hospital, No. 99 Longcheng Street, Taiyuan 030032, Shanxi, China.

References

1. Ilias I, Pacak K. A clinical overview of pheochromocytomas/paragangliomas and carcinoid tumors. Nucl Med Biol. 2008;35(Suppl 1):S27-34.
2. Sarveswaran V, Kumar S, Kumar A, Vamseedharan M. A giant cysticpheochromocytoma mimicking liver abscess an unusual presentation—a case report. Clin Case Rep. 2015;3(1):64–8.
3. Salgaonkar H, Behera RR, Sharma PC, Chadha M, Katara AN, Bhandarkar DS. Laparoscopic resection of a large paraganglioma arising in the organ of Zuckerkandl: report of a case and review of the literature. J Minim Access Surg. 2016;12(4):378–81.
4. Kravarusic D, Pinto-Rojas A, Al-Assiri A, Sigalet D. Laparoscopic resection of extra-adrenal pheochromocytoma—case report and review of the literature in pediatric patients. J Pediatr Surg. 2007;42(10):1780–4.
5. Thapar PM, Dalvi AN, Kamble RS, Vijaykumar V, Shah NS, Menon PS. Laparoscopic transmesocolic excision of paraganglioma in the organ of Zuckerkandl. J Laparoendosc Adv Surg Tech A. 2006;16(6):620–2.
6. Cozzupoli P, Veneziano D, Sicuro O, Carbone L, Sgrò E. Laparoscopic resec tion of a large functional paraganglioma in the organ of Zuckerkandl. Urology. 2011;71:S168.
7. Joshi CJ, Bhat S. 2018 Organ of Zuckerkandl: laparoscopic excision of a rarity. Indian J Surg. 2018;9486:1.
8. Gill T, Adler K, Schrader A, Desai K, Wermers J, Beteselassie N. Extra-adrenal pheochromocytoma at the organ of Zuckerkandl: a case report and literature review. Radiol Case Rep. 2017;12(2):343–7.
9. Hodin R, Lubitz C, Phitayakorn R, Stephen A. Diagnosis and management of pheochromocytoma. Curr Prob Surg. 2014;51(4):151–87.
10. Shen SJ, Cheng HM, Chiu AW, Chou CW, Chen JY. Perioperative hypertensive crisis in clinically silent pheochromocytomas: report of four cases. Chang Gung Med J. 2005;28(1):44–50.

10. Shen SJ, Cheng HM, Chiu AW, Chou CW, Chen JY. Perioperative hypertensive crisis in clinically silent pheochromocytomas: report of four cases. Chang Gung Med J. 2005;28(1):44–50.
11. Kota SK, Kota SK, Panda S, Modi KD. Pheochromocytoma: an uncommon presentation of an asymptomatic and biochemically silent adrenal incidentaloma. Malays J Med Sci. 2012;19(2):86–91.
12. Yoshida K, Sasaguri M, Kinoshita A, Ideishi M, Ikeda M, Arakawa K. A case of a clinically "silent" pheochromocytoma. Pheochromocytoma. Jpn J Med. 1990;29(1):27–31.
13. Havekes B, Pacak K. Pheochromocytoma. Nat Clin Pract Cardiovasc Med. 2008;5:E1.
14. Munakomi S, Rajbanshi S, Adhikary PS. Case report: a giant but silent adrenal pheochromocytoma—a rare entity. F1000Res . 2016;5:290.
15. Li C, Chen Y, Wang W, Teng L. A case of clinically silent giant right pheochromocytoma and review of literature. Can Urol Assoc J. 2012;6(6):E267–9.
16. Wang HL, Sun BZ, Xu ZJ, Lei WF, Wang XS. Undiagnosed giant cystic pheochromocytoma: a case report. Oncol Lett. 2015;10(3):1444–6.
17. Peyrin L, Cottet-Emard JM, Cottet-Emard RM, Vouillarmet A. The diagnosis of atypical pheochromocytoma: a challenge for the biologist as well. Pathol Biol (Paris). 2001;49(3):247–54.
18. Zhu GD, Tang C, Song WB, Yang ZS, Zhang Y, Fan JH, et al. Surgical treatment of 137 cases of pheochromocytoma/paraganglioma: outcome analysis and clinical experience from a single institution. J Mod Urol. 2017;08:36–40.
19. Costa MH, Ortiga-Carvalho TM, Violante AD, Vaisman M. Pheochromocytomas and paragangliomas: clinical and genetic approaches. Front Endocrinol (Lausanne). 2015;6:126.
20. Lodish MB, Adams KT, Huynh TT, Prodanov T, Ling A, Chen C, Shusterman S, Jimenez C, Merino M, Hughes M, et al. Succinate dehydrogenase gene mutations are strongly associated with paraganglioma of the organ of Zuckerkandl. Endocr Relat Cancer. 2010;17(3):581–8.
21. Chen H, Sippel R, O'dorisio S, Vinik A, Lloyd R, Pacak K. Pheochromocytoma, paraganglioma, and medullary thyroid cancer. The North American Neuroendocrine Tumor Society Consensus Guideline for the diagnosis and management of neuroendocrine tumors. Pancreas. 2010;39(6):775–83.
22. Shuch B, Ricketts CJ, Metwalli AR, Pacak K, Linehan WM. The genetic basis of pheochromocytoma and paraganglioma: implications for management. Urology. 2014;83(6):1225–32.

6

Intravesical prostatic protrusion may affect early postoperative continence undergoing robot-assisted radical prostatectomy

Katsuya Hikita*, Masashi Honda, Shogo Teraoka, Ryoma Nishikawa, Yuske Kimura, Panagiota Tsounapi, Hideto Iwamoto, Shuichi Morizane and Atsushi Takenaka

Abstract

Background: In this study, we investigated the effect of preoperative prostate morphology, especially intravesical prostatic protrusion (IPP), on continence after robot-assisted radical prostatectomy (RARP).

Methods: Retrospective analysis was applied to patients who underwent RARP between October 2010 and July 2014. The following parameters were assessed in all patients: age, body mass index (BMI), prostate-specific antigen, magnetic resonance imaging and pressure-flow studies findings. The impact of preoperative and intraoperative factors on postoperative urinary incontinence (UI) was assessed using multivariate logistic regression analysis. To evaluate the effects of IPP, the patients were divided into groups according to the IPP length: Group 1, < 5 mm and Group 2, ≥ 5 mm. The International Prostate Symptom Score (IPSS), Overactive Bladder Symptom Score, Quality of Life index and the number of pads used were assessed.

Results: A total of 119 patients were eligible for this study. Multivariate analyses showed that IPP (odds ratio (OR) 1.14, 95% confidence interval (CI) 1.02–1.28, $p < 0.05$) and nerve-sparing (NS) (OR 0.23, 95% CI 0.18–0.61, $p < 0.01$) were significant factors related to UI in the first month after RARP. Twelve months after RARP, multivariate analyses revealed that only NS is a factor related to postoperative UI (OR 0.23, 95% CI 0.18–0.61, $p < 0.01$). The comparison of Groups 1 and 2 indicated significant differences in age ($p < 0.01$), prostate volume ($p < 0.01$), total IPSS and voiding symptom score ($p < 0.05$), compliance ($p < 0.01$), and detrusor pressure at maximum flow ($p < 0.01$). Group 1 had a higher continence rate (38.0%) than Group 2 (20.8%) in the first month after RARP ($p < 0.05$), but the difference was no longer significant from the third month after RARP. The total IPSS and voiding symptom scores were significantly different between the two groups before RARP, however, the significant difference disappeared from the first month after RARP.

Conclusions: The data suggest that IPP affects early postoperative UI. Although NS was strongly involved in UI in the early and later stages after RARP, IPP had no effect on UI in the later stages.

Keywords: Prostate/diagnostic imaging, Prostatectomy/adverse effects, Urinary incontinence/surgery, Robotic surgical procedures/adverse effects, Quality of life

Background

To date there is a variety of treatments for localized prostate cancer (PCa) that can be performed, including active surveillance, radiation therapy and radical prostatectomy. In particular, the robot-assisted laparoscopic radical prostatectomy (RARP) has become a widely performed type of treatment in patients with PCa due to low blood

*Correspondence: k-hikita@tottori-u.ac.jp
Division of Urology, Department of Surgery, Faculty of Medicine, Tottori University, 36-1 Nishicho, Yonago, Japan

loss and transfusion rates, shorter hospital stay, and fine surgical manipulation [1]. Although RARP is less invasive than conventional open radical prostatectomy (ORP) or laparoscopic radical prostatectomy (LRP), there is post-operative urinary incontinence (UI), as with other procedures. UI after radical prostatectomy has a negative effect on patient's quality of life (QOL) and has a higher impact in sexual function [2]. So far various surgical techniques have been reported to reduce postoperative UI after RARP [3].

Several studies reported that RARP provides earlier urinary continence compared to ORP and LRP [1]. It has been reported that 17.3% of patients undergoing RARP had urinary continence immediately after catheter removal. The 12-month urinary recovery after RARP ranged from 84 to 97% better than after ORP, where urinary recovery ranged from 60 to 93% and after LRP ranged from 66 to 95% [1, 4].

On the other hand, patient's factors have also been noted regarding UI after surgery. Several studies have suggested that age, body mass index (BMI), preoperative International Prostate Symptom Score (IPSS) and prostate volume (PV) affect early UI after RARP [1]. Patients with severe lower urinary tract symptoms (LUTS) showed improvement in their subjective symptoms after RARP [5]. Alternatively, reports have investigated the association between benign prostatic hyperplasia (BPH) patterns and early continence after RARP [6]. Currently, several markers have been identified as significant in the clinical progression of BPH. Intravesical prostatic protrusion (IPP) predicts the extent of bladder outlet obstruction in pressure-flow studies (PFS). However, there is limited knowledge on the effects of RARP on LUTS, especially in men with both BPH and PCa. RARP is used to treat both BPH and PCa, and opt for radical surgical removal of the prostate. This study investigates the associations between preoperative BPH patterns, preoperative LUTS and UI after RARP. In particular, the impact of preoperative IPP on preoperative and postoperative UI were examined in detail.

Methods

Ethics

This study was conducted at the Division of Urology, Tottori University Hospital, Yonago, Japan. The study was approved by the Tottori University Ethics Committee (No. 2545).

Patients

Patients who underwent RARP for PCa (stages cT1c–cT3b N0 M0) between October 2010 and July 2014 at our department were included in this study. All patients were signed up after being fully briefed in accordance with the institutional ethics committee. Approved informed consent was obtained and patients were informed that the data would be used anonymously for clinical research purposes. All study data were prospectively collected and retrospectively analysed. The age, BMI, prostate-specific antigen (PSA), Gleason score (GS) and clinical stage were recorded. All patients underwent PFS and magnetic resonance imaging (MRI) before RARP. IPSS, Overactive Bladder Symptom Score (OABSS), QOL index and the number of pads used per day were evaluated before RARP and 1-, 3-, 6-, 9- and 12-months after RARP.

Surgical procedures

All surgical procedures were performed by six surgeons. The four grades of postero-lateral resection of the prostate were the guide for performing the nerve-sparing (NS) techniques. These included: grade 1, intrafascial dissection; grade 2, interfascial dissection; grade 3, extrafascial dissection and grade 4, wide dissection [7]. The NS grade which was used, was based on the MRI findings and GS from the biopsy. The surgeon decided the NS grade preoperatively and intraoperatively. In this study, NS was defined as at least unilateral NS grade 1 or 2, while non-NS was defined as a NS grade of 3 or 4.

Definition of continence and patient questionnaire

In this study, continence was defined as using no pads, and was assessed in the physician's interview with the patient at each outpatient visit before RARP and 1-, 3-, 6-, 9- and 12-months after RARP. Urinary symptom status was analysed using the IPSS, OABSS and QOL index. The IPSS consists of seven questions to assess voiding symptoms (incomplete emptying, intermittency, weak stream and straining to void) and storage symptoms (frequency, urgency and nocturia) [8].

PFS

PFS was performed by a single examiner using the standard method prescribed by the International Continence Society, using a Solar Gold urodynamic system (MMS USA Inc., Dover, NH, USA) [9]. An 8-Fr double lumen catheter was inserted into bladder and normal saline was injected at 50 ml/min. A balloon catheter was placed into the rectum and abdominal pressure was measured. Detrusor pressure was defined as the intravesical pressure minus abdominal pressure. The first desire to void (FDV), maximum cystometric capacity (MCC), bladder compliance, detrusor pressure at maximum flow (PdetQmax) and presence of detrusor overactivity (DO) were recorded.

MRI measurements

The PV, IPP, membranous urethra length (MUL), membranous urethra width (MUW) and levator thickness (LT) were measured using MRI. The PV was calculated as height × width × length × π/6 (axial and mid-sagittal T2-weighted image). The IPP was measured from the tip of the protruding prostate to the base of the bladder (mid-sagittal T2-weighted image). The MUL was measured as the distance from the prostatic apex to the level of the urethra at the penile bulb on coronal T2-weighted image. The MUW was defined as the maximum diameter of the membranous urethra (axial T2-weighted images). LT was calculated as (the outer levator distance minus the inner levator distance)/2 on axial T2-weighted image (Fig. 1).

The effect of IPP

The effect of IPP was investigated by stratifying the IPP into two levels. The patients were subsequently categorised into two groups based on the IPP length: Group 1 (< 5 mm) and Group 2 (≥ 5 mm). To confirm the difference between the two groups, we compared the pad-free rate, IPSS, OABSS and QOL index before RARP and at 1-, 3-, 6-, 9- and 12-months after RARP.

Statistical analysis

The data were presented as median values and interquartile range (IQR) and evaluated using the Mann–Whitney U test and Yates chi-square test, where a p -value of less than 0.05 was considered significant. Logistic regression analysis was performed to determine independent predictive values of the main risk factors of UI that have been reported in previous studies (age, BMI, PV, IPSS, OABSS, bladder compliance, NS, MUL, LT and IPP) in the first month and 12 months after RARP [10–14]. The predictors were investigated using multivariate analysis to determine which ones were affected by early and long-term UI. The 95% confidence interval (CI) was calculated for each odds ratio (OR). A p-value of less than 0.05 was considered significant. Statistical analysis was performed using the Statistical Package for the Social Sciences version 19 (IBM, Armonk, NY) software package.

Results

A total of 119 patients were eligible for this study. The number of patients who did not use pads at 1-, 3-, 6-, 9- and 12-months after RARP were 37 (31.0%), 63 (52.9%), 82 (68.9%), 85 (71.4%) and 91 (76.5%), respectively.

The median values of patient age, BMI and PSA before RARP were 66 (48–76) years, 23.5 (18.0–30.6) kg/m^2 and 7.8 (3.2–37.1) ng/mL, respectively. The MRI evaluation

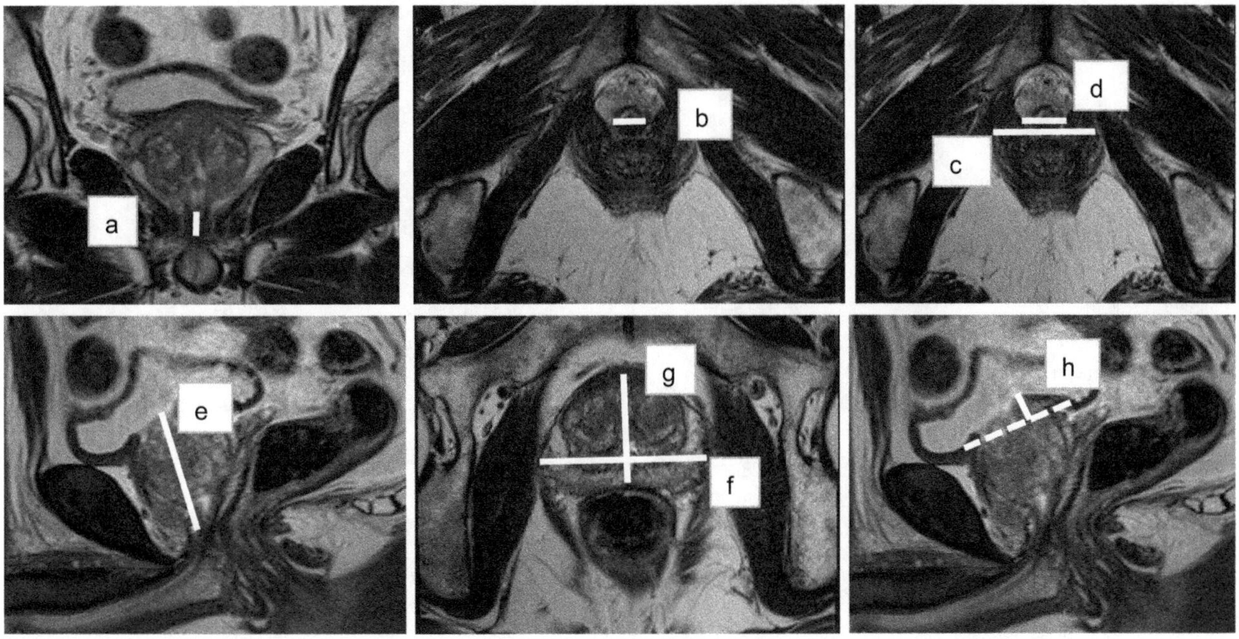

Fig. 1 MRI measurements. *a* is the MUL. MUL was measured as the distance of the apex of the prostate to the base of the bulbous urethra. *b* is the MUW. MUW was defined as the maximum diameter of the membranous urethra. LT was calculated as (*c* − *d*)/2. *c* stands for the outer levator distance and *d* stands for the inner levator distance. PV was calculated as *e* × *f* × *g* × π/6/1000. *e* is the maximum height of the prostate, *f* is the maximal prostate width and *g* is the maximal prostate length. Intravesical prostatic protrusion [*h* (mm)], which is measured from the tip of the protruding prostate to the base of the bladder (mid-sagittal T2-weighted image)

revealed that the median values of PV, MUL, MUW, LT and IPP before RARP were 26.0 (9.6–66.1) mL, 12.1 (8.9–16.1) mm, 10.6 (9.8–13.5) mm, 11.1 (7.9–15.1) mm, and 3.8 (0.0–16.5) mm, respectively. In terms of the clinical stage, 108 patients had ≤ T2c, 10 patients had T3a and one patient had T3b disease. Twenty-one patients had a GS of 6, 50 patients had a score of 7 and 48 patients had scores ≥ 8. According to NCCN risk stratification, 14 patients were considered at low risk, 53 patients were at intermediate risk and 52 patients were at high risk. A NS procedure was performed bilaterally or unilaterally in 51 patients. Lymph node dissection was performed in 105 patients.

The median total IPSS score, IPSS voiding symptom score, storage symptom score, OABSS and QOL index were 6 (0–28), 4 (0–18), 4 (0–12), 3 (0–10) and 3 (0–6), respectively. The median compliance, FDV, MCC and PdetQmax were 49.8 (5.0–290.2) ml/cmH$_2$O, 144 (47–400) ml, 277 (55–470) ml and 45 (6–90) cmH$_2$O, respectively. DO was identified in 10 patients (Table 1).

Multivariate analysis was performed using the risk factors reported in previous studies (age, BMI, PV, IPSS, OABSS, compliance, NS, MUL, LT and IPP) as being linked to UI in the first month and 12 months after RARP, showed that the IPP (OR 1.14, 95% CI 1.02–1.28, $p < 0.05$) and NS (OR 0.23, 95% CI 0.18–0.61, $p < 0.01$) remained

Table 1 Patients' characteristics

	Overall population	Group 1	Group 2	*p* value
Number of patients	119	71	48	
Median age, years (IQR)	66 (48–76)	64 (48–76)	69 (53–76)	< 0.05
Median BMI, kg/m^2 (IQR)	23.5 (18.0–30.6)	23.6 (18.1–28.9)	22.9 (18.0–30.6)	0.8
Median PSA, ng/mL (IQR)	7.8 (3.2–37.1)	7.8 (3.2–34.6)	7.7 (4.3–37.1)	0.45
Clinical stage				
<T2c	108	64	44	0.96
T3a	10	6	4	
T3b	1	1	0	
T4	0	0	0	
GS of biopsy				
<6	21	13	8	0.46
7	50	25	25	
>8	48	33	15	
Risk class (NCCN)				
Low	14	9	5	0.54
Intermediate	53	27	26	
High	52	35	17	
Lymph node dissection (%)	105 (88.2)	62 (87.3)	43 (89.6)	0.75
Nerve sparing (%)	51 (42.8)	28 (39.4)	23 (47.9)	0.15
Median PV, mL (IQR)	26.0 (9.6–66.1)	24.8 (11.1–53.2)	32.8 (9.6–66.1)	<0.01
Median MUL, mm (IQR)	12.1 (8.9–16.1)	12.1 (9.1–15.3)	12.9 (8.9–16.1)	0.53
Median MUW, mm (IQR)	10.6 (9.8–13.5)	10.8 (9.9–13.4)	10.3 (9.8–13.5)	0.76
Median LT, mm (IQR)	11.1 (7.9–15.1)	11.0 (8.3–15.1)	11.3 (7.9–15.1)	0.66
Median IPP, mm (IQR)	3.8 (0.0–16.5)	1.0 (0.0–4.9)	7.8 (6.2–16.5)	<0.01
Median IPSS Total score (IQR)	6 (0–28)	6 (0–22)	8 (0–28)	<0.05
Median IPSS voiding symptom score (IQR)	4 (0–18)	3 (0–15)	5 (0–18)	<0.01
Median IPSS storage symptom score (IQR)	4 (0–12)	3 (0–12)	4 (0–12)	0.55
Median OABSS score (IQR)	3 (0–10)	2 (0–10)	4 (2–10)	0.45
Median QOL index (IQR)	3 (0–6)	3 (0–6)	3 (0–6)	0.35
Median compliance, mL/cmH$_2$O (IQR)	49.8 (5.0–290.2)	55.9 (5.0–290.2)	42.4 (5.4–153.9)	<0.01
Median FDV, mL (IQR)	144 (47–400)	144 (81–400)	134 (47–301)	0.62
Median MCC, mL (IQR)	277 (55–470)	282 (120–470)	264 (55–431)	0.96
Median PdetQmax, cmH$_2$O (IQR)	45 (6–90)	41 (6–89)	48 (28–90)	<0.01
DO (%)	10 (8.4)	7 (9.8)	3 (6.2)	0.22

as significant factors in the first month after RARP. At 12 months after RARP, the only factor that remained significantly associated with UI on multivariate analysis was NS (OR 0.88, 95% CI 0.78–0.99, $p < 0.05$) (Table 2).

The patients were stratified into two groups according to IPP length: Group 1 (<5 mm: n=71) and Group 2 (≥5 mm: n=48). The comparison of the two groups indicated significant differences in age ($p < 0.01$), PV ($p < 0.01$), total preoperative IPSS score ($p < 0.05$), preoperative IPSS voiding symptom score ($p < 0.01$), bladder compliance ($p < 0.01$) and PdetQmax ($p < 0.01$) (Table 1).

With respect to the total IPSS and voiding symptom score, a significant difference was observed between the two groups before RARP ($p < 0.01$), but the significant difference disappeared from the first month after RARP. The IPSS storage symptom score, QOL index and OABSS were not significantly different between groups 1 and 2 both before and after RARP (Fig. 2).

The evaluation of UI in Group 1 showed that the number of patients who did not use pads at 1-, 3-, 6-, 9- and 12-months after RARP were 27 (38.0%), 40 (56.3%), 50 (70.4%), 53 (74.6%) and 55 (77.5%), respectively. In Group 2, the number of patients who did not use pads at 1-, 3-, 6-, 9- and 12-months after RARP were 10 (20.8%), 23 (47.9%), 32 (66.7%), 32 (66.7%) and 36 (75.0%), respectively. Group 1 had a higher continence rate than Group 2 in the first month after RARP ($p < 0.05$); however, the significant difference disappeared 3 months onward after RARP (Fig. 2).

Discussion

The post-RARP UI is influenced by the preoperative patient's characteristics as well as the surgical technique. In a systematic review, the 12-month UI rates ranged from 4 to 31% with a mean value of 16% after RARP [1]. In our study, the number of patients who did not use pads at 1-, 3-, 6-, 9- and 12-months after RARP were 37 (31.0%), 63 (52.9%), 82 (68.9%), 85 (71.4%) and 91 (76.4%), respectively. The incontinence rate in this study was higher than in the previous reports. One possible reason for the high UI rate in this study was the older age of patients than in the previous reports [1, 15]. It might also be related to the surgical technique used. Studies that evaluated the impact of different surgical techniques on UI after RARP found that posterior musculofascial reconstruction with or without anterior reconstruction was associated with a small advantage in the recovery from urinary continence 1 month after RARP [1, 16]. In our study, both anterior and posterior reconstruction was performed in all cases. Therefore, the effects of the reconstruction could not be assessed. Although bladder neck preservation was not evaluated in this study, it was previously reported to be associated with a higher continence rate after RARP [12, 13]. With respect to NS, this procedure has been known to favour continence. Retrospective studies showed that better continence rates at 9–12 months after LRP or RARP were achieved in patients with at least one completely spared neurovascular bundle [11]. In our study, NS is a solid factor associated with a higher preserved continence rate from the early to the long-term postoperative period. NS was performed in only 51 cases (42.9%), which might have contributed to the high rate of UI observed in this study [16].

Besides the surgical technique, several other factors related to UI after RARP have been mentioned. Some reports show that patient age, BMI, MUL, LT, IPP, race, OABSS and severity of preoperative IPSS score are factors associated with the continence rate after RARP [5, 10–12, 19, 20]. Therefore, we performed multivariate analysis based on these factors in this study. NS and IPP

Table 2 Multivariate analyses to identify significant predictors of postoperative urinary incontinence at 1 and 12 months in patients undergoing RARP

Predictors	1 month after RARP			12 months after RARP		
	OR	95% CI	*p*	OR	95% CI	*p*
Age, years	1.04	0.97–1.12	0.23	1.03	0.95–1.12	0.43
BMI, kg/m^2	0.89	0.75–1.01	0.23	0.97	0.81–1.16	0.72
Nerve sparing, yes/no	0.23	0.18–0.61	0.003	0.88	0.78–0.99	0.03
PV, mL	1	0.96–1.05	0.96	1	0.96–1.05	0.9
MUL, mm	0.91	0.82–1.00	0.06	0.95	0.85–1.10	0.39
LT, mm	1.05	0.92–1.20	0.45	0.98	0.87–1.10	0.74
IPP, mm	1.14	1.02–1.28	0.02	0.99	0.87–1.14	0.96
IPSS Total score	0.95	0.82–1.06	0.33	1.04	0.87–1.14	0.39
OABSS score	1.07	0.79–1.44	0.65	1.06	0.82–1.37	0.66
Compliance, mL/cmH_2O	0.99	0.99–1.01	0.65	1.01	0.99–1.02	0.2

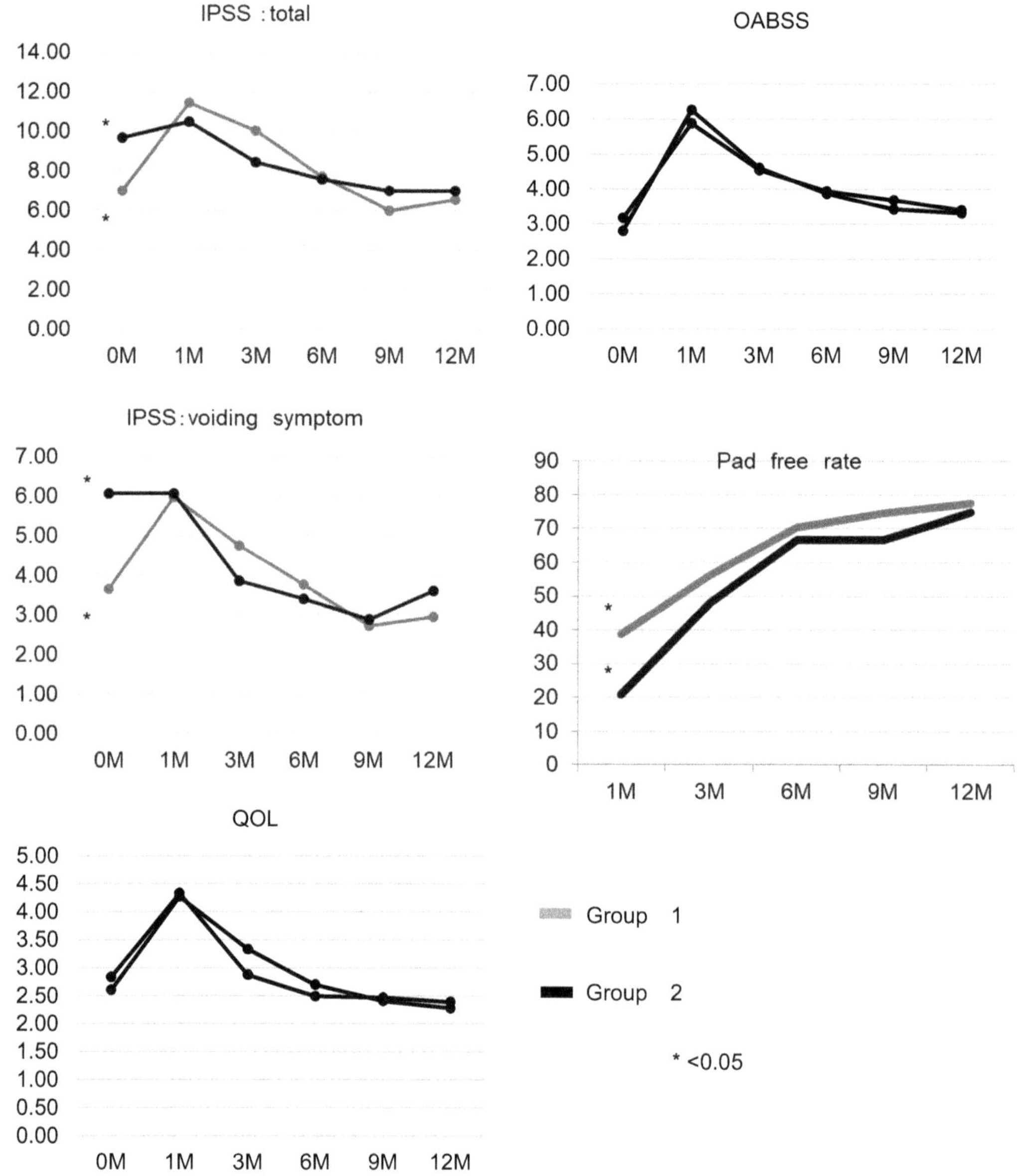

Fig. 2 The distribution of the total International Prostate Symptom Score (IPSS), voiding symptom score, QOL index, OABSS score, and pad-free rate between groups 1 and 2 preoperatively and at 1-, 3-, 6-, 9-, and 12-month follow-ups

were significant factors for UI during the first month post-RARP. As for NS, as reported by Suardi et al., this factor has an early effect on UI rates and is still a significant factor 12 months postoperatively [16]. However, although IPP affected early postoperative UI, this effect disappeared at 12 months postoperatively.

In this study, we focused on and examined the impact of IPP on UI after RARP. In a previous study, the impact of IPP on the effects of the therapy for BPH was extensively evaluated [21]. RARP provides treatment for both BPH and PCa; opt for radical surgical removal of the prostate. Therefore, the effect of IPP on preoperative urinary status also affects the urinary status after RARP. Additionally, as Grivas et al. reported that IPP predicts the extent of bladder outlet obstruction seen in PFS, it is understandable that IPP affects both preoperative and post-RARP urinary states [6]. However, Grivas et al. also reported that IPP was not a significant factor affecting the continence rate, although their study evaluated outcomes at only 6 and 12 months after RARP [6]. Alternatively, this study is more detailed with evaluations before RARP and at 1-, 3-, 6-, 9- and 12-months after RARP. In this study, IPP was not a significant factor related to the continence rate 12 months after RARP, but was only linked to UI at the first month after surgery. Furthermore, previous reports have also shown that IPP affects UI, with significant differences in the recovery of continence at 3-, 6- and 12-months after surgery [15]. Our study showed that postoperative UI was affected by preoperative IPP at an earlier stage.

Besides the impact of IPP on early post-RARP UI, there were also significant differences between the two groups in bladder compliance, PdetQmax, IPSS total score, IPSS voiding symptom score and PV. A higher grade of IPP would result in a higher degree of subclinical bladder dysfunction before RARP, resulting in a lower rate of urinary continence after RARP. Yamada et al. reviewed 272 patients after RARP. Multivariable analysis showed that the presence of an unstable bladder preoperatively was an independent negative predictor of the recovery of continence within 12 months after surgery [13]. In our study, although IPP affected bladder compliance, there were no significant differences in FDV, MCC, OABSS and IPSS storage symptom score between the two groups. Thus, although IPP potentially have an impact on urinary storage symptoms, no significant difference was found in this study because there were only few cases with a high IPP grade. Hence, different results might have been obtained if the number of cases was higher.

In this study, the total IPSS score and voiding symptom score were preoperatively significantly different between the two groups. However, there was no significant difference after surgery. Therefore, patients with severe preoperative voiding symptoms benefit from RARP.

The limitations of this study were the small number of cases, few cases of severe IPP and lack of evaluation of bladder neck preservation. Since it was difficult to perform bladder neck preservation in high-grade IPP patients, the assessment of bladder neck preservation in cases of IPP facilitates the evaluation of its effect on UI in the future.

Thus, future studies assessing the effect of IPP on UI should include a larger number of severe cases of IPP to enable more detailed study.

Conclusions

The results of this study suggest that IPP affects urinary continence in the early postoperative period. Although NS was strongly involved in urinary continence in both early and later stages after RARP, IPP had no effect in the later stages. Various preoperative factors are involved in continence after RARP, and IPP is one of those factors. More detailed evaluation of a larger number of cases in the future will help shed more light on this topic.

Abbreviations

PCa: Prostate cancer; RARP: Robot-assisted radical prostatectomy; ORP: Open radical prostatectomy; UI: Urinary incontinence; QOL: Quality of life; LRP: Laparoscopic radical prostatectomy; BMI: Body mass index; IPSS: International Prostate Symptom Score; PV: Prostate volume; LUTS: Lower urinary tract symptoms; BPH: Benign prostatic hyperplasia; IPP: Intravesical prostatic protrusion; PFS: Pressure-flow study; PSA: Prostate-specific antigen; GS: Gleason score; MRI: Magnetic resonance imaging; OABSS: Overactive Bladder Symptom Score; NS: Nerve-sparing; DO: Detrusor overactivity; FDV: First desire to void; MCC: Maximum cystometric capacity; Pdet Qmax: Detrusor pressure at peak urinary flow rate; MUL: Length of the membranous urethra; MUW: Width of the membranous urethra; LT: Levator thickness; IQR: Interquartile range; CI: Confidence interval; OR: Odds ratios.

Acknowledgements

The authors would like to thank Enago for the English language review.

Authors' contributions

KH: Project development, data analysis, manuscript writing; HI and SM: Project development, data collection, data analysis; PT, ST, RN and YK: data analysis; MH and AT: Project development, Manuscript Revision; YN: Manuscript Revision. All authors read and approved the final manuscript.

Competing interests

The authors declare that they have no competing interests.

References

1. Ficarra V, Novara G, Rosen RC, Artibani W, Carroll PR, Costello A, et al. Systematic review and meta-analysis of studies reporting urinary continence recovery after robot-assisted radical prostatectomy. EUR Urol. 2012;62:405–17. https://doi.org/10.3349/ymj.2016.57.5.1165.
2. van der Poel HG, Tillier C, de Blok WM, Acar C, van Muilekom EH, van den Bergh RC. Interview-based versus questionnaire-based quality of life outcomes before and after prostatectomy. J Endourol. 2013;11:1411–6. https://doi.org/10.1089/end.2012.0735.
3. Lei Y, Alemozaffar M, Williams SB, Hevelone N, Lipsitz SR, Plaster BA, et al. Altermal division and selective suture ligation of the dorsal vein complex during robot-assisted laparoscopic radical prostatectomy: description of technique and outcomes. EUR Urol. 2011;59:235–43. https://doi.org/10.1016/j.eururo.2010.08.043.
4. Sammon JD, Sharma P, Trinh QD, Ghani KR, Sukumar S, Menon M. Predictors of immediate continence following robot-assisted radical prostatectomy. J Endourol. 2013;27:442–6. https://doi.org/10.1089/end.2012.0312.
5. Gordon A, Skarecky DW, Ahlering T. Long-term outcomes in severe lower urinary tract symptoms in men undergoing robotic-assisted radical prostatectomy. Urology. 2014;84(4):826–31. https://doi.org/10.1016/j.urolo gy.2014.05.052
6. Grivas N, van der Roest R, Tillier C, Schouten D, van Muilekom E, Schoots I, van der Poel H, Heijmink S. Patterns of benign prostate hyperplasia based on magnetic resonance imaging are correlated with lower urinary tract symptoms and continence in men undergoing a robot-assisted radical prostatectomy for prostate cancer. Urology. 2017;107:196–201. https://doi.org/10.1016/j.urology.2017.05.047.
7. Tewari AK, Srivastava A, Huang MW, Robinson BD, Shevchuk MM, Durand M, Sooriakumaran P, Grover S, Yadav R, Mishra N, Mohan S, Brooks DC, Shaikh N, Khanna A, Leung R. Anatomical grades of nerve sparing: a risk-stratified approach to neural-hammock sparing during robot-assisted radical prostatectomy (RARP). BJU Int. 2011;108:984–92. https://doi.org/10.1111/j.1464-410X.2011.10565.x.
8. Steele GS, Sullivan MP, Sleep DJ, Yalla SV. Combination of symptom score, flow rate and prostate volume for predicting bladder outflow obstruction in men with lower urinary tract symptoms. J Urol. 2000;164:344–8. https://doi.org/10.1016/S0022-5347(05)67356-9.
9. Abrams P, Cardozo L, Fall M, Griffiths D, Rosier P, Ulmsten U, van Kerrebroeck P, Victor A, Wein A. The standardisation of terminology of lower urinary tract function: report from the Standardisation Sub-committee of the International Continence Society. Neurourol Urodyn. 2002;21(2):167–78. https://doi.org/10.1002/nau.10052.

10. Lavigueur-Blouin H, Noriega AC, Valdivieso R, Hueber PA, Bienz M, Alhathal N, et al. Predictors of early continence following robot-assisted radical prostatectomy. CUAJ. 2015;9:e93–7. https://doi.org/10.5489/cuaj.2086.
11. Honda M, Kawamoto B, Morizane S, Hikita K, Muraoka K, Sejima T, Takenaka A. A prognostic model for predicting urinary incontinence after robot-assisted radical prostatectomy. Int J Med Robot. 2017;13:e1780. https://doi.org/10.1002/rcs.1780.
12. Jo JK, Hong SK, Byun SS, Zargar H, Autorino R, Lee SE. Urinary continence after robot-assisted laparoscopic radical prostatectomy: the impact of intravesical prostatic protrusion. Yonsei Med J. 2016;57(5):1145–451. https://doi.org/10.3349/ymj.
13. Yamada Y, Fujimura T, Fukuhara H, et al. Overactive bladder is a negative predictor of achieving continence after robot-assisted radical prostatectomy. Int J Urol. 2017;24:749–56. https://doi.org/10.1111/iju.13411.
14. Barnoiu OS, Garcia Galisteo E, Baron Lopez F, Vozmediano Chicharro R, Soler Martinez J, Del Rosal Samaniego JM, Machuca Santacruz J, Baena GV. Prospective urodynamic model for prediction of urinary incontinence after robot-assisted radical prostatectomy. Urol Int. 2014;92(3):306–9. https://doi.org/10.1159/000354352.
15. Kaye DR, Hyndman ME, Segal RL, Mettee LZ, Trock BJ, Feng Z, et al. Urinary outcomes are significantly affected by nerve sparing quality during radical prostatectomy. Urology. 2013;82(6):1348–53. https://doi.org/10.1016/j.urology.2013.06.067.
16. Suardi N, Moschini M, Gallina A, Gandaglia G, Abdollah F, Capitanio U, Bianchi M, et al. Nerve-sparing approach during radical prostatectomy is strongly associated with the rate of postoperative urinary continence recovery. BJU Int. 2013;111:717–22. https://doi.org/10.1111/j.1464-410X.2012.11315.x.
17. Friedlander DF, Alemozaffar M, Hevelone ND, et al. Stepwise description and outcomes of bladder neck sparing during robot-assisted laparoscopic radical prostatectomy. J Urol. 2012;188:1754–60. https://doi.org/10.1016/j.juro.2012.07.045.
18. Nyarangi-Dix JN, Radtke JP, Hadaschik B, et al. Impact of complete bladder neck preservation on urinary continence, quality of life and surgical margins after radical prostatectomy: a randomized, controlled, single blind trial. J Urol. 2013;189:891–8. https://doi.org/10.1016/j.juro.2012.09.082.
19. Smolski M, Esler RC, Turo R, Collins GN, Oakley N, Brough R. Bladder neck sparing in radical prostatectomy. Indian J Urol. 2013;29(4):338–44. https://doi.org/10.4103/0970-1591.
20. Song W, Kim CK, Park BK, et al. Impact of preoperative and postoperative membranous urethral length measured by 3 Tesla magnetic resonance imaging on urinary continence recovery after robotic-assisted radical prostatectomy. Can Urol Assoc J. 2017;11:E93-99. https://doi.org/10.5489/cuaj.4035.
21. Lim KB, Ho H, Foo KT, Wong MY, Fook-Chong S. Comparison of intravesical prostatic protrusion, prostate volume and serum prostatic-specific antigen in the evaluation of bladder outlet obstruction. Int J Urol. 2006;13:1509–13. https://doi.org/10.1111/j.1442-2042.2006.01611.x.

7

Effects of pre-emptive pregabalin and multimodal anesthesia on postoperative opioid requirements in patients undergoing robot-assisted laparoscopic prostatectomy

K. Sisa[1†], S. Huoponen[1†], O. Ettala[3], H. Antila[1,2], T. I. Saari[1,2] and P. Uusalo[1,2*]

Abstract

Background: Previous findings indicate that pre-emptive pregabalin as part of multimodal anesthesia reduces opioid requirements compared to conventional anesthesia in patients undergoing robot-assisted laparoscopic prostatectomy (RALP). However, recent studies show contradictory evidence suggesting that pregabalin does not reduce postoperative pain or opioid consumption after surgeries. We conducted a register-based analysis on RALP patients treated over a 5-year period to evaluate postoperative opioid consumption between two multimodal anesthesia protocols.

Methods: We retrospectively evaluated patients undergoing RALP between years 2015 and 2019. Patients with American Society of Anesthesiologists status 1–3, age between 30 and 80 years and treated with standard multimodal anesthesia were included in the study. Pregabalin (PG) group received 150 mg of oral pregabalin as premedication before anesthesia induction, while the control (CTRL) group was treated conventionally. Postoperative opioid requirements were calculated as intravenous morphine equivalent doses for both groups. The impact of pregabalin on postoperative nausea and vomiting (PONV), and length of stay (LOS) was evaluated.

Results: We included 245 patients in the PG group and 103 in the CTRL group. Median (IQR) opioid consumption over 24 postoperative hours was 15 (8–24) and 17 (8–25) mg in PG and CTRL groups ($p = 0.44$). We found no difference in postoperative opioid requirement between the two groups in post anesthesia care unit, or within 12 h postoperatively ($p = 0.16$; $p = 0.09$). The length of post anesthesia care unit stay was same in each group and there was no difference in PONV Similarly, median postoperative LOS was 31 h in both groups.

Conclusion: Patients undergoing RALP and receiving multimodal analgesia do not need significant amount of opioids postoperatively and can be discharged soon after the procedure. Pre-emptive administration of oral pregabalin does not reduce postoperative opioid consumption, PONV or LOS in these patients.

Keywords: Robot-assisted laparoscopic prostatectomy, Multimodal analgesia, Anesthesia

Background

Prostate cancer is the second most frequent malignancy among males worldwide [1]. Robotic-assisted laparoscopic radical prostatectomy (RALP) has evolved into the predominant surgical approach in localized prostate cancer. Due to its minimally invasive nature, RALP is

*Correspondence: pijuus@utu.fi
†K. Sisa and S. Huoponen have contributed equally to this work
[1] Perioperative Services, Intensive Care and Pain Medicine, Turku University Hospital, Turku, Finland

associated with decreased pain levels compared to open prostatectomy (ORP) [2]. Despite its minimally invasiveness, patients undergoing RALP experience mild to moderate postoperative pain and often need opioids perioperatively [3, 4].

Standardized, multimodal analgesic regimen with non-opioid agents aims to minimize the use of opioids and thereby decrease opioid-related adverse effects [5]. A recent review concluded that multimodal analgesia is readily available and the evidence to support its efficiency is strong [6]. However, the effect of current analgesia regimen is poorly studied and to our knowledge, there is only one study evaluating the multimodal analgesic regimen in patients undergoing RALP [7]. A recent systematic review on the perioperative pain regimen for radical prostatectomy surgery concluded a need to develop an optimal pain management protocol in this patient population [8].

Pregabalin is a gamma-aminobutyric acid analogue that binds to voltage-gated calcium channels and decreases pain sensation by inhibiting calcium influx and the subsequent release of excitatory neurotransmitters in the central nervous system. Previously, multiple systematic reviews and meta-analyses have concluded pregabalin to cause an opioid sparing effect during the perioperative period in several patient groups [9–11]. Pregabalin has been used for as premedication in patients undergoing RALP [7]. However, recent studies have brought up concerns about respiratory depression in patients that received pregabalin in combination with opioids and/ or general anesthetics [12, 13]. While pregabalin predisposes analgesic effects, the use of pregabalin as a routine component of premedication has been challenged due to the imbalance of clinical advantages and possible side effects [14]. Thus, re-evaluation of the effect of pregabalin on RALP is justified.

The primary objective of our study was to evaluate the impact of single dose of pre-emptive pregabalin on postoperative opioid consumption of RALP patients receiving multimodal analgesia. We hypothesized that the cumulative consumption of opioids after RALP is modest and pregabalin would cause no meaningful effect on postoperative opioid consumption. Our secondary aim was also to evaluate the efficacy of our perioperative multimodal analgesic regimen of RALP.

Methods

Patient population

Eligible patients were identified from the RALP register of Department of Urology, Turku University Hospital. Patient data were retrieved from patient database and anesthesia reports of the hospital. Patients scheduled for RALP under multimodal anesthesia in Turku University Hospital (tertiary hospital), South-West Finland between 2015 and 2019 were retrospectively screened and patients with ASA status 1–3, age between 35 and 80 years, weight between 50 and 100 kg were included in the study.

Exclusion criteria included: patients receiving other adjuvant analgesics such as clonidine or tricyclic antidepressants pre-, intra- or postoperatively, patients with chronic opioid or gabapentinoid use, patients with history of chronic pain syndrome, perioperative abnormalities or patients with kidney failure (creatinine clearance < 90 ml/min), patients with abnormal liver function tests or patients with clinically significant abnormalities in preoperative medical examination, ECG or laboratory values and patients undergoing total intravenous anesthesia.

Consecutive patients who met the inclusion criteria and received 150 mg of pregabalin for premedication were identified between January 2015 and December 2017 (pregabalin group; PG). Based on controversial reports regarding use of pregabalin [13, 14] this premedication was discontinued in the beginning of 2018 and consecutive patients who met the inclusion criteria and did not receive any pregabalin during their treatment were identified between between January 2018 and August 2019 (control group; CTRL).

ERAS protocol

Patients were allowed to take clear liquids until 2 h before the procedure. Multimodal anesthesia with restricted fluid protocol (app. 5 ml/kg/h) was used. Nasogastric tubes were used intraoperatively and removed before the extubation. Perioperative pain was managed with several non-opioid agents (see "Anesthesia management" and "Management of postoperative pain and nausea" sections) Opioids were given only on demand only for stronger pain. Patients were allowed to take normal diet starting from 4 h after discharge from the PACU and encouraged to walk in the evening of the operation day.

Surgical technique

RALPs were performed by four experienced urologists all performing at least 50 prostatectomies a year. The procedure were done per routine using a technique originally introduced by Abbou et al. [15]. If feasible, bladder neck was preserved and/ or a uni- or bilateral nerve sparing was performed. Also, extended lymphadenectomy was performed in selected cases [16]. For reconstruction, a Rocco stich was used [17]. Also, in the end of the surgery, all patients received an infiltration anesthesia with 40 ml of 0.75% Ropivacaine to troacar openings. Blood loss was measured intraoperatively by taking account the amount of blood in suction and the weight of the cloths.

Anesthetic management

All patients received preoperatively 1500 to 2000 mg of paracetamol orally and 90 to 120 mg of etoricoxib orally according to their weight. Higher dose for patients over 90 kg and lower dose for patients less than 90 kg. PG group received additional 150 mg of pregabalin orally one hour before the anesthesia induction. The fixed dose of pregabalin was based on previous study on pre-emptive multimodal analgesia of RALP [7]. General anesthesia was induced with intravenous propofol and intravenous fentanyl and maintained with volatile anesthetics (sevoflurane or desflurane). Patients received intraoperatively 8 mg of intravenous betamethasone, 25 mg of intravenous esketamine, 0.75 mg of intravenous dehydrobenzperidol and 2500/10 mg of intravenous metamizole-pitofenone combination (Litalgin®). Neuromuscular blockade was induced with rocurone and reversed with neostigmine-glycopyrrollate. We monitored the depth of anesthesia with entropy (GE B850 Monitor Entropy Module, Helsinki, Finland) and our aim was to keep the target state entropy (SE) between 35 and 45. Intraoperative mean arterial pressure (MAP) target was between 65 and 75 mmHg depending on the patients age and disease history.

Management of postoperative pain and nausea

In postoperative anesthesia care unit (PACU) a standard pain therapy regimen based on intravenous oxycodone was used. Oxycodone was administered at the dose of 0.03–0.05 mg/kg if patient reported moderate or intense pain (Visual Analog Scale; VAS > 3). Postoperative nausea and vomiting (PONV) was treated with 4 mg of intravenous ondansetron. If patients received antiemetics postoperatively, it was considered as PONV, and if patients received repeated doses of ondansetron or other antiemetics, it was considered as severe PONV.

In the ward all patients received 1000 mg of paracetamol three times a day for postoperative pain. More intense pain (VAS > 3) was managed with 0.05–0.1 mg/kg of oral oxycodone.

Time to discharge

Time to the discharge was defined as the period of time between the end of surgery and the time of discharge of the patient from the urologic inpatient ward. Clock times were obtained from the hospital's patient information system.

Statistics

The primary outcome variable was the cumulative amount of opioids administered to the patients (mean equivalent dose; MED) in PACU and within 12 and 24 h after the end of surgery [17]. A 25% reduction in opioid use was considered clinically feasible. For a study power of 80% ($\alpha = 0.05$, $\beta = 0.2$), the required sample size per group was calculated to be at least 75. Secondary outcomes were the incidence of PONV and severe PONV, PACU time, LOS, duration of surgery (including docking time), intraoperative fentanyl consumption and intraoperative blood loss. The Shapiro–Wilks test ($p > 0.05$) and Q–Q-plots were used to assess normality assumptions. Student's t test was used to compare the groups with normally distributed data, and Wilcoxon's rank sum test was used to test non-normally distributed data. Nominal data were tested using chi-square analysis. $P < 0.05$ (two-tailed) was considered statistically significant. The results are expressed as mean values with standard deviations (SD), and as medians with interquartile ranges (IQR) when the normality assumption was not met. The covariate effect on postoperative opioid consumption was modelled using linear mixed model for repeated measurements. Time effect was handled as continuous to compare the slope of cumulative opioid dose between the groups (group * time interaction) adjusted with age, BMI, intraoperative fentanyl requirement, operative time as continuous covariate; pelvic lymph node dissection and group as categorical explanatory variables. Compound symmetry was selected for covariance-variance structure in the model. To fulfill assumption for normality a square root transformation was used and the normal distribution assumption was checked using studentized residuals. The analyses were performed with JMP Pro 13.0 and SAS® System programs, version 9.4 for Windows (SAS Institute Inc., Cary, NC, USA).

Results

245 consecutive patients were included in the PG group and 103 consecutive in the CTRL group (Additional file 1: Fig. S1). There was no difference in the patient characteristics (Table 1).

There was no difference in postoperative opioid consumption between the groups. Median (IQR) opioid consumption was in 11 (5–20) versus 12 (5–20) mg in PACU (median difference 1.5 mg, 95% CI − 3.0 to 4.5 mg, $p = 0.16$), 14 (6–21) versus 15 (8–24) within 12 postoperative hours (median difference 1.5 mg, 95% CI − 1.0 to 6.0 mg, $p = 0.09$), and 15 (8–24) versus 17 (8–25) mg within 24 postoperative hours in PG and CTRL groups respectively (median difference 1.5 mg, 95% CI − 1.0 to 7.5 mg, $p = 0.44$) (Fig. 1).

There was no difference in PONV ($p = 0.34$), severe PONV ($p = 0.84$), PACU stay ($p = 0.18$), LOS ($p = 0.62$), time of anesthesia ($p = 0.22$), intraoperative fentanyl consumption ($p = 0.06$), intraoperative blood loss

Table 1 Patient characteristics

	PG-group (n=245)	CTRL-group (n=103)	*p* value
Age (y)[a]	66 (61–69)	66 (61–69)	0.96
Weight (kg)[b]	85 (12)	84 (11)	0.79
BMI (kg/m^2)[b]	26 (3)	26 (3)	0.83
Gleason			0.57
6 (n (%))	49 (20)	17 (17)	
7–8 (n (%))	165 (67)	75 (73)	
9–10 (n (%))	31 (13)	11 (11)	
T-class			0.41
T1 (n (%))	91 (37)	37 (36)	
T2 (n (%))	103 (42)	48 (47)	
T3 (n (%))	49 (20)	17 (17)	
T4 (n (%))	2 (1)	1 (1)	
Duration of surgery (min)[a]	163 (143–195)	169 (146–198)	0.22
Intraoperative blood loss (ml)[a]	81 (50–150)	100 (50–150)	0.497
Lymph node extraction (n (%))	108 (44.1)	45 (43.7)	0.94

[a] Median and interquartile range (IQR)

[b] Mean and SD

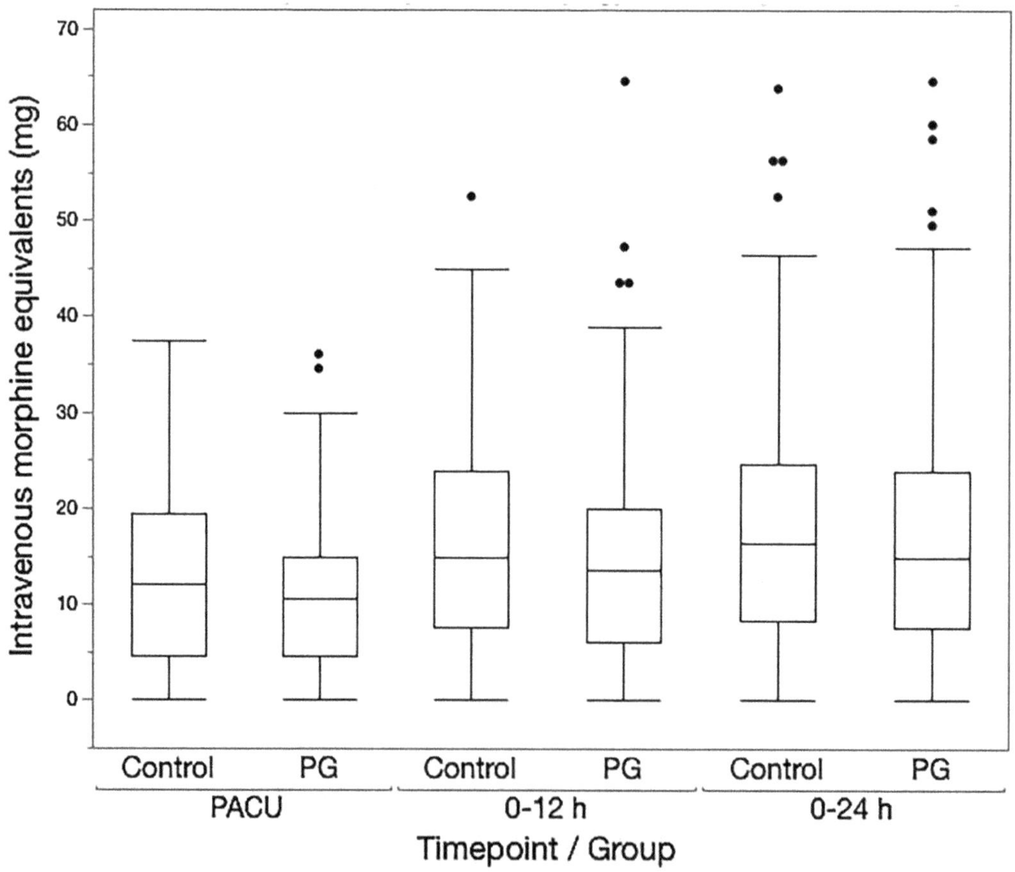

Fig. 1 Postoperative opioid consumption in oral morphine equivalents (mg) within three postoperative time periods

Table 2 Outcomes of the study

	PG-group (n = 245)	CTRL-group (n = 103)	*p* value
Intraoperative fentanyl requirement (mg)[a]	400 (350–450)	350 (300–400)	0.06
Postoperative opioid consumption in PACU (mg)[a]	11 (5–20)	12 (5–20)	0.16
Postoperative opioid consumption 0–12 h (mg)[a]	14 (6–21)	15 (8–24)	0.09
Postoperative opioid consumption 0–24 h (mg)[a]	15 (8–24)	17 (8–25)	0.44
PACU time (min)[a]	128 (108–152)	126 (103–145)	0.18
LOS (h)[a]	31 (28–49)	31 (28–48)	0.62
PONV (n (%))	19 (7.6)	7 (6.6)	0.34
Severe PONV (n (%))	4 (1.6)	2 (1.9)	0.84
Opioid requirement on first postoperative day (n (%))[b]	79 (32.2)	37 (35.9)	0.36

[a] Median and interquartile range (IQR)

[b] mean and SD

Table 3 Summary of final repeated-measures mixed models of the effect of group

	Postoperative opioid consumption		
Independent variable	DF	F value	*p* value
Age	339	28.03	< 0.001
Group	383	2.51	0.11
Timepoint	690	289.11	< 0.001
Timepoint*Group	690	0.88	0.35
BMI	339	1.24	0.27
Intraoperative fentanyl	339	0.72	0.4
Intraoperative time	339	4.20	0.04
Lymph node extraction	339	1.12	0.29

Data show the effect of group on postoperative opioid consumption taking into account age, BMI, intraoperative fentanyl consumption, intraoperative time and lymph node extraction. Models were run using linear mixed model for repeated measurements

($p = 0.497$) or in opioid requirement on first postoperative day between the two groups (Table 2).

In a subgroup analysis of patients undergoing lymph node extraction, there was no difference in the opioid requirement 0–48 h postoperatively in the CTRL group compared with the CTRL group ($p = 0.94$). Similarly, in a subgroup analysis of patients not undergoing lymph node extraction, there was no difference in the opioid requirement 0–24 h postoperatively in the PG group compared with the CTRL group ($p = 0.34$).

In a multivariate analysis intraoperative time was associated with postoperative opioid consumption and age was negatively associated with postoperative opioid consumption. There was no association between postoperative opioid consumption and BMI, intraoperative fentanyl consumption or lymph node extraction. There was no difference in the postoperative opioid consumption between the groups (Table 3).

Adverse events

There were no adverse events recorded.

Discussion

Our results indicate that pre-emptive administration of oral pregabalin does not reduce postoperative opioid consumption, PONV, PACU time or LOS in patients undergoing RALP. Considering the possible side effects related to use of pregabalin [14], our results do not encourage to use pregabalin in patients undergoing RALP. Instead we were able to demonstrate the feasibility of a new multimodal analgesic protocol that has not been earlier introduced for patients undergoing RALP. Patients receiving this regimen needed only small amount of opioids for postoperative pain and can be discharged soon after the procedure.

The groundwork of multimodal analgesic regimen is formed by paracetamol in combination with a non-steroidal anti-inflammatory drug (NSAID) or a cyclooxygenase 2 (COX2) inhibitors, when no contraindications are encountered, and local anesthesia—a combination proposed by the guidelines from the American Society of Anesthesiologists task force on acute pain management [18] Ketamine, a traditional anesthetic, has been shown to be an effective adjunct for postoperative analgesia at low doses [19]. Systemic corticosteroids, like dexamethasone are often used for the prevention of PONV, but have also been shown to reduce postoperative pain in many types of surgery [20].

Trabulsi et al. [7] demonstrated in their retrospective study a positive effect of multimodal analgesia on postoperative opioid consumption after RALP. In addition to paracetamol and celecoxib (COX2-inhibitor), their regimen included 150 mg single-dose of pregabalin as premedication. Compared to conventional analgesic regimen use of above-mentioned premedication decreased postoperative opioid consumption. In more recent meta-analyses pregabalin as a component of postoperative acute pain management protocol has been generally questioned. While pregabalin may have a minimal opioid-sparing effect, the risk of serious adverse effects seems to be increased and a routine use of pregabalin for postoperative pain treatment cannot be recommended [14, 21].

Our multimodal analgesia regimen included esketamine, betamethasone and metamizole-pitofenone. Preemptive use of esketamine for postoperative pain has been studied in several patient groups and there is strong evidence suggesting its use intraoperatively [22]. Use of glucocorticoids as an adjunct to general anesthesia has been shown to decrease postoperative pain, but glucocorticoids have previously studied mainly in orthopedic patients [23]. There is also evidence that intraoperative use of betamethasone decreases PONV after general anesthesia [24]. Single dose metamizole has been shown to have good analgesic effects on postoperative pain [25] and it is often administered together with a spasmolytic compound pitofenone. The above mentioned intraoperative multimodal analgesia has been used in Turku University Hospital for RALP patients over 8 years.

Multimodal analgesia often includes also utilization of local anesthetic-based regional analgesic techniques. In our multimodal analgesia protocol patients received local anesthetic infiltration to the troacar openings. Transversus abdominis plane block (TAP) has been recently introduced as part of multimodal anesthesia and analgesia of RALP [26]. TAP has been shown to reduce pain and opioid consumption after RALP [27] and may be done by the surgeon under visual control or by anesthesiologist under ultrasound guidance. However, to reach a high success rate, this procedure requires training [28].

Due to its minimally invasive nature, the RALP is associated with decreased pain levels compared to open prostatectomy [3]. Immediately after RALP, the main source of pain/discomfort is abdominal, followed by catheter related, penile and bladder-spasm-related discomfort. With current analgesic regimens, abdominal pain after RALP is mild to moderate—on average rated 3 to 4 of 10 on a pain scale [4]. A recent systematic review on the optimal perioperative pain regimen for radical prostatectomy concluded that there is a lack of evidence to develop an optimal pain management protocol in this patient population and specific studies comparing pain and analgesic requirements for open and minimally invasive surgical procedures are warranted [8]. In the face of current opioid crisis, an attempt to minimize the use of opioids perioperatively should become a part of standard care for all surgical patients [29, 30].

The majority of patients undergoing RALP at high-volume centers are discharged on the first postoperative day [31]. In our study the median of LOS was 31 h, which is in line with earlier findings. Postoperative pain was well controlled and major part of patients did require opioids on first postoperative day. The main reasons for discharge later than on the first postoperative day were logistical i.e. patient living in the rural areas needing a special means of transportation or suspicion of acute postoperative complication such as bleeding or infection.

Perioperative dosing of pregabalin has been recently surveyed in various laparoscopic surgery patient populations. In a very recent randomized controlled trial patients undergoing laparoscopic colorectal surgery and receiving two doses of oral pregabalin had lower postoperative opioid consumption but similar pain scores compared to control group [32]. A prospective study with patients undergoing laparoscopic living donor nephrectomy receiving two doses of oral pregabalin had lower postoperative opioid consumption but similar pain scores compared to the control group [33]. Contrary to these, a recent randomized controlled trial with similar setting to our study concluded that pregabalin together with celecoxib offered no analgesic superiority over standard opioid care in postoperative pain therapy following laparoscopic cholecystectomy. Recent large systematic review including 39 trials on endoscopic abdominal surgery found no clinically significant analgesic effect for perioperative used gabapentinoids. Use of perioperative pregabalin was associated with greater risk of adverse events [34]. Our findings together with this systematic review suggest that routine use of pregabalin for patients undergoing laparoscopic surgery cannot be recommended.

Our retrospective study has some limitations. First, while patients after RALP experience mild to modest pain and the amounts of opioids are modest as well, it is difficult to demonstrate meaningful difference. Furthermore, owing to the lack of data, we were not able to reliably assess the postoperative pain scores, or the amount of opioid use after discharge. For the same reason, we were not able to assess the incidence of chronic pain and hyperesthesia in the long term. The retrospective design of the study could have also affected the results, even when only consecutive patients were included to avoid any selection bias. On the other hand all patients in our study received a standardized multimodal anesthesia and only few experienced surgeons were involved in the procedure. Moreover, we were able to demonstrate an effective multimodal anesthesia protocol associated with few side effects and a short LOS.

To strengthen the findings of our study, the effect of pregabalin on postoperative opioid consumption and pain of patients undergoing RALP could be studied in a prospective manner. Another medication worth giving an opportunity as a part of multimodal analgesic regimen would be alpha-2-agonist clonidine, which has been shown to reduce postoperative opioid consumption [35, 36], but has not been studied in patients undergoing RALP. While deep Trendelenburg position during RALP often comes with a rise in mean arterial blood pressure [37], clonidine's ability to provide perioperative hemodynamic stability could be of use.

According to our findings, patients undergoing RALP that receive paracetamol and etoricoxib as premedication, esketamine, betamethasone, metamizole-pitofenone, fentanyl and local infiltration anesthesia intraoperatively, and paracetamol for postoperative pain need only small amounts of opioids postoperatively. While our findings demonstrated that routine use of pre-emptive pregabalin does not decrease postoperative opioid consumption in patients undergoing RALP, perioperative use of pregabalin may still have potential benefits in patients with a history of neuropathic or chronic pain.

Conclusion

Pre-emptive administration of oral pregabalin does not reduce postoperative opioid consumption, PONV, PACU time or LOS in patients undergoing RALP. Our findings indicate that patients receiving multimodal analgesia can be discharged soon after the procedure and require less opioids for postoperative pain.

Abbreviations

RALP: Robot-assisted laparoscopic prostatectomy; PG: Pregabalin group; CTRL: Control group; PONV: Postoperative nausea and vomiting; LOS: Length of stay; ORP: Open prostatectomy; PACU: Post anesthesia care unit; NSAID: Non-steroidal anti-inflammatory drug; COX2: Cyclooxygenase 2 inhibitor; VAS: Visual analog scale; MED: Mean equivalent dose of morphine.

Acknowledgements

We thank Ms. Eliisa Löyttyniemi for assisting with the statistical analysis of this manuscript.

Authors' contributions

All authors are accountable for all aspects of the accuracy and integrity of the manuscript in accordance with ICMJE criteria and provided their consent for publication. KS, SH, HA and PU designed and planned the study, analyzed the data wrote the paper. KS, SH and PU recruited patients from hospital database, PU was responsible for statistical analyses and OE, HA and TS participated writing. All authors read and approved the final manuscript.

Competing interests

This was a non-commercial, investigator-initiated study, and it has not received any funding from the industry. T. Saari and P. Uusalo have received honoraria for speaking at symposia organized by Orion Pharma. The other authors declare that they have no conflicts of interest.

Author details

[1] Perioperative Services, Intensive Care and Pain Medicine, Turku University Hospital, Turku, Finland. [2] Department of Anaesthesiology and Intensive Care, University of Turku, Kiinamyllynkatu 4-8, P.O. Box 51, 20521 Turku, Finland. [3] Department of Urology, University of Turku, Turku, Finland.

References

1. Bray F, Ferlay J, Soerjomataram I, Siegel RL, Torre LA, Jemal A. Global cancer statistics 2018: GLOBOCAN estimates of incidence and mortality worldwide for 36 cancers in 185 countries. CA Cancer J Clin. 2018;68:394–424.
2. Coughlin GD, Yaxley JW, Chambers SK, Occhipinti S, Samaratunga H, Zajdlewicz L, Teloken P, Dunglison N, Williams S, Lavin MF, Gardiner RA. Robot-assisted laparoscopic prostatectomy versus open radical retropubic prostatectomy: 24-month outcomes from a randomised controlled study. Lancet Oncol. 2018;19:1051–60.
3. D'Alonzo RC, Gan TJ, Moul JW, Albala DM, Polascik TJ, Robertson CN, Sun L, Dahm P, Habib AS. A retrospective comparison of anesthetic management of robot-assisted laparoscopic radical prostatectomy versus radical retropubic prostatectomy. J Clin Anesth. 2009;21:322–8.
4. Woldu SL, Weinberg AC, Bergman A, Shapiro EY, Korets R, Motamedinia P, Badani KK. Pain and analgesic use after robot-assisted radical prostatectomy. J Endourol. 2014;28:544–8.
5. Helander EM, Menard BL, Harmon CM, Homra BK, Allain AV, Bordelon GJ, Wyche MQ, Padnos IW, Lavrova A, Kaye AD. Multimodal analgesia, current concepts, and acute pain considerations. Curr Pain Headache Rep. 2017;21:3. https://doi.org/10.1007/s11916-017-0607-y.
6. Wick EC, Grant MC, Wu CL. Postoperativemultimodal analgesia pain management with nonopioid analgesics and techniques a review. JAMA Surg. 2017;152:691–7.
7. Trabulsi EJ, Patel J, Viscusi ER, Gomella LG, Lallas CD. Preemptive multimodal pain regimen reduces opioid analgesia for patients undergoing robotic-assisted laparoscopic radical prostatectomy. Urology. 2010;76:1122–4.
8. Joshi GP, Jaschinski T, Bonnet F, Kehlet H, Barrie H, Fischer J, Hill A, Lirk P, Neugebauer EAM, Rawal N, Schug SA, Simanski CJP, Van de Velde M, Vercauteren M. Optimal pain management for radical prostatectomy surgery: what is the evidence? BMC Anesthesiol. 2015;15:1–10. https://doi.org/10.1186/s12871-015-0137-2.
9. Mishriky BM, Waldron NH, Habib AS. Impact of pregabalin on acute and persistent postoperative pain: a systematic review and meta-analysis. Br J Anaesth. 2015;114:10–31.
10. Lam DMH, Choi SW, Wong SSC, Irwin MG, Cheung CW. Efficacy of pregabalin in acute postoperative pain under different surgical categories a meta-analysis. Med (United States). 2015;94:e1944.
11. Eipe N, Penning J, Yazdi F, Mallick R, Turner L, Ahmadzai N, Ansari MT. Perioperative use of pregabalin for acute pain-a systematic review and meta-analysis. Pain. 2015;156:1284–300.
12. Ohnuma T, Krishnamoorthy V, Ellis AR, Yan R, Ray ND, Hsia HL, Pyati S, Ste fan M, Bryan WE, Pepin MJ, Lindenauer PK, Bartz RR, Raghunathan K. Asso ciation 'between gabapentinoids on the day of colorectal surgery and adverse postoperative respiratory outcomes. Ann Surg. 2019;270:e65–7.
13. Myhre M, Diep LM, Stubhaug A. Pregabalin has analgesic, ventilatory, and cognitive effects in combination with remifentanil. Anesthesiology. 2016;124:141–9.
14. Fabritius ML, Strøm C, Koyuncu S, Jæger P, Petersen PL, Geisler A, Wetterslev J, Dahl JB, Mathiesen O. Benefit and harm of pregabalin in acute pain treatment: a systematic review with meta-analyses and trial sequential analyses. Br J Anaesth. 2017;119:775–91.
15. Abbou CC, Hoznek A, Salomon L, Olsson LE, Lobontiu A, Saint F, Cicco A, Antiphon P, Chopin D. Laparoscopic radical prostatectomy with a remote controlled robot. J Urol. 2017;197:S210–2.
16. Briganti A, Larcher A, Abdollah F, Capitanio U, Gallina A, Suardi N, Bianchi M, Sun M, Freschi M, Salonia A, Karakiewicz PI, Rigatti P, Montorsi F. Updated nomogram predicting lymph node invasion in patients with

prostate cancer undergoing extended pelvic lymph node dissection: the essential importance of percentage of positive cores. Eur Urol. 2012;61:480–7.
17. Rocco F, Carmignani L, Acquati P, Gadda F, Dell'Orto P, Rocco B, Casellato S, Gazzano G, Consonni D. Early continence recovery after open radical prostatectomy with restoration of the posterior aspect of the Rhabdosphincter. Eur Urol. 2007;52:376–83.
18. Chou R, Gordon DB, De Leon-Casasola OA, Rosenberg JM, Bickler S, Brennan T, Carter T, Cassidy CL, Chittenden EH, Degenhardt E, Griffith S, Manworren R, McCarberg B, Montgomery R, Murphy J, Perkal MF, Suresh S, Sluka K, Strassels S, Thirlby R, Viscusi E, Walco GA, Warner L, Weisman SJ, Wu CL. Management of postoperative pain: A clinical practice guideline from the American pain society, the American society of regional anesthesia and pain medicine, and the American society of anesthesiologists' committee on regional anesthesia, executive commi. J Pain. 2016;17:131–57.
19. Laskowski K, Stirling A, McKay WP, Lim HJ. A systematic review of intravenous ketamine for postoperative analgesia. Can J Anesth. 2011;58:911–23.
20. Waldron NH, Jones CA, Gan TJ, Allen TK, Habib AS. Impact of perioperative dexamethasone on postoperative analgesia and side-effects: systematic review and meta-analysis. Br J Anaesth. 2013;110:191–200.
21. Momon A, Verdier B, Dolomie JO, Gardette M, Pereira B, Curt I, Duale C. A single preoperative administration of dexamethasone, low-dose pregabalin, or a combination of the 2, in spinal surgery, does not provide a better analgesia than a multimodal analgesic protocol alone. Clin J Pain. 2019;35:594–601.
22. Brinck ECV, Tiippana E, Heesen M, Bell RF, Straube S, Moore RA, Kontinen V. Perioperative intravenous ketamine for acute postoperative pain in adults. Cochrane Database Syst Rev. 2018. https://doi.org/10.1002/14651858.CD012033.pub4.
23. Yang Q, Zhang Z, Xin W, Li A. Preoperative intravenous glucocorticoids can decrease acute pain and postoperative nausea and vomiting after total hip arthroplasty: a PRISMA-compliant meta-analysis. Med (United States). 2017. https://doi.org/10.1097/MD.0000000000008804.
24. Olanders KJ, Lundgren GAE, Johansson AMG. Betamethasone in prevention of postoperative nausea and vomiting following breast surgery. J Clin Anesth. 2014. https://doi.org/10.1016/j.jclinane.2014.02.006.
25. Hearn L, Derry S, Moore RA. Single dose dipyrone (metamizole) for acute postoperative pain in adults. Cochrane Database Syst Rev. 2016. https://doi.org/10.1002/14651858.CD011421.pub2.
26. Shahait M, Lee DI. Application of TAP block in laparoscopic urological surgery: current status and future directions. Curr Urol Rep. 2019;20(5):20. https://doi.org/10.1007/s11934-019-0883-7.
27. Rogers T, Bhat KRS, Moschovas M, Onol F, Jenson C, Roof S, Gallo N, Sandri M, Gallo B, Patel V. Use of transversus abdominis plane block to decrease pain scores and narcotic use following robot-assisted laparoscopic prostatectomy. J Robot Surg. 2020. https://doi.org/10.1007/s11701-020-01064-9.
28. Taninishi H, Matsusaki T, Morimatsu H. Transversus abdominis plane block reduced early postoperative pain after robot-assisted prostatectomy: a randomized controlled trial. Sci Rep. 2020;10(1):3761. https://doi.org/10.1038/s41598-020-60687-y.
29. Alam A, Juurlink DN. L'épidémie de prescription d'opioïdes: une vue d'ensemble destinée aux anesthésiologistes. Can J Anesth. 2016;63:61–8.
30. Susan O. A flood of opioids, a rising tide of deaths. N Engl J Med. 2010;363:1981–5.
31. Patel HRH, Linares A, Joseph JV. Robotic and laparoscopic surgery: cost and training. Surg Oncol. 2009;18:242–6.
32. Baloyiannis I, Theodorou E, Sarakatsianou C, Georgopoulou S, Perivoliotis K, Tzovaras G. The effect of preemptive use of pregabalin on postoperative morphine consumption and analgesia levels after laparoscopic colorectal surgery: a controlled randomized trial. Int J Colorectal Dis. 2020;35(2):323–31. https://doi.org/10.1007/s00384-019-03471-3
33. Myhre M, Romundstad L, Stubhaug A. Pregabalin reduces opioid consumption and hyperalgesia but not pain intensity after laparoscopic donor nephrectomy. Acta Anaesthesiol Scand. 2017;61(10):1314–24. https://doi.org/10.1111/aas.12963.
34. Verret M, Lauzier F, Zarychanski R, Perron C, Savard X, Pinard AM, Leblanc G, Cossi MJ, Neveu X, Turgeon AF. Perioperative use of Gabapentinoids for the management of postoperative acute pain: a systematic review and meta-analysis. Anesthesiology. 2020;133(2):265–79.
35. Sung CS, Lin SH, Chan KH, Chang WK, Chow LH, Lee TY. Effect of oral clonidine premedication on perioperative hemodynamic response and postoperative analgesic requirement for patients undergoing laparoscopic cholecystectomy. Acta Anaesthesiol Sin. 2000;38:23–9.
36. Loayza Hidalgo MP, Szimanski Auzani JA, Carpenedo Rumpel L, Lemos Moreira N, Costa Cursino AW, Caumo W. The clinical effect of small oral clonidine doses on perioperative outcomes in patients undergoing abdominal hysterectomy. Anesth Analg. 2005;100:795–802.
37. Lestar M, Gunnarsson L, Lagerstrand L, Wiklund P, Odeberg-Wernerman S. Hemodynamic perturbations during robot-assisted laparoscopic radical prostatectomy in 45° trendelenburg position. Anesth Analg. 2011;113:1069–75.

8

Analysis of risk factors of bladder neck contracture following transurethral surgery of prostate

Yi-Zhong Chen[1], Wun-Rong Lin[1,2], Yung-Chiong Chow[1,2], Wei-Kung Tsai[1,2], Marcelo Chen[1,2,3*] and Allen W. Chiu[1,2,4]

Abstract

Backgrounds: The aim of the present study was to investigate the perioperative parameters associated with bladder neck contracture (BNC) after transurethral surgery of the prostate and to compare the incidence of BNC after transurethral resection of the prostate (TURP) or Thulium vaporesection (resection group) versus Thulium vapoenucleation or enucleation of the prostate (enucleation group).

Methods: Between March 2008 and March 2020, 2363 patients received TURP and 1656 patients received transurethral surgery of the prostate with Thulium laser (ThuP) at Mackay Memorial Hospital. A total of 62 patients developed BNC. These BNC patients were age-and operation-matched to 124 randomly sampled TURP/ThuP controls without BNC. A 1:1 propensity score matching model was used to evaluate the difference in incidence of BNC.

Results: Our study demonstrated that a greater proportion of BNC patients had history of cerebrovascular accidents (11/62 vs. 7/124, $p=0.009$), coronary artery disease (14/48 vs. 16/108, $p=0.03$), chronic kidney disease (14/62 vs. 11/124, $p=0.01$), and two or more comorbidities (29/62 vs. 27/124, $p=0.001$) compared with NBNC patients. Multivariate analysis showed that smaller prostate volume (OR 0.96 (0.94–0.99), $p=0.008$) and recatherization (OR 5.6 (1.02–30.6), $p=0.047$) were significantly associated with BNC. A ROC curve predicted that a prostate volume $<42.9\ cm^3$ was associated with a notably higher rate of BNC. The propensity score matching model reported there was no difference in incidence between resection and enucleation groups.

Conclusion: This study demonstrated that incidence of BNC was the same in different surgical techniques and that low prostate volume, recatherization and ≥ 2 comorbidities were positively correlated with the development of BNC after TURP or ThuP.

Keywords: Transurethral resection of prostate, Bladder neck contracture, Benign prostate hypertrophy, Thulium enucleation/vaporesection/vapoenucleation of prostate

Introduction

Benign prostate hyperplasia (BPH) is a common problem among older males. As life expectancy increases, BPH has become a common problem [1]. BPH with lower urinary tract symptoms has a notable impact on daily life and can lead to severe genitourinary problems. When surgically indicated, bipolar transurethral resection of prostate (TURP) and transurethral surgery of the prostate with Thulium laser (ThuP), which are the major endoscopic surgery options, are typically performed, and they have been shown to have favorable outcomes.

*Correspondence: mchen4270@yahoo.com
[1] Department of Urology, MacKay Memorial Hospital, No. 92, Sec. 2, Zhongshan N. Rd., Zhongshan Dist., Taipei 104, Taiwan

Improvement in surgical instruments and technology have resulted in decreased intra-operative and post-operative complications. Bleeding is the most commonly observed intra-operative complication, while dysuria is a bothersome post-operative complication [2, 3]. Post-operative dysuria can often be caused by urethra stricture or bladder neck contracture (BNC). The incidence of BNC in the medical literature has been reported to range from 2.2 to 9.8% [4].

The underlying mechanism of BNC is not currently well understood [5]. Many risk factors have been associated with BNC, such as untreated preoperative urinary tract infection, small prostate volume, unsuitable resectoscope diameter, long operative time, history of prostatitis and recatherization after surgery [5–7]. The aim of the current study was to investigate the perioperative parameters associated with the occurrence of BNC after TURP or ThuP, and the difference in BNC incidence rates between different techniques, resection and enucleation.

Methods

We retrospectively reviewed the medical records of patients who underwent either TURP or ThuP at Mackay Memorial Hospital between March 2008 and March 2020. 16 surgeons performed the surgery and they were all experience in transurethral surgery. A total of 2363 patients underwent TURP and 1656 patients ThuP. Among ThuP, 458 patients received Thulium vaporesection (ThuVap) and 1158 patients received Thulium vapoenucleaiton of the prostate (ThuVep) and Thulium enucleation of the prostate (ThuEp). Patients with primary bladder neck stenosis, active infection before surgery, history of previous endoscopic surgery of the urinary tract, or incomplete data were excluded from this study. A total of 66 patients found to have BNC after the procedure and a total of 3953 patients didn't have BNC after the procedure. Four were excluded due to lack of PSA data, and therefore a total of 62 patients were included in the study. BNC occurred after TURP in 35 patients and after ThuP in 27 patients. They all subsequently received bladder neck incision at a later date. BNC was suspected if patients complained of progressive dysuria or gradually decreasing maximal urinary flow (less than 10 mL/s in the urodynamic study). Definite diagnosis was made by cystoscopy. Upon confirmation of the diagnosis of BNC, bladder neck incision was performed using bipolar instruments (energy set at 160 J for cutting and 80 J for coagulation). Due to low incidence rate (1.6%, 66/4019) of BNC, we designed a 1:2 case control cohort. These 62 BNC patients (BNC group, 35 TURP 10 ThuVap and 17 ThuVep or ThuEp) were age- and operation-matched to 124 randomly sampled controls without BNC (NBNC group, 70 TURP, 20 ThuVap and 34 ThuVep or ThuEp). There was no statistically significance in age and operation between BNC and NBNC group (Table 1; Additional file 1: Table S1). Propensity score matching model was used to minimize the bias in patients between resection group (N = 135, 105 TURP and 30 ThuVap) and enucleation group (N = 51, ThuVep or ThuEp). We conducted a 1:1 propensity score matching model and propensity score was set at 0.01.

The standard procedures for TURP and ThuP was: 1) urethral sounding from 16 French (Fr) to 32 Fr. 2) Insertion of a 24 Fr resectoscope in a 26 Fr sheath. 3) Resection of the prostate piece by piece using bipolar instruments (energy set at 160 J for cutting and 80 J for coagulation) or vaporesection or enucleation of the prostatic adenoma with a 120 W-Thulium laser (Vela XL or RevoLix 120, energy set at 20–40 W for enucleation and 60–80 W for resection). 4) Resected tissue was then morcellated or evacuated. 5) Final hemostasis was achieved with bipolar instruments (160 J for cutting and 80 J for coagulation). During TURP and ThuP, normal saline was used as the flushing fluid during surgery. A 22 Fr urethral triple-lumen Foley catheter was placed for traction for 8 h post-operation and for continuous irrigation with sterile saline for 24 h post-operation. The Foley was removed in 48–72 h post-operatively. Antibiotic prophylaxis with first generation cephalosporin was administered pre-operatively and 12 h post-operatively. Patients were then prescribed oral first-generation cephalosporin for a week.

We reviewed patient medical records to obtain the preoperative prostate specific antigen (PSA) level, smoking history, complete hemochemical data (including white blood cell count, red blood cell count, platelet count, renal and liver function, and electrolytes), prostate volume (measured by transrectal ultrasound), pathology, surgical time, uroflowmetry, comorbidities (hypertension, diabetes mellitus, coronary artery disease, cerebrovascular accident, chronic kidney disease and other malignancy), concomitant endoscopic cystolithotripsy (ESCL), capsule perforation during surgery, the whether or not a Foley was inserted before surgery, postoperative complication (urinary tract infection according to urine culture and epididymitis/orchitis, prostate bleeding and blood transfusion), postoperative pathology (benign prostate hyperplasia or prostate cancer), recatherization after surgery. The percentage of prostate resection was defined as the prostate specimen weight/prostate volume. Resection speed was defined as prostate specimen/surgical time (g/minutes) in patients receiving TURP. Resection speed could not be evaluated because a significant amount of time was spent in morcellation during ThuP. Chronic kidney disease was defined as an eGFR < 60 ml/min/1.73 m^2 or creatinine > 1.2 mg/dl.

Table 1 Patients' characteristics between the BNC and NBNC groups

	TURP		P value	ThuP		P value	Total		P value
	BNC (N=35)	NBNC (N=70)		BNC (N=27)	NBNC (N=54)		BNC (N=62)	NBNC (N=124)	
Age (years)	68.95±11.04	68.47±10.80	0.83	71.96±7.92	71.44±7.82	0.78	70.26	69.67	0.746
Prostate volume (ml)	40.46±20.29	55.05±18.40	0<0.001*	46.37±16.83	60.03±21.42	<0.001*	43.0±18.95	57.2±19.84	0<0.001*
PSA (ng/ml)	5.17±7.02	9.69±15.5	0.10	11.76±22.92	8.12±11.85	0.35	8.04±16.19	9.0±14.02	0.67
Maximal urinary flow (ml/s)	11.24±10.20	7.89±6.01	0.04*	9.43±7.01	8.79±5.87	0.67	10.4±8.84	8.28±5.94	0.05
Post-voiding residual urine (ml)	154.6±194.94	141.51±177.94	0.73	110.25±147.49	97.71±150.84	0.72	135.29±175.91	122.43±167.45	0.39
Foley insertion before TURP or ThuP (yes/no)	9/26	13/57	0.40	5/22	9/45	0.84	14/48	22/102	0.43
Preoperative Hemoglobin (gm/dl)	14.05±1.14	14.16±1.58	0.73	13.63±0.99	14.10±1.30	0.12	13.87±1.09	14.12±1.45	0.22
Postoperative Hemoglobin (gm/dl)	13.41±1.37	13.54±1.56	0.68	13.00±0.90	13.32±1.29	0.23	13.22±1.20	13.44±1.44	0.65
Hemoglobin change (gm/dl)	0.67±0.56	0.62±0.67	0.70	0.59±0.50	0.76±0.76	0.29	0.64±0.53	0.68±0.71	0.65
Prostate resection weight (g)	11.09±16.0	16.0±10.86	0.02*	12.37±14.94	17.65±15.09	0.14	11.64±11.75	16.67±12.84	0.01*
Percentage of prostate resected (%)	29.2±15.63	27.98±13.96	0.69	24.76±23.42	27.01±16.67	0.62	27.2±19.36	27.5±15.13	0.91
Surgical time (min)	85.11±100.93	100.93±31.69	0.01*	93.63±35.20	111.94±37.11	0.04*	43.0±30.9	57.2±34.5	0.001*
Resection speed (g/min)	0.12±0.06	0.15±0.09	0.04*	–	–	–	–	–	–
Hospital stay (days)	3.14±0.49	3.19±0.57	0.71	3.00±0.28	3.13±0.48	0.20	3.08±0.42	3.16±0.53	0.30
Smoking (yes/no)	17/18	25/45	0.21	7/20	9/45	0.32	24/38	34/90	0.12
Hypertension (yes/no)	18/17	32/38	0.58	17/10	24/30	0.12	35/27	56/68	0.15
Diabetes mellitus (yes/no)	7/28	10/60	0.45	7/20	8/46	0.23	14/48	18/106	0.17
Cerebrovascular accidents (yes/no)	7/28	5/65	0.05	4/23	2/52	0.07	11/51	7/117	0.009*
Coronary artery disease (yes/no)	6/29	10/60	0.70	9/18	6/48	0.02*	14/48	16/108	0.09
Chronic kidney disease (yes/no)	5/30	8/62	0.68	9/18	3/51	0.001*	14/48	11/113	0.01*

Table 1 (continued)

	TURP		P value	ThuP		P value	Total		P value
	BNC (N=35)	NBNC (N=70)		BNC (N=27)	NBNC (N=54)		BNC (N=62)	NBNC (N=124)	
Number of comorbidities (≥2/≤1)	14/21	16/54	0.07	15/12	11/43	0.001*	29/33	27/97	0.001*
Prostate cancer (yes/no)	6/69	6/64	0.193	2/25	4/50	1	8/54	10/114	0.29
Other malignancy (yes/no)	5/30	3/67	0.07	1/26	1/53	0.61	6/56	4/54	0.09
Concurrent ESCL (yes/no)	2/33	4/66	1	0/27	4/50	–/–	2/60	8/116	0.36
Recatherization after surgery (yes/no)	4/31	0/70	–/–	3/24	2/52	0.19	7/55	2/122	0.004*
Post-opertion urinary tract infection (yes/no)	1/34	1/69	0.61	2/25	0/54	–/–	3/59	1/123	0.11

* means $p < 0.05$

All data in the case control study between BNC and NBNC were compared using Student's t-tests, chi-squared tests, univariate and multivariate logistic regression analysis. All data in the propensity score matching model between resection and enucleation groups were compared using paired t test, McNemar's test and logistic regression analysis. IBM SPSS Statistics 25.0 was used for data analysis. Statistical significance was set at $p<0.05$.

Use of the data in the current study was approved by the Institutional Review Board of Mackay Memorial Hospital. All personal information was de-identified prior to data analysis, thus ensuring patient confidentiality.

Results

Our study showed that 66 patients developed BNC between 2008 and 2020. The incidence of BNC was 1.7% (39/2363) after TURP and 1.6% (27/1656) after ThuP (2.2% after ThuVap (10/458), and 1.4% (17/1198) after ThuVep). The average time to a diagnosis of BNC was 21.3 months (range from 2 to 130 months, IQR: 19 months).

Sixty-two BNC patients with complete data (35 TURP, 10 ThuVap and 17 ThuVep or ThuEp) were randomly age- and operation-matched in a 1:2 ratio with 124 patients without BNC (70 TURP, 20 ThuVap and 34 ThuVep or ThuEp). The average age of BNC group and NBNC group was 70.2 and 69.7 years old respectively ($p=0.746$) and general patients' characteristic were listed in Table 1 and Additional file 1: Table S1. Three patients with BNC and one patient with NBNC had postoperative urinary tract infection and received oral antibiotics. One patient after ThuVep without BNC developed post-operative bleeding and blood clot retention and received further surgery.

Univariate analysis showed that when compared with patients without BNC, those with BNC had significantly smaller prostates (43.0 ± 18.95 ml vs. 57.2 ± 19.84 ml, $p<0.001$), lower resection weight (11.64 ± 11.75 g vs. 16.67 ± 12.84 g, $p=0.01$), shorter operative times (43.0 ± 30.9 min vs. 57.2 ± 34.5 min, $p=0.001$) and recatherization after surgery [yes/no, 7/55 vs. 2/122, $p=0.01$, OR 5.6 (1.02–30.6)] (Table 2). Multivariate logistic analysis showed those with BNC had significant smaller prostate volume (OR 0.96 (0.94–0.99), $p=0.008$) and high incidence of recatherization (OR 5.6 (1.02–30.6), $p=0.047$) compared with those without BNC (Table 3). There were no significant differences in percentage of prostate resected, initial PSA, preoperative hemoglobin, postoperative hemoglobin, hemoglobin change, hospital stay, smoking history, current ESCL, maximal flow rate, post-voiding residual urine, post-operative urinary tract infection, and whether or not a Foley was inserted preoperatively. In subgroup analysis, those with BNC after TURP had significant smaller prostate volume and slower resection speed compared with NBNC group (Table 1). A ROC curve predicted that

Table 2 Univariate logistic regression analysis of incidence of BNC

	TURP OR (95% interval)	P value	ThuP OR (95% interval)	P value	Total OR (95% interval)	P value
Prostate volume (ml)	0.95 (0.92–0.99)	0.007*	0.96 (0.94–0.99)	0.008*	0.96 (0.94–0.98)	< 0.001*
Maximal urinary flow (ml/s)	1.06 (1.001–1.12)	0.046*				
Prostate resection weight (g)	0.94 (0.89–0.99)	0.04*			1.02 (0.93–0.99)	0.01*
Surgical time (min)	0.98 (0.96–0.99)	0.01*	0.98 (0.97–0.99)	0.04*	0.98 (0.97–0.99)	0.02*
Resection speed (g/min)	0.002 (0.001–0.94)	0.048*	–	–	–	–
Cerebrovascular accidents (yes/no)					3.6 (1.3–9.8)	0.01*
Coronary artery disease (yes/no)			4 (1.2–12.8)	0.02*		
Chronic kidney disease (yes/no)			8.5 (2.1–34.9)	0.003*	3 (1.3–7.0)	0.007*
Number of comorbidities (≥ 2/ ≤ 1)			4.9 (1.7–13.4)	0.002*	3.2 (1.6–6.1)	0.001*
Recatherization after surgery (yes/no)					5.6 (1.6–38.6)	0.01*

* means p < 0.05

Table 3 Multivariate logistic regression analysis of incidence of BNC

	TURP OR (95% interval)	P value	ThuP OR (95% interval)	P value	Total OR (95% interval)	P value
Prostate volume (ml)	0.95 (0.92–0.99)	0.007*	0.96 (0.92–1)	0.07	0.96 (0.94–0.99)	0.008*
Maximal urinary flow (ml/s)	1.04 (0.98–1.1)	0.20				
Prostate resection weight (g)	1.04 (0.82–1.3)	0.74			1.02 (0.98–1.1)	0.67
Surgical time (min)	0.99 (0.96–1.03)	0.97	0.99 (0.97–1)	0.65	0.99 (0.98–1)	0.38
Resection speed (g/min)	0.027 (–)	0.78	–	–	–	–
Cerebrovascular accidents (yes/no)					1.6 (0.5–5.4)	0.42
Coronary artery disease (yes/no)			3 (0.6–14)	0.17		
Chronic kidney disease (yes/no)			7.3 (1.1–49.4)	0.04*	2.7 (0.9–7.9)	0.08
Number of comorbidities (≥ 2/ ≤ 1)			1.1 (0.2–5.2)	0.92	1.6 (0.7–3.8)	0.28
Recatherization after surgery (yes/no)					5.6 (1.02–30.6)	0.047*

* means p < 0.05

a prostate volume < 42.9 cm^3 (AUC: 0.718, sensitivity: 0.766, specificity: 0.409) had a higher rate of BNC (Fig. 1).

Analysis of comorbidities showed that a greater proportion of BNC patients had history of cerebrovascular accidents [11/62 vs. 7/124, p = 0.009, OR 3.6 (1.3–9.8)], chronic kidney disease [14/62 vs. 11/124, p = 0.01, OR 3.0 (1.3–7.0)], and two or more comorbidities [29/62 vs. 27/124, p = 0.001, OR 3.2 (1.6–6.1)] (Tables 1 and 2). The presence of prostate cancer or other malignancies was not associated with risk of BNC. In ThuP subgroup analysis, a greater proportion of BNC patients had history of coronary artery disease [9/18 vs. 6/48, p = 0.02, OR 4.0 (1.2–12.8)], chronic kidney disease [9/18 vs. 3/51, p = 0.001, OR 8.5 (2.1–34.9)], and two or more comorbidities [15/12 vs. 11/43, p = 0.001, OR 4.9 (1.6–13.4)] (Tables 1 and 2). However, multivariate logistic regression analysis showed no significant difference in comorbidities. In ThuP subgroup analysis, a greater portion of BNC patients had history of chronic kidney disease [p = 0.04, OR 7.3 (1.1–49.4)] (Table 3).

In order to evaluate whether different surgical techniques were associated with the incidence of BNC, a 1:1 propensity score matching model according to age, prostate volume and comorbidity was built and propensity score was set at 0.01 (Table 4). 49 matched pairs were evaluated and there was no significant difference in all parameters (p > 0.05). Logistic regression analysis showed there was no significant difference in incidence of BNC between resection and enucleation group (p = 0.5).

In our study, six patients after TURP, three patients after ThuVap and two patients after ThuVep or ThuEp had recurrent BNC and received bladder neck incision two times. One patient after TURP and one patient after ThuVap had recurrent BNC and received bladder neck incision three times.

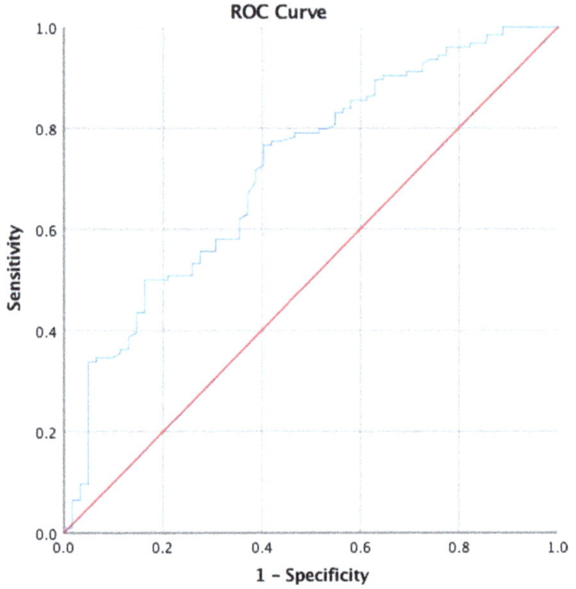

Fig. 1 ROC curve for prostate volume to determine the cutoff value that predicts the occurrence of BNC after TURP or ThuP. Red line, reference line; blue line, prostate volume in cm^3. Threshold: prostate volume: 42.9 cm^3, AUC: 0.718, sensitivity: 0.766, specificity: 0.409

Discussion

BPH with lower urinary tract symptoms is a common problem in older males. TURP is still considered the gold standard surgical treatment, and ThuP and Holmium laser enucleation of prostate (Holep) have recently been incorporated into national and international guidelines due to their noninferior efficacy and safety [8]. BNC is a common postoperative complication that typically occurs early within the first 2 years post-operation [9]. Our study showed average time to a diagnosis of BNC was 21.3 months. A meta-analysis reported that the incidence of BNC was 2% [10]. Another study showed that TURP resulted in BNC rates between 1% and 12.3% [2]. The incidence of BNC reported after ThuVeP ranges from 0 to 2.4% [11, 12]. The incidence of BNC after Holep is between 1.3 and 2.1% [13–15]. Our study results were comparable with these previous studies as the incidence of BNC was 1.5% after TURP and 1.6% after ThuP (2.2% after ThuVap (10/458), and 1.4% (17/1198) after ThuVep or ThuEp).

BNC after prostate surgery is a well-known complication but its underlying cause is not well understood. Many risk factors, including small prostate volume, higher International Prostate Symptom Score storage scores, preoperative uncontrolled infection, unsuitable resectoscope, large resection loop, extensive resection of the bladder neck, long surgical time and recatherization after surgery have been shown to be associated with the risk of BNC [6–8]. The most reported risk factor is small prostate volume with over-resection of the bladder neck. Over-resection of the bladder neck can lead to fibrosis or scarring of the bladder neck, which in turn leads to BNC. Chiu et al.reported that the incidence of BNC increased to 16% in patients with a prostate volume < 20 g [16]. Our study showed that a prostate volume < 42.9 cm^3 had a higher rate of BNC. Low volume of prostate resected and short surgical time were positively correlated with small prostate volume during TURP. Resection speed is a better parameter as it adjusts for resected prostate weight and surgical time. We hypothesized slow resection speed was correlated with unfavorable surgical processes, such as hemorrhage, poor endoscopic vision, prolonged operative time and perforation of the prostatic fossa or bladder neck. In these cases, more meticulate and extensive hemostasis using a bipolar resection loop will likely be performed and this can lead to a higher chance of thermal injury of the bladder neck, which increases the risk of bladder neck scarring. However, our study showed a lower resection speed in BNC group compared to NBNC group in TURP (OR 0.002 (0.001–0.94), $p = 0.048$) but no significant difference in pre- and post-operative hemoglobin and hemoglobin change (Tables 1 and 2).

A randomized controlled study reported that ThuEp significantly reduced the risk of BNC compared with ThuVap [17]. Another study reported that the incidence of BNC after plasmakinetic enucleation of prostate was only 0.9% [18]. Qian et al. suggested that enucleation of the prostate can keep the bladder neck intact and prevent injury caused by laser energy, which in turn reduces scar formation and decreases the development of BNC [17]. In our study, the propensity score matching model showed no difference in the incidence of BNC between resection and enucleation groups, which could be related to the use of bipolar devices for final hemostasis in both TURP and ThuP.

We hypothesized that preoperative comorbidities and smoking history are potential risk factors for BNC. Microvascular disease may be associated with BNC due to poor healing and local ischemia [19]. Development of microvascular disease, such as diabetes mellitus, coronary artery disease, cerebrovascular disease, hypertension, chronic kidney disease and smoking history could theoretically alter the microvascular blood supply in the bladder neck, and accompanied by local ischemia and the wounds caused by TURP or ThuP, could lead to scar formation. In the current study, chronic kidney disease ($p = 0.007$) and cerebrovascular accidents ($p = 0.01$) were associated with increased BNC risk. In addition, the presence of ≥ 2 comorbidities was a significant risk factor ($p = 0.001$) and 3.2 for BNC, which could indicate that there is a correlation between microvascular disease and BNC (Table 2).

Table 4 Propensity score match-controlled (1:1) cohort by age, prostate volume and comorbidity

	All patients			Cohort		
	Resection group (N = 135)	Enucleation group (N = 51)	P value	Resection group (N = 49)	Enucleation group (N = 49)	P value
Age (years)	68.8 ± 10.3	72.9 ± 7.4	0.049*	71.6 ± 8.1	72.5 ± 7.2	0.44
Prostate volume (ml)	51.02 ± 20.72	56.37 ± 19.90	0.72	57.40 ± 23.59	54.90 ± 18.87	0.42
PSA (ng/ml)	8.77 ± 15.22	8.47 ± 13.51	0.57	8.08 ± 7.90	7.88 ± 13.4	0.88
Maximal urinary flow (ml/sec)	9.44 ± 7.33	8.47 ± 13.51	0.58	8.46 ± 5.83	8.10 ± 6.41	0.79
Post-voiding residual urine (ml)	129.28 ± 171.40	119.94 ± 167.55	0.45	124.20 ± 156.88	119.88 ± 170.97	0.20
Foley insertion before TURP or ThuP (yes/no)	26/109	10/41	0.96	9/40	9/40	1.0
Pre-operation hemoglobin (ng/ml)	14.06 ± 1.43	13.99 ± 1.11	0.12	14.06 ± 1.60	14.02 ± 1.11	0.49
Post-operation Hemoglobin (ng/ml)	13.41 ± 1.47	13.29 ± 1.08	0.01*	13.28 ± 1.68	13.31 ± 1.07	0.86
Hemoglobin change (ng/ml)	0.66 ± 0.64	0.68 ± 0.71	0.82	0.77 ± 0.74	0.69 ± 0.72	0.13
Prostate resection weight (g)	14.64 ± 11.69	16.10 ± 15.10	0.045*	17.81 ± 13.65	15.33 ± 14.33	0.14
Percentage of prostate resected (%)	27.77 ± 14.93	26.65 ± 20.57	0.015*	30.10 ± 14.75	26.21 ± 20.45	0.71
Surgical time (min)	95.71 ± 32.76	111.69 ± 35.43	0.49	102.67 ± 29.92	110.33 ± 35.47	0.75
Hospital stay (days)	3.13 ± 0.50	3.14 ± 0.49	0.31	3.06 ± 0.48	3.14 ± 0.50	0.80
Smoking (yes/no)	48/87	10/41	0.036*	15/34	10/39	0.33
Hypertension (yes/no)	65/70	26/25	0.73	25/24	24/25	1.0
Diabetes mellitus (yes/no)	25/110	7/44	0.44	9/40	7/42	0.79
Cerebrovascular accidents (yes/no)	12/123	6/45	0.55	5/44	5/44	1.0
Coronary artery disease (yes/no)	22/113	9/42	0.83	10/39	8/41	0.82
Chronic kidney disease (yes/no)	16/119	9/42	0.30	8/41	8/41	1.0
Number of comorbidities (≥2/≤1)	38/97	18/33	0.34	15/34	16/33	1.0
Prostate cancer (yes/no)	15/120	3/48	0.28	5/44	3/46	0.73
Other malignancy (yes/no)	9/126	1/50	0.20	3/46	1/48	0.63
Concurrent ESCL (yes/no)	9/126	1/50	0.20	3/46	1/48	0.63
Recatherization after surgery (yes/no)	4/131	5/46	0.052	1/48	5/44	0.22
Postopertive urinary tract infection (yes/no)	3/132	1/50	0.91	1/48	1/48	1
BNC (yes/no)	45/90	17/34	1	13/36	16/33	0.69

* means $p < 0.05$

Foley insertion before surgery, postoperative urinary tract infection and repeated catherization after surgery could be possible unfavorable factors related to inflammation or trauma in the urinary tract, which can cause scar formation in the urethra and bladder neck. Tao et al. reported that post-operative urinary tract infection and recatherization were correlated to urethra stricture and not correlated to BNC [7]. Grechenkov et al. reported that repeated postoperative drainage of bladder [6]. Our study reported that recatherization was related to BNC (OR 5.6 (1.02–30.6), $p < 0.047$) while Foley insertion before surgery and postoperative urinary tract infection were not correlated to BNC.

A prophylactic incision of the bladder neck using a bipolar loop or laser at the end of surgery, may reduce the incidence of BNC [7]. Incision of the bladder neck by laser is preferred [20]. Dysuria is the primary symptom of BNC, and a positive diagnosis is confirmed by cystoscopy. Urethral dilation is a potential management tool for BNC but repeat urethral dilation due to recurrent BNC was observed in 90% of patients in the first two years [21]. BNC is managed by bladder neck incision, which has a 72% success rate [22]. In our study, 62 patients with BNC received bladder neck incision via bipolar instruments, which has a 79% (49/62) success rate. 13 patients had recurrent bladder neck contracture and received bladder neck incision. Refractory BNC presents as recurrent dysuria in a short time and may require repeat bladder neck incision. Another technique combines bladder neck incision with a transurethral irrigation agent or transurethral injection of a cytotoxic agent. Eltahawy et al. reported an 83% success rate for the combination of bladder neck incision via Holmium laser and irrigation with triamcinolone, while Redshaw et al. showed a 75% success rate for bladder neck incision using a cold-knife and transurethral injection of mitomycin C [23, 24].

This study had several limitations. First, we did not use the International Prostate Symptom Score as a parameter in the study due to incomplete medical records. Preoperative Foley status, maximal flow rates and post-voiding residual urine were not significant different between the BNC and NBNC patients ($p=0.43$, $p=0.05$ and $p=0.39$). Second, it was a single center, retrospective study, the number of patients was small and selection bias would be existent. Third, some patients were lost to follow-up years after TURP or ThuP, which could lead to an underestimation of the BNC incidence rates. There was the same size of resectoscope, resection loop and energy settings, and no previous endourological interventions, all of which minimized bias in the present study.

Our study demonstrated that low prostate volume, recatherization and the presence of ≥ 2 comorbidities were positively correlated with the development of BNC after TURP or ThuP and the incidence was the same in resection and enucleation groups. Low resection speed was positively correlated with the development of BNC after TURP. A small prostate volume less than < 42.9 cm^3 had a higher rate of BNC. However, larger studies are needed to verify these results. Our study may serve as reference for clinical urologists and our results can be used during the explanation of BNC risks before surgery.

Abbreviations

PSA: Prostate specific antigen; BPH: Benign prostate hyperplasia; TURP: Bipolar transurethral resection of prostate; ThuVap: Thulium vaporesection; ThuVep: Thulium vapoenucleation of the prostate; ThuEp: Thulium enucleation of the prostate; ThuP: Transurethral surgery of the prostate with Thulium laser; BNC: Bladder neck contracture; ESCL: Concomitant endoscopic cystolithotripsy; Holep: Holmium laser enucleation of prostate.

Acknowledgements

There is no potential financial and non-financial funding.

Authors' contributions

YZC: project development, data collection, data analysis, and manuscript writing. WRL: data collection and data analysis. YCC: data collection and data analysis. WKT: data collection and data analysis. MC: project development, data analysis, and manuscript editing. AWC: manuscript editing. All authors have read and approved the manuscript.

Competing interests

The authors declare that they have no competing interests.

Author details

[1] Department of Urology, MacKay Memorial Hospital, No. 92, Sec. 2, Zhongshan N. Rd., Zhongshan Dist., Taipei 104, Taiwan. [2] School of Medicine, MacKay Medical College, New Taipei City, Taiwan. [3] Department of Cosmetic Applications and Management, MacKay Junior College of Medicine, Nursing and Management, Taipei, Taiwan. [4] School of Medicine, National Yang-Ming University, Taipei, Taiwan.

References

1. Cindolo L, Marchioni M, Emiliani E, et al. Bladder neck contracture after surgery for benign prostatic obstruction. Minerva Urol Nefrol. 2017;69(2):133–43.
2. Rassweiler J, Teber D, Kuntz R, Hofmann R. Complications of transurethral resection of the prostate (TURP)—incidence, management, and prevention. Eur Urol. 2006;50(5):969–79 (**discussion 980**).
3. Lin Y, Wu X, Xu A, et al. Transurethral enucleation of the prostate versus transvesical open prostatectomy for large benign prostatic hyperplasia: a systematic review and meta-analysis of randomized controlled trials. World J Urol. 2016;34(9):1207–19.
4. Lee YH, Chiu AW, Huang JK. Comprehensive study of bladder neck contracture after transurethral resection of prostate. Urology. 2005;65(3):498–503 (**discussion 503**).
5. Doluoglu OG, Gokkaya CS, Aktas BK, et al. Impact of asymptomatic prostatitis on re-operations due to urethral stricture or bladder neck contracture developed after TUR-P. Int Urol Nephrol. 2012;44(4):1085–90.
6. Grechenkov A, Sukhanov R, Bezrukov E, et al. Risk factors for urethral stricture and/or bladder neck contracture after monopolar transurethral resection of the prostate for benign prostatic hyperplasia. Urologia. 2018;85(4):150–7.
7. Tao H, Jiang YY, Jun Q, et al. Analysis of risk factors leading to postoperative urethral stricture and bladder neck contracture following transurethral resection of prostate. Int Braz J Urol. 2016;42(2):302–11.
8. Gravas SCJN, Gacci M, Gratzke C, Herrmann TRW, Mamoulakis C, Rieken M, Speakman MJ, Tikkinen KAO. Management of non-neurogenic Male LUTS. 2020. https://uroweb.org/guideline/treatment-of-non-neurogenic-male-luts/-1_3.
9. Young BW. The retropubic approach to vesical neck obstruction in children. Surg Gynecol Obstet. 1953;96(2):150–4.
10. Ahyai SA, Gilling P, Kaplan SA, et al. Meta-analysis of functional outcomes and complications following transurethral procedures for lower urinary tract symptoms resulting from benign prostatic enlargement. Eur Urol. 2010;58(3):384–97.

11. Netsch C, Bach T, Herrmann TR, Gross AJ. Thulium:YAG VapoEnucleation of the prostate in large glands: a prospective comparison using 70- and 120-W 2-microm lasers. Asian J Androl. 2012;14(2):325–9.
12. Netsch C, Pohlmann L, Herrmann TR, Gross AJ, Bach T. 120-W 2-microm thulium:yttrium-aluminium-garnet vapoenucleation of the prostate: 12-month follow-up. BJU Int. 2012;110(1):96–101.
13. Primiceri G, Castellan P, Marchioni M, Schips L, Cindolo L. Bladder neck contracture after endoscopic surgery for benign prostatic obstruction: incidence, treatment, and outcomes. Curr Urol Rep. 2017;18(10):79.
14. Ibrahim A, Alharbi M, Elhilali MM, Aube M, Carrier S. 18 Years of holmium laser enucleation of the prostate: a single center experience. J Urol. 2019;202(4):795–800.
15. Elzayat EA, Elhilali MM. Holmium laser enucleation of the prostate (HoLEP): long-term results, reoperation rate, and possible impact of the learning curve. Eur Urol. 2007;52(5):1465–71.
16. Chiu AW, Chen MT, Chang LS, et al. Prophylactic bladder neck incision in the treatment of small benign prostatic hyperplasia. Zhonghua Yi Xue Za Zhi (Taipei). 1990;45(1):22–5.
17. Sun Q, Guo W, Cui D, et al. Thulium laser enucleation versus thulium laser resection of the prostate for prevention of bladder neck contracture in a small prostate: a prospective randomized trial. World J Urol. 2019;37(5):853–9.
18. Chen SS, Lin MJ, Weng MF, et al. Influence of prostate size on the perioperative and postoperative outcome of transurethral plasmakinetic enucleation of the prostate: Results of 892 patients with 3 years of follow-up. Kaohsiung J Med Sci. 2018;34(10):576–82.
19. Borboroglu PG, Sands JP, Roberts JL, Amling CL. Risk factors for vesicourethral anastomotic stricture after radical prostatectomy. Urology. 2000;56(1):96–100.
20. Madersbacher S, Marberger M. Is transurethral resection of the prostate still justified? BJU Int. 1999;83(3):227–37.
21. Kaynar M, Gul M, Kucur M, Celik E, Bugday MS, Goktas S. Necessity of routine histopathological evaluation subsequent to bladder neck contracture resection. Cent Eur J Urol. 2016;69(4):353–7.
22. Herschorn S, Elliott S, Coburn M, Wessells H, Zinman L. SIU/ICUD consultation on urethral strictures: posterior urethral stenosis after treatment of prostate cancer. Urology. 2014;83(3 Suppl):S59-70.
23. Eltahawy E, Gur U, Virasoro R, Schlossberg SM, Jordan GH. Management of recurrent anastomotic stenosis following radical prostatectomy using holmium laser and steroid injection. BJU Int. 2008;102(7):796–8.
24. Redshaw JD, Broghammer JA, Smith TG 3rd, et al. Intralesional injection of mitomycin C at transurethral incision of bladder neck contracture may offer limited benefit: TURNS study group. J Urol. 2015;193(2):587–92.

9

Ureteral distal ends combined and inserted into the ileum: A novel anastomotic technique for urinary diversion

Qi Wang, Liang Tang, Liangkuan Bi, Jie Min, Lu Fang, Wei Sun and Dexin Yu*

Abstract

Background: This study aimed to introduce a novel method for ureteroileal anastomosis, explore its clinical effectiveness, observe the incidence of postoperative anastomotic stricture, and compare the postoperative complications with those of other types of ureteroileal anastomosis reported in the literature.

Methods: Both ureters were first anastomosed at their distal ends and then inserted into the proximal end of the ileal loop. A postoperative follow-up analysis was performed to evaluate major complication indicators, including anastomotic stricture, anastomotic leak, and hydroureteronephrosis.

Results: We successfully performed ureteral distal ends anastomosis combined with end-to-end insertion into the ileum for 143 patients. The mean postoperative follow-up lasted 37 months (range: 10–68 months). There was no occurrence of an anastomotic leak. The incidence of anastomotic stricture combined with hydronephrosis, ileal conduit stones, urinary tract infection, and renal dysfunction were 2.1%, 0.7%, 2.1%, and 4.2%, respectively.

Conclusion: Ureteral distal ends combined and inserted into the ileum were simple to perform and helped achieve precise anastomosis with fewer postoperative complications.

Background

Since Bricker first developed ileal conduit in 1950, it has been popularized in urinary diversion following surgical treatment of muscle-invasive bladder cancer. Given its convenience, safety, and technical maturity, it has currently become the most common method of urinary diversion for incontinent diversions [1]. Ureteroileal anastomosis is a crucial procedure in ileal conduit and a key factor affecting the quality of life and prognosis after surgery. Some patients may experience different postoperative complications, including urinary tract obstruction, urinary leakage, symptomatic infection, which are most likely related to ureteroileal anastomosis instead of cystectomy [2, 3].

There have been many methods regarding ureteroileal anastomosis in ileal conduit, including anti-refluxing or refluxing anastomosis as well as anastomotic type selection [4]. Many managements intended to reduce postoperative complications have not been improved. In recent years, our research group has improved ureteroileal anastomosis, an essential procedure in which both ureters are first anastomosed at their ends and then inserted into the ileum in an end-to-end manner. This article presented the clinical experience and efficacy of applying this technique to ileal conduit reconstruction and provided a literature review on ureteroileal anastomosis techniques and their complications.

Methods

The present study retrospectively analyzed the clinical data of 143 patients who underwent laparoscopic radical cystectomy and ileal conduit in our hospital from 2014 to

*Correspondence: yudx_urology@126.com
Department of Urology, The Second Affiliated Hospital of Anhui Medical University, Hefei, China

2019. Ileal conduit reconstruction involved ureteral anastomosis at the ends of both ureters combined with end-to-end insertion into the proximal end of the ileal loop. According to the modified Clavien classification system [5], all surgical complications were recorded. The present study focused on evaluating the long-term postoperative complications after surgery, especially the incidence of anastomotic stricture and hydroureteronephrosis.

A Urinary diversion was performed following laparoscopic radical cystectomy and pelvic lymph node dissection. First, an infraumbilical trocar incision next to the right rectus abdominis was extended longitudinally, measuring 4 cm, at which a specimen was taken out, followed by pulling the ileum out. A 10-cm-long pedicled loop of ileum was cut 15 cm away from the ileocecal region. After intestinal continuity was restored, the mesenteric hiatus was closed. The remained mesenteric length depended on the thickness of the abdominal wall to ensure adequate mesenteric blood flow. The left ureter was transposed under the mesosigmoid, pre sacredly. The distal ends of both ureters were trimmed. The nourishing blood vessels and fat surrounding the ureters were preserved as much as possible, and it was not recommended to remove too much fat attached to the ends of the ureters (Fig. 1a). The medial edge of each ureteral end was slitted longitudinally to 15 mm in length (Fig. 2a). The anterior and posterior edges of one slitted ureteral wall were separately sutured to the corresponding anterior and posterior edges of the other slitted ureteral wall with interrupted stitches using 4–0 absorbable suture, which formed a lumen. After the distal lumens of both ureters were anastomosed into one lumen, two stitches were placed on the serosal layers of the right and left ureters above the anastomotic lumen to reinforce them together, which were localized 10 mm from the upper edge of the anastomotic ureter (Figs. 1b, 2b).

A 7-Fr single J-stent was placed in each ureter and led out from the distal end of the ileal loop (Fig. 1c).

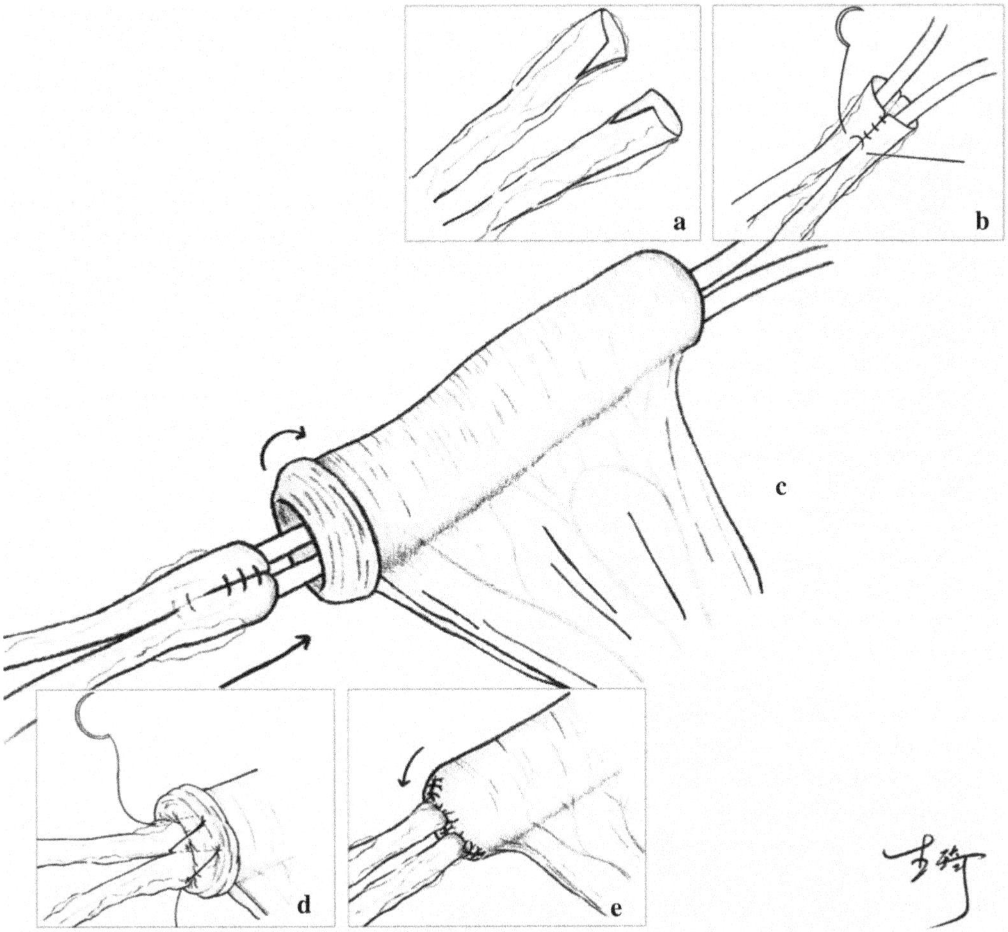

Fig. 1 **a, b** The ends of both ureters were trimmed and combined. **c** A 7-Fr single J-stent was placed in each ureter and led out from the ileal loop. **d, e** The ureters were inserted into the ileal loop and the proximal end of the ileal loop was closed

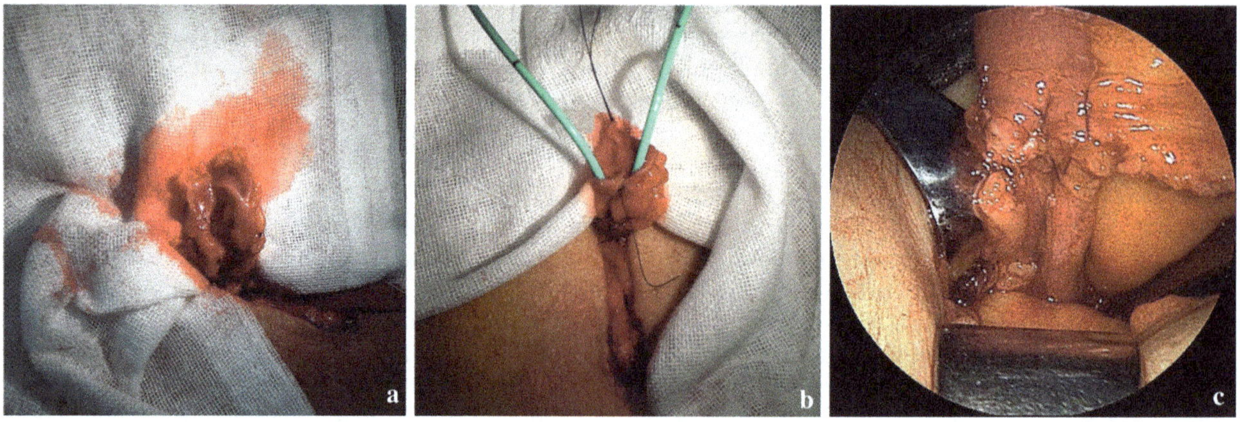

Fig. 2 **a** Both ureters were trimmed and adipose tissue was attached to the ends. **b** After the suture of the ends of both ureters, a uniform lumen has been formed. **c** Successfully complete the ureteral anastomosis combined with end-to-end insertion into the ileum

The intestinal mucosa of the ileal loop's proximal end was everted like a cuff, with an eversion length of 15 mm. The distal end of the anastomotic ureter was wholly inserted into the lumen of the proximal end of the ileal loop, with the insertion length similar to the intestinal mucosa's eversion length (15 mm). Continuous stitches with a 4-0 absorbable suture were used to suture the ureteral serosa longitudinally and the ileal mucosa at the junction between the ileum and the upper edge of the inserted ureter, requiring 4–5 stitches for one circumference of the anastomosis (Fig. 1d). Deep insertion of the needle was avoided when suturing ureteral serosa, and the ureter lumen was brought slowly to the ileal mucosa upon pulling the suture. Excessive suture of the ureter tissue was avoided to prevent changes in the blood supply. Excessive traction of the ureter was avoided when pulling the suture so as to prevent ureter avulsion or ureteral wall compression. After the everted ileal mucosa was restored, continuous stitches with a 3-0 absorbable suture were used to close the proximal end of the ileal loop. When suturing around both ureters, squeezing of the intestinal wall due to excessive tightening of the suture was avoided to prevent ureter stricture (Figs. 1e, 2c). At the incision site, The ileal loop was pulled out at the incision site 4–6 cm and left outside of the body, followed by the closure of its surrounding peritoneum with a 1-0 silk suture. The external oblique aponeurosis was sutured around the lower part of the ileal loop for fixation (usually 6 stitches), which prevented retraction of the ileum. The distal end of the ileal loop formed a nipple 20 mm above the skin level, fixed with a 1-0 silk suture, completing the creation of an abdominal stoma for the ileal conduit.

Results

A total of 143 patients were enrolled in this study, aged 63–82 years. The postoperative pathological results of all patients showed urothelial carcinoma. Pathological staging of the tumors performed using the TNM staging system. The surgery lasted ~187 to 263 min, and the intraoperative blood loss was ~50 to 280 ml (Table 1). The postoperative bowel function recovery took ~1 to 5 days to complete, and the patients could get out of bed ~1 to 3 days after the surgery. Fourteen days after the surgery, the single J-stents were removed. Postoperative hospital stays lasted ~5 to 13 days, with an average of 9 days.

Table 1 Characteristics of the studied population

Mean (SD)/Percentage (%)	
Demographic and pathological characteristics	
Age (years)	70.7 (14.13)
BMI, kg/m^2, mean (SD)	23.5 (3.3)
Follow-up time, mean (SD)	37 (6.7)
Male, n (%)	106 (74.1)
Female, n (%)	37 (25.9)
ASA score, n (%)	
2	118 (83)
≥3	25 (27)
Pathologic stage, n (%)	
pT2	77 (54)
pT3	50 (35)
pT4	16 (11)
Operative time (min.), SD	223 (25.34)
Ureteroileal anastomosis time (min.), SD	22 (4.7)
Estimated blood loss (mL), SD	180 (66.7)

The patients whose pathology showed positive lymph nodes or staged pT3-4 began to undergo re-examination combined with adjuvant chemotherapy 1 month after surgery. The other patients were followed up from the third month after surgery. Routine follow-up items included urinary system color Doppler ultrasonography, CT and blood routine, and renal function and electrolytes, focusing on whether the patient had developed hydronephrosis (and its degree), ureteroileal anastomotic stricture, anastomotic leak, ileal conduit stones, upper urinary tract stones, urinary tract infection, and renal dysfunction.

The median follow-up time of the patients was 37 months (10–68 months). Local recurrence and metastasis occurred in 7 cases (4.9%) after surgery, and 6 died, of which 3 died of bladder tumors. Postoperative complications and treatment were (Tables 2, 3): (1) 3 cases of anastomotic stricture (2.1%), all occurring to the left side and within 12–24 months after surgery, combined with varying degrees of hydroureteronephrosis; (2) the treatment was via the ileal conduit to locate the joint opening of the ureters to enter the narrowed lumen of the left ureter for balloon dilation and insertion of a double-J stent. A postoperative review showed that the stricture was relieved, and the hydroureteronephrosis was relieved. One patient with ileal conduit stones was treated with ureteroscopic holmium laser lithotripsy, and there was no recurrence of stones in the 1-year follow-up. There were 3 patients with apparent signs of urinary tract infection: (1) 1 patient presented with anastomotic stricture, and the infection was controlled after surgical treatment; (2) 2 patients presented with no obstructive factors and no obvious hydronephrosis as confirmed with the examination. The infection was controlled with anti-infection and symptomatic treatment; (3) 6 patients presented with renal dysfunction and slightly increased creatinine levels (< 200 umol/L). Among them, 1 was treated with surgery, and 5 were given symptomatic treatment for kidney preservation, after which the renal function was improved. The reasons for early renal dysfunction may be caused by temporary hydronephrosis or transient ureteral edema after removal of single J-stents. There was no incidence of urinary anastomotic leak.

Table 2 Major postoperative complications in 143 patients

Anastomotic stricture (%)	Anastomotic leak (%)	Ileal conduit stones (%)	Urinary tract infection (%)	Renal dysfunction (%)
3 (2.1)	0	1 (0.7)	3 (2.1)	6 (4.2)

Discussion

Radical cystectomy combined with urinary diversion is the primary surgical method for treating muscle-invasive bladder tumors, among which urinary diversion has a decisive impact on the quality of life of patients after surgery. Ileal conduit surgery is the gold standard procedure for incontinent diversions. For patients who are not suitable for orthotopic neobladder reconstruction, the ileal conduit is the first choice. Due to its short surgical duration and simple formation steps, the ileal conduit is more suitable for patients with more serious underlying diseases and elderly patients [6–8].

Whether the patients present with postoperative renal ureteral dilatation, urinary leakage, or symptomatic upper urinary tract infections such as pyelonephritis, the root cause is ureteroileal anastomotic stricture or anastomotic leak. Such ureteroileal anastomosis-related complications are most common, accounting for 25%-60% of all complications [9, 10]. The most common methods for

Table 3 Treatment of postoperative complications

No	Complications	Time from cystectomy to diagnosis	Treatment
1	Anastomotic stricture Urinary tract infection Renal dysfunction	12 mo	Balloon dilation and insertion of a double-J stent + anti-infective therapy
2	Anastomotic stricture	15 mo	Balloon dilation and insertion of a double-J stent
3	Anastomotic stricture	20 mo	Balloon dilation and insertion of a double-J stent
4	Ileal conduit stone	10 mo	URSL + Insertion of a double-J stent
5	Urinary tract infection	7 mo	anti-infective therapy
6	Urinary tract infection	3 mo	anti-infective therapy
7	Renal dysfunction	5 mo	Protection of renal function
8	Renal dysfunction	3 mo	Protection of renal function
9	Renal dysfunction	24 mo	Protection of renal function
10	Renal dysfunction	18 mo	Protection of renal function
11	Renal dysfunction	34 mo	Protection of renal function

anastomotic construction are: (1) the end-to-side ureteroileal anastomosis (Bricker anastomosis), which generally involves inserting the ureteral ends through the sidewall of the ileum into the intestinal segment to a depth of about 1 cm and then suturing around the insertion site. Therefore, the anastomotic stoma is prone to angulation, the inserted ureter has a short free length, and scars from around the anastomotic stoma; (2) the end-to-end ureteroileal anastomosis (Wallace anastomosis), which involves slitting the medial wall of the distal end of each ureter for approximately 3 cm, laying both ureters adjacent to each other, suturing the two medial edges to form a single lumen, and anastomosing the lateral edges of the single lumen to the ileal end. This procedure is prone to cause the excessive free length of the lower ureters, which reduces the distal blood flow, causes an excessive anastomotic tension, and results in an extensive anastomosis range. Before the formation of an ileal conduit in these two surgical procedures, the free length of the middle and lower part of the left ureter (which was moved to the right) should be longer than that of the right ureter, thereby resulting in a higher degree of traction injuries and blood flow decrease, as well as a higher suture tension. Therefore, stricture and urinary leakage are relatively common in the left ureteroileal anastomosis [4, 11, 12].

The documentary on applying different ureteroileal anastomosis techniques in recent years was reviewed, focusing on anastomotic leak and stricture compared with the present results (Table 4). Despite modifications, the Bricker anastomosis is still prone to anastomotic stricture, while the Wallace anastomosis is more likely to cause anastomotic leak [5, 9, 11, 13]. The present anastomosis procedure led to a significantly lower incidence of anastomotic stricture (2.1%) than the two anastomosis techniques above and did not result in anastomotic leak in any patient.

During the ureter and ileum's anastomosis, the ends of both ureters were slitted, reconstructed, and sutured together to form a single lumen. Next, the reshaped lumen was entirely inserted into the proximal end of the ileal loop with an insertion length of about 1.5 cm. The ureteral serosa and the ileal mucosa at the junction between the ileum and the upper edge of the inserted lumen were anastomosed, and the proximal end of the ileal loop was closed. This anastomosis procedure avoided two problems: (1) the stricture, angulation, and concealment of ureteral anastomosis due to large amounts of ileal mucosal folds in the immediate proximity of the ureteral anastomosis; (2) the difficulty of locating the opening under direct vision in later reexamination and thus the failure to explore the ureters. The advantages of ureteral anastomosis combined with end-to-end insertion into the ileum were mainly manifested in four aspects. (1) The longitudinal slitting and reconstruction of the distal ends of both ureters enlarged the ureteral diameter and eliminated the contraction of the circular muscle in the ureteral wall, minimizing the incidence of luminal stricture. The slit length was only 15 mm, and thus this method was superior to the Wallace method in protecting the distal blood vessels. (2) Anastomotic stricture is generally attributed to the scar tissues formed at the anastomosis site. At the same time, there was no direct anastomosis between the distal opening of the conjoined ureters and the ileal mucosa and no contact between the distal end and the ileal mucosal folds, thereby avoiding the stricture and obstruction at the distal ureteral opening that would otherwise be present due to surgical scars and fold occlusion. (3) In the end-to-end insertion mode, the free length was long without anastomosis angulation, and there was no apparent high-tension anastomosis during surgery, so the anastomosis was more exact, thereby reducing the probability of urinary leakage. (4) Even in postoperative anastomotic stricture, it was easy to locate the joint distal opening of both ureters at the proximal end of the ileal conduit under a ureteroscope and explore each ureter to locate the narrowed segment and conduct treatment accordingly (Fig. 3a, b). Such a procedure is safe and convenient, even applicable in the case of urinary tract stones. It should be noted that the key to the successful implementation of the ureteral anastomosis combined with end-to-end insertion into the ileum is to maintain sufficient blood flow when freeing the ureters and to ensure that the anastomosis

Table 4 Summary of literature reporting late complications related to ureteroileal anastomosis in bladder cancer patients after ileal conduit surgery

Reference	Technique	Total (cases)	Anastomotic leak	Anastomotic stricture
Christoph et al. [11]	Bricker	75	–	19 (25.3)
	Wallace	65	–	5 (7.7)
Kavaric et al. [5]	Modified Wallace	70	6 (8.5)	2 (3)
Li et al. [9]	Modified Bricker	145	4 (2.8)	5 (3.4)
The present study	Combined with end-to-end insertion	143	0 (0)	3 (2.1)

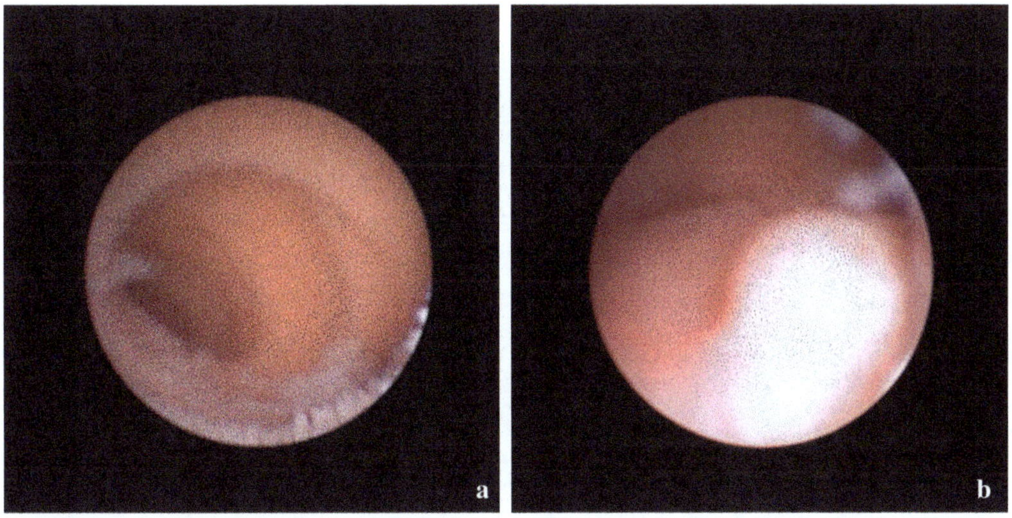

Fig. 3 **a**, **b** The ureteroscopy entered the ileal conduit, and the common opening of bilateral ureters was found at its proximal end

is performed in the absence of significant tension. Otherwise, ureteral insertion into the ileum can result in a certain degree of tension and affect the distal blood flow, which in turn can increase the incidence of postoperative anastomotic leak and stricture.

This anastomosis method allows the ureters and the ileum to be conjoined in their respective physiological peristaltic directions so that the peristaltic path of the ureter and the ileum are consistent without noticeable deviation and angulation, thereby forming a peristaltic flow to promote urinary excretion [14]. The normal peristalsis of the ureters after surgery can stimulate and drive the ileal peristalsis to a certain extent, which effectively removes the intestinal mucus produced by the goblet cells in the intestinal wall thereby reducing the risk of intestinal mucus accumulation obstructing the urethral opening. Moreover, the normal peristalsis facilitates timely and thorough drainage of urine in the ileal conduit into an ostomy bag, reducing the residence time of bacteria in the ileal conduit, and avoiding prolonged contact of urine with mucus due to poor drainage and thereby inflammatory changes, which in turn reduces the incidence of retrograde upper urinary tract infection after surgery [15].

As a retrospective clinical study, the present study had certain limitations, especially the absence of a control group for comparison. More research is needed to prove further the feasibility of this technique based on more clinical data. However, the present results have shown that this technique is safe and effective. As indicated by the follow-up data, the present anastomosis technique has better clinical outcomes than the traditional techniques, achieving a significantly lower incidence of anastomotic stricture and urinary leakage as the primary complications.

Conclusion

Ureteral distal ends combined with end-to-end insertion into the ileum is more favorable for reducing the incidence of postoperative anastomotic stricture, anastomotic leak, and urinary tract infection. It is also convenient to use for dealing with postoperative complications such as hydroureteronephrosis, ureteral stricture, and stone formation, thereby making it worthy of wide clinical application. Considering that there is no clinical standard for ureteroileal anastomosis, further studies are needed to explore better anastomosis methods for the patients.

Acknowledgements

All authors conducted the conception and design of the study, acquisition and interpretation of data, drafting the article, final approval of the version to be published.

Authors' contributions

Each author has participated sufficiently in the work and takes public responsibility for appropriate portions of the content. The authors have agreed to be accountable for all aspects of the work and ensure that questions related to the accuracy or integrity of any part of the work are appropriately investigated and resolved. YDX created the design and concept of the study together with WQ and TL. Supported by BLK and MJ they acquired the data and implemented the clinical trial. Literature research was conducted by FL and SW. The manuscript was prepared by WQ. Statistical analysis was carried out by WQ and TL. All authors reviewed and edited the manuscript.

Competing interests

The authors declare that they have no competing interests.

References

1. Hautmann R, Abol-Enein H, Lee T, et al. Urinary diversion: how experts divert. Urology. 2015;85:233–8.
2. Barbieri CE, Schwartz MJ, Boorjian SA, et al. Ureteroileal anastomosis with intraluminal visualization: technique and outcomes. Urology. 2010;76:1496–500.
3. Shah S, Movassaghi K, Sinner D, et al. Ureteroenteric strictures after open radical cystectomy and urinary diversion: the University of Southern California experience. Urology. 2015;86:87–91.
4. Ficarra V, Giannarini G, Crestani A, et al. Retrosigmoid versus traditional ileal conduit for urinary diversion after radical cystectomy. Eur Urol. 2019;75:294–9.
5. Kavaric P, Eldin S, Nenad R, et al. Modified wallace anastomotic technique reduces ureteroenteric stricture rates after ileal conduit urinary diversion. IBJU. 2020;46:446–55.
6. Davis N, Burke J, McDermott T, et al. Bricker versus Wallace anastomosis: a meta-analysis of ureteroenteric stricture rates after ileal conduit urinary diversion. Can Urol Assoc J. 2015;9:E284–90.
7. Westermann M, Parker W, Viers B, et al. Malignant ureteroenteric anastomotic stricture following radical cystectomy with urinary diversion: Patterns, risk factors and outcomes. Urol Oncol. 2016;34(485):e1-6.
8. Packiam V, Agrawal V, Cohen A, et al. Lessons from 151 ureteral reimplantations for postcystectomy ureteroenteric strictures: a single center experience over a decade. Urol Oncol. 2017;35(112):e19-25.
9. Li Z, Liu Z, Yao K, et al. An improved ileal conduit surgery for bladder cancer with fewer complications. Cancer Commun. 2019;39:19–28.
10. Donahue TF, Bochner BH, Sfakianos JP, Kent M, Bernstein M, Hilton WM, et al. Risk factors for the development of parastomal hernia after radical cystectomy. J Urol. 2014;191:1708–13.
11. Christoph F, Herrmann F, Werthemann P, et al. Ureteroenteric strictures: a single center experience comparing Bricker versus Wallace ureteroileal anastomosis in patients after urinary diversion for bladder cancer. BMC Urol. 2019;19:100.
12. Baten E, Akand M, Floyd MS Jr, et al. Evaluation of conservative approach in the management of ureteroenteric strictures following radical cystectomy with Bricker ileal conduit: a single-center experience. Scand J Urol. 2016;50:439–44.
13. Movassaghi K, Shah SH, Cai J, et al. Incisional and parastomal hernia following radical cystectomy and urinary diversion: the University of Southern California Experience. J Urol. 2016;196:777–81.
14. Ahmadi N, Ashrafi AN, Hartman N, et al. Use of indocyanine green to minimise uretero-enteric strictures after robotic radical cystectomy. BJU Int. 2019;124:302–7.
15. Shah SH, Movassaqhi K, Skinner D, et al. Ureteropenteric strictures after open radical cystectomy and urinary diversion: the university of Southern California experience. Urology. 2015;86:87–91.

10

Endoscopic urethrotomy versus open urethroplasty for men with bulbar urethral stricture: The OPEN randomised trial cost-effectiveness analysis

Jing Shen[1], Luke Vale[1*], Beatriz Goulao[2], Paul Whybrow[3], Stephen Payne[4] and Nick Watkin[5] on behalf of OPEN trial investigators

Abstract

Background: Bulbar urethral stricture is a common cause for urinary symptoms in men and its two main treatment options both have drawbacks with little evidence on their relative cost-effectiveness. Current guidelines on the management of recurrent bulbar urethral stricture have been predominantly based on expert opinion and panel consensus.

Objective: To assess the relative cost-effectiveness of open urethroplasty and endoscopic urethrotomy as treatment for recurrent urethral stricture in men.

Methods: Set in the UK National Health Service with recruitment from 38 hospital sites, a randomised controlled trial of open urethroplasty and endoscopic urethrotomy with 6-monthly follow-up over 24 months was conducted. Two hundred and twenty-two men requiring operative treatment for recurrence of bulbar urethral stricture and having had at least one previous intervention for stricture were recruited. Effectiveness was measured by quality- adjusted life years (QALYs) derived from EQ-5D 5L. Cost-effectiveness was measured by the incremental cost per QALY gained over 24 months using a within trial analysis and a Markov model with a 10-year time horizon.

Results: In the within trial, urethroplasty cost on average more than urethrotomy (cost difference: £2148 [95% CI 689, 3606]) and resulted in a similar number of QALYs on average (QALY difference: − 0.01 [95% CI − 0.17, 0.14)] over 24 months. The Markov model produced similar results. Sensitivity analyses using multiple imputation, suggested that the results were robust, despite observed missing data.

Conclusions: Based on current practice and evidence, urethrotomy is a cost-effective treatment compared with urethroplasty.

Keypoints: Urethrotomy and urethroplasty both led to symptom improvement for men with bulbar urethral stricture—a common cause for urinary symptoms in men; Urethroplasty appeared unlikely to offer good value for money compared to urethrotomy based on current evidence.

Trial registration: ISRCTN: 98009168 (date: 29 November 2012) and it is also in the UK NIHR Portfolio (reference 13507).

*Correspondence: luke.vale@newcastle.ac.uk

[1] Population Health Sciences Institute, Newcastle University, Newcastle upon Tyne, UK

Keywords: Cost-effectiveness, Economic model, Randomised controlled trial, Urethral stricture, Urethroplasty, Urethrotomy

Introduction

Bulbar urethral stricture is a common cause for urinary symptoms (typically difficulty in passing urine) in men. Initial treatment is usually by endoscopic urethrotomy, a procedure that produces widening of the narrowed urethral segment by incising the stricture internally under vision. In about 50% of the cases the stricture will recur requiring re-treatment [1]. This can be via a repeat endoscopic urethrotomy, graduated dilatation or formally repaired by urethroplasty with either excision of the stricture and anastomosis, or augmentation using a graft such as buccal mucosa.

Urethrotomy is most commonly performed for recurrent bulbar stricture because it is minimally invasive, does not require specialist surgical expertise, and has a short period of urethral catheterisation and recovery. However, further recurrence is likely [2]. Open urethroplasty is more invasive, requires specialist expertise, a longer period of catheterisation and a more protracted return to normal activities. Nevertheless, urethroplasty may offer the prospect of long-term cure without the need for further interventions [3, 4]. When men are choosing between these two options, they have to make a trade-off between the invasiveness and effectiveness of each operation [1, 5–8]. Current decision-making is therefore determined by the availability of local expertise, clinician guidance, patient co-morbidity, and patient preferences.

The guidelines from the American Urological Association (AUA) and Société Internationale d'Urologie (SIU) recommend treatment with endoscopic techniques for first time bulbar strictures [1]. For recurrent strictures the guideline recommendations differ, with the AUA recommending urethroplasty and the SIU recommending endoscopic approaches *or* urethroplasty if symptomatic recurrence is after more than 3 months [1]. The reviews underpinning published guidelines, sponsored jointly by the SIU, the International Consultation on Urologic Disease [1, 5] and by the AUA [7], included non-randomised studies, predominantly of retrospective cohort design. Consequently the formulation of the guideline recommendation subsequent to these reviews was predominantly based on expert opinion and panel consensus rather than any robust evidence of the relative effectiveness or cost-effectiveness of these two treatment options.

To address this evidence gap, a randomised controlled trial (RCT) was conducted to compare the clinical and cost-effectiveness of urethroplasty versus endoscopic urethrotomy for the alleviation of urinary symptoms in men with recurrent bulbar stricture over 24 months (the OPEN (open urethroplasty versus endoscopic urethrotomy) Trial [6]). Clinical results of the OPEN trial are presented elsewhere [9]. This paper presents the cost-effectiveness analysis results.

Methods

OPEN was a pragmatic patient-randomised two-arm superiority trial, which recruited across 38 National Health Service (NHS) secondary care providers in the UK. The algorithm allocated participants to each intervention in a 1:1 ratio with recruitment site and time since last procedure (< 12 months or ≥ 12 months) as minimisation covariates. Trial procedures and statistical analysis are described elsewhere [6, 9].

The OPEN trial's economic analysis comprised a within trial cost-effectiveness analysis and Markov model with a 10-year time horizon. The within trial analysis estimated the costs from a societal perspective, quality adjusted life years (QALYs) gained and incremental cost per QALY of open urethroplasty compared to endoscopic urethrotomy over a 24-month period. As urethroplasty was a priori expected to be both more effective and more costly than endoscopic urethrotomy, with its benefits persisting beyond 24 months, Markov modelling [10] was conducted to examine the relative efficiency with a 10-year time horizon. Costs were reported as pound Sterling for the price year 2017. Where costs came from different years they were converted to 2017 values using the Consumer Price Index [11], as this was the last full year when unit costs were available before the analysis was conducted. All costs and QALYs were appropriately discounted using the recommended discount rate (3.5% per annum) [12]. Sensitivity analysis [13] was conducted to address uncertainty in study parameters and multiple imputation [14] was adopted to deal with missing data.

Resource use and cost

Micro costing methods [15] were used to estimate the cost of the two interventions on a per patient basis. The cost of the interventions included the staff involved, the use of reusable and disposable equipment and use of the theatre suite. Data that varied by participant were collected on the trial's Case Report Form, whilst other data came from communications with clinicians at the main trial site (Freeman hospital, Newcastle upon Tyne, UK). The unit costs of these resources came from standard sources [16–18].

When trial participants had a re-intervention during the trial's follow-up period, the same process of micro costing used to cost the index procedure was invoked. Other use of primary and secondary NHS services, medications and participants' out-of-pocket expenses relating to the condition came from the Case Report Form and a bespoke participant cost questionnaire completed at six-monthly intervals. Unit costs came from standard sources and participant cost questionnaire.

Quality-adjusted life years

QALYs were based on responses to the EQ-5D-5L collected at baseline, immediately prior to surgery, 1 week after catheter removal, 3, 6, 9, 12, 24 months following surgery, 18 and 24 months after randomisation and at the end of study. The responses to the EQ-5D-5L questionnaire were scored using UK population tariffs [19] to produce a health state utility score for each participant in each of the treatment groups using the area under the curve (AUC) method [20].

Given the large number of time points for EQ-5D-5L data and to align with the primary effectiveness analysis [9], it was decided that to be included in the AUC analysis as a complete case, the participant must have at least three EQ-5D-5L observations with one at the start of the assessment period, one at the mid-range and one at the end. The specific requirements depended on whether the participants had an initial intervention and the type of analysis conducted (details in the note under Table 2).

For all calculations of QALYs, the first observation used was set at time point zero and the actual date of completion for each individual EQ-5D-5L questionnaire was used to calculate the number of days from the first observation. In the sensitivity analyses, QALYs were rescaled to the nominal data collection points, i.e. 730 days, to account for difference in waiting times between the two interventions (note that cost data did not require rescaling in the same way as the recall period, because it was pre-defined within the data collection tools). Additionally, multiple imputation for EQ-5D-5L at all missing time points was conducted to calculate QALYs for all participants.

Within trial cost-utility analysis

The cost-utility analysis used an intention-to-treat principle. The incremental cost-effectiveness ratio (ICER) was calculated by dividing the difference in mean costs by the difference in mean QALYs for each group. Results were presented as point estimates of the mean incremental costs, QALYs and cost per QALY, estimated using seemingly unrelated regression [21], controlling for dichotomised time since last procedure (less than 12 months, 12 months or more), allocated treatment arm and baseline utility. Multiple imputation was performed to complete any missing data and used in the sensitivity analysis. Stochastic uncertainty in parameter estimates was addressed through the application of bootstrapping and the estimation of cost-effectiveness acceptability curves.

Markov model

The Markov model consisted of three health states—symptom-free, symptomatic and deceased—in care pathways describing the process of care and disease incidence and progression. The base case analysis used parameters that were estimated based on information given by study participants who were allocated and received the allocated treatment. Both probabilistic and deterministic sensitivity analyses were conducted to address uncertainty. Deterministic sensitivity analyses included basing model parameters on those who received the same treatment procedure regardless of their allocated intervention group (due to cross-over in the trial) and varying the probabilities of follow-up intervention conditional on the previous intervention. The parameters used to populate the Markov model are reported in supplementary material (Additional file 1: Table S1). Model structure is shown in supplementary material (Additional file 1: Figure S3).

Results

A total of 222 men were randomised, two of whom were excluded from analysis post-randomisation because further assessment prior to intervention found them to be ineligible. 108 were in the urethroplasty group and 112 in the urethrotomy group.

Costs

Total costs combining NHS resource use costs (intervention, re-intervention and health service use during follow-up) and patients' out-of-pocket costs are presented in Table 1. The cost of urethroplasty was statistically significantly higher over 24 months post randomisation than that of urethrotomy, with the cost difference ranging between £1333 and £2123 depending on whether follow-up care and patient costs were included for the base care and sensitivity analyses.

Quality-adjusted life years

Estimates of QALYs for the base case analysis and all the sensitivity analyses are presented in Table 2. Urethrotomy in general appears to generate higher QALYs than urethroplasty. However, the difference was not statistically significant apart from evidence of a slight difference for the rescaled QALYs at 24 months after surgery ($p < 0.1$) and the rescaled QALYs with imputation ($p < 0.1$).

Within trial cost-utility analysis

In the base case, urethroplasty costed more than urethrotomy while generating a lower QALY, therefore, was dominated by urethrotomy (Table 3). The base case results appeared robust as they were similar in the sensitivity analyses (Table 3). The cost-effectiveness acceptability curve (Fig. 1) and incremental cost and QALY plots (Additional file 1: Figure S1) are presented for the base case.

Markov model

In the base case analysis, urethroplasty is unlikely to be considered cost-effective under current society's willingness to pay threshold for a QALY and this is supported by the sensitivity analyses results (Table 4 and Figs. 2 and Additional file 1: Figure S2). This is mainly due to the higher cost of urethroplasty compared to urethrotomy, whilst both of the treatment options produce similar QALY gains. This is despite those receiving urethroplasty

Table 1 Total cost (£) for each trial group

Total cost	Urethroplasty		Urethrotomy	
	Mean (SD) £	N	Mean (SD) £	N
Base case				
Total intervention and re-intervention cost	4332 (3151)	89	2209 (2368)	91
Total NHS cost (intervention and re-intervention with follow-up)	4455 (3191)	89	2657 (3476)	91
Total societal cost (NHS and patient costs)	4480 (3218)	89	2730 (3713)	91
Sensitivity analysis with data imputation				
Total intervention and re-intervention cost	4559 (3061)	108	2911 (2713)	112
Total NHS cost (intervention and re-intervention with follow-up)	4674 (3135)	108	3310 (3552)	112
Total societal cost (NHS and patient costs)	4704 (3155)	108	3371 (3755)	112

Table 2 Utility values at each time point and QALYs over the trial follow-up

EQ-5D 5L	Urethroplasty		Urethrotomy	
	Mean (SD)	N	Mean (SD)	N
QALYs at 24 months after randomisation	1.75 (0.40)	55	1.76 (0.35)	54
QALYs at 24 months after randomisation (rescaled to 730 days)	1.66 (0.34)	55	1.70 (0.34)	54
QALY at 24 months after surgery	1.73 (0.54)	44	1.77 (0.34)	56
QALY at 24 months after surgery (rescaled to 730 days)	1.42 (0.40)	44	1.58 (0.30)	56
QALY at 24 months after randomisation with imputation	1.73 (0.32)	108	1.76 (0.28)	112
QALY at 24 months after randomisation with imputation (rescaled to 730 days)	1.67 (0.29)	108	1.72 (0.27)	112
QALY at 24 months after surgery with imputation	1.75 (0.37)	108	1.76 (0.29)	112
QALY at 24 months after surgery with imputation (rescaled to 730 days)	1.67 (0.30)	108	1.72 (0.26)	112

QALY calculations For those participants who did not receive an initial intervention, to be included in the AUC analysis without imputation, they must have complete EQ-5D-5L data on all of the three time points: baseline, 18 months and 24 months after randomisation. For those participants who received an initial intervention, the base case analysis examined QALY over the period from baseline to 24 months after randomisation, therefore, the base case AUC analysis required complete EQ-5D-5L data at baseline and 24 months after randomisation, and at one of the data collection points of 3, 6, 9, 12 following surgery and 18 months following randomisation. Given the differences in the time lengths between randomisation and undergoing an intervention between urethroplasty and urethrotomy, sensitivity analyses also examined QALY over the period from the time prior to surgery to 24 month post-surgery, in which case the AUC analysis required complete EQ-5D-5L data at prior to surgery and 24 months after surgery, and at one of the data collection points of 3, 6, 9, 12 following surgery and 18, 24 months following randomisation

Table 3 Cost-effectiveness analysis (within trial)

Investigation strategy	Cost (£) mean (95% CI)	Incremental Cost (£) mean (95% CI)	QALY mean (95% CI)	Incremental effect mean (95% CI)	ICER (£)	Probability of each treatment strategy is cost-effective for different threshold values for society's willingness to pay				
						£0 k (%)	£10 k (%)	£20 k (%)	£30 k (%)	£50 k (%)
Base case, 24 months post randomisation										
Urethroplasty (n = 46)	4869 (4123, 5614)	2148 (689, 3606)	1.74 (1.61, 1.86)	− 0.01 (− 0.17, 0.14)		0	0	1	3	13
Urethrotomy (n = 46)	2721 (1444, 3999)		1.75 (1.65, 1.85)		Dominant	100	100	99	97	87
24 months post randomisation (rescaled QALY)										
Urethroplasty (n = 46)	4869 (4123, 5614)	2148 (689, 3606)	1.65 (1.55, 1.76)	− 0.04 (− 0.18, 0.11)		0	0	0	1	4
Urethrotomy (n = 46)	2721 (1444, 3999)		1.69 (1.59, 1.79)		Dominant	100	100	100	99	96
24 months post surgery										
Urethroplasty (n = 37)	4963 (3977, 5949)	1672 (− 65, 3409)	1.73 (1.54, 1.92)	− 0.04 (− 0.24, 0.16)		0	0	4	9	15
Urethrotomy (n = 48)	3291 (1947, 4636)		1.77 (1.67, 1.87)		Dominant	100	100	96	91	85
24 months post surgery (rescaled QALY)										
Urethroplasty (n = 37)	4963 (3977, 5949)	1672 (− 65, 3409)	1.42 (1.28, 1.56)	− 0.16 (− 0.31, − 0.01)		0	0	0	0	0
Urethrotomy (n = 48)	3291 (1947, 4636)		1.58 (1.49, 1.67)		Dominant	100	100	100	100	100
24 months post randomisation with imputation										
Urethroplasty (n = 108)	4704 (4102, 5305)	1333 (410, 2256)	1.73 (1.67, 1.79)	− 0·03 (− 0.11, 0.05)		0	0	0	0	1
Urethrotomy (n = 112)	3371 (2667, 4074)		1.76 (1.71, 1.81)		Dominant	100	100	100	100	99
24 months post randomisation with imputation (rescaled QALY)										
Urethroplasty (n = 108)	4704 (4102, 5305)	1333 (410, 2256)	1.67 (1.62, 1.73)	− 0.05 (− 0.13, 0.02)		0	0	0	0	0
Urethrotomy (n = 112)	3371 (2667, 4074)		1.72 (1.67, 1.77)		Dominant	100	100	100	100	100
24 months post surgery with imputation										
Urethroplasty (n = 108)	4704 (4102, 5305)	1333 (410, 2256)	1.75 (1.68, 1.82)	− 0.02 (− 0.10, 0.07)		0	0	0	0	3
Urethrotomy (n = 112)	3371 (2667, 4074)		1.76 (1.71, 1.82)		Dominant	100	100	100	100	97
24 months post surgery with imputation (rescaled QALY)										
Urethroplasty (n = 108)	4704 (4102, 5305)	1333 (410, 2256)	1.67 (1.61, 1.73)	− 0.05 (− 0.12, 0.02)		0	0	0	0	0
Urethrotomy (n = 112)	3371 (2667, 4074)		1.72 (1.67, 1.77)		Dominant	100	100	100	100	100

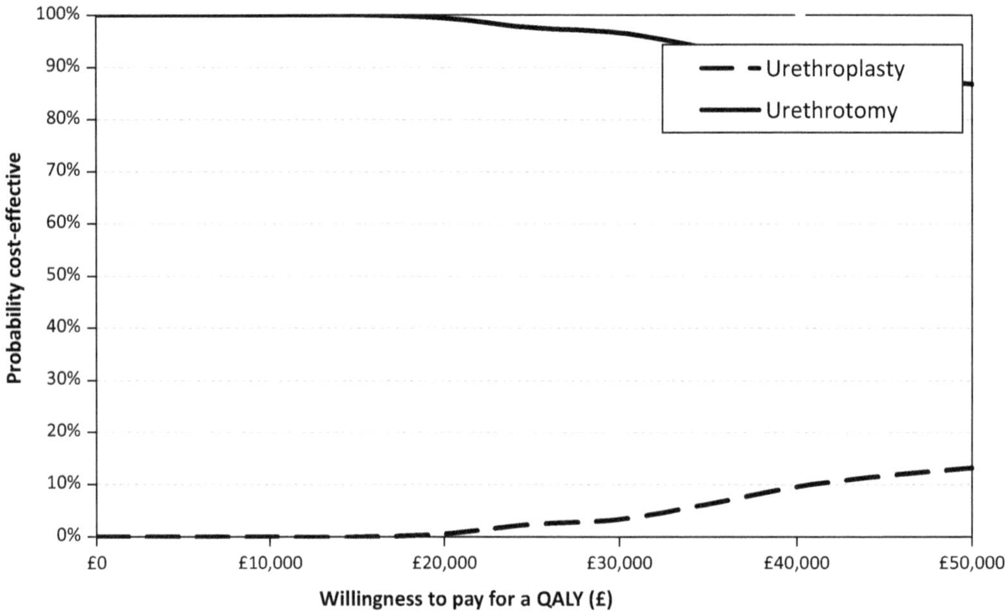

Fig. 1 Cost-effectiveness acceptability curve (Base case)

Table 4 Markov model result over 10 years

Analyses	Treatment strategy	Cost (£)	QALY	ICER (£)	Probability of each treatment strategy is cost-effective for different threshold values for society's willingness to pay for a QALY				
					£0 k (%)	£10 k (%)	£20 k (%)	£30 k (%)	£50 k (%)
Base case	Urethroplasty	8026	7.61	301,073	0	0	0	0	2
	Urethrotomy	6553	7.60		100	100	100	100	98
Parameters based on treatment received	Urethroplasty	7987	7.61	307,328	0	0	0	0	1
	Urethrotomy	6490	7.60		100	100	100	100	99
Always receive the same treatment at recurrence	Urethroplasty	9026	7.61	476,162	0	0	0	0	0
	Urethrotomy	4059	7.60		100	100	100	100	100
Always receive the other treatment at recurrence	Urethroplasty	8076	7.61	263,383	0	0	1	2	4
	Urethrotomy	7054	7.60		100	100	99	98	96

having a lower chance of recurrence compared to those receiving urethrotomy.

Discussion

Relative efficiency within the trial follow-up and over a 10-year time horizon was found to favour urethrotomy compared with urethroplasty. Effectiveness as measured by QALYs appeared to be broadly equivalent between the two trial arms of the OPEN trial, and this was in line with the primary clinical outcome finding showing no statistically significant difference in the primary patient reported outcome between trial arms [9]. Costs were higher in the urethroplasty arm than the urethrotomy arm. Therefore, urethroplasty had a higher cost whilst producing similar QALY gain, making it unlikely to be cost-effective, despite having a lower chance of recurrence compared to urethrotomy.

The relatively high cost of urethroplasty is the main reason that it was not as cost-effective. It may be possible to reduce the cost of urethroplasty by using day-care surgery [22], a shorter period of catheterisation [23] or by rationalising follow-up to those most likely to need it and discharging symptom stable patients at an early stage [24]. Length of stay following urethroplasty within the trial was 1.34 (SD 0.95) days vs 0.52 (SD 1) for urethrotomy [25]. Therefore, scope to substantially reduce length of stay is limited and even if length of

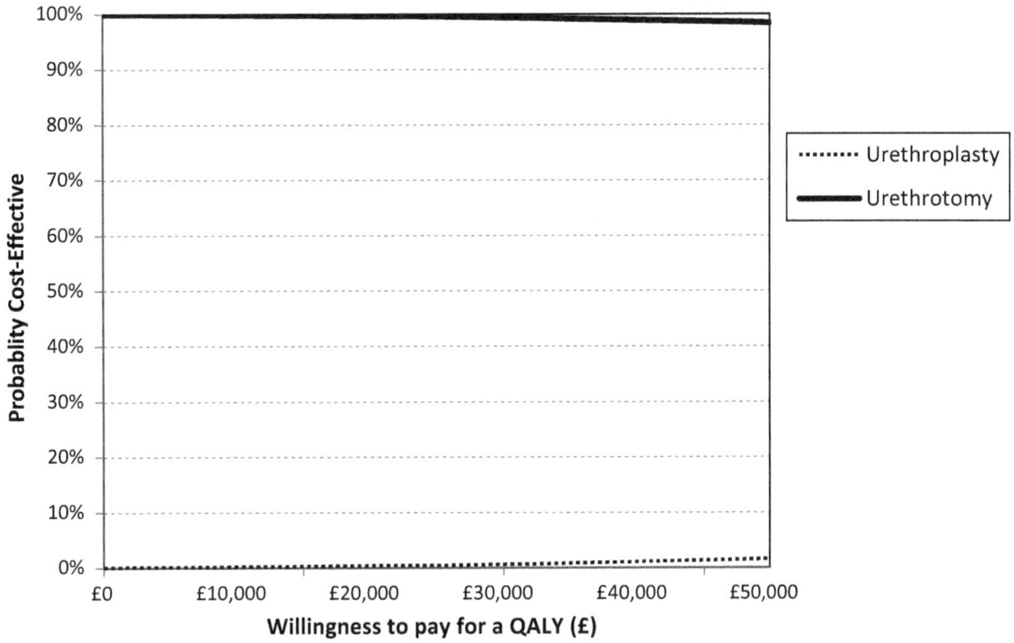

Fig. 2 Cost-effectiveness acceptability curve (Markov model base case)

stay was reduced to zero this would be insufficient to reduce the cost of urethroplasty to close to the cost of urethrotomy.

However, the higher cost of urethroplasty is driven by the higher theatre procedure and it is unlikely that theatre time could be reduced significantly to alleviate the increased costs of urethroplasty. Hospitalisation accounts for around 15% of the total intervention cost. Strategies to reduce length of stay could be explored as a way of lowering the cost of urethroplasty. In Europe, practice varies widely with length of stay ranging from 2 to 7 days in high volume centres exaggerating the difference between the two procedures costs. The mean length of stay in the UK trial was 2 days. It is unlikely that further substantial reductions in length of stay would be possible, although pre-operative counselling, improved perioperative analgesia and discharge education could help reduce this to 1.5 days.

Although the study showed no difference in effectiveness as measured by QALYs, it is worth noting that the loss of quality of life during recovery from subsequent procedures was not taken into consideration. Given the likelihood of recurrence requiring repeated treatments, this decrement in quality of life could make a difference in total QALYs between the two treatments. Patients undergoing urethroplasty are also less likely to have recurrence in the long-term based on the observation during the trial's follow-up period and consequently suffer less loss in quality of life and hence may accrue more QALYs over time. However, there was no obvious signal of reductions in quality of life caused by differences in recurrent rates [25]. However, this requires further study. Additionally, EQ-5D as a generic quality of life measure may not be sensitive enough to capture changes in health-related quality of life among patients with bulbar urethral stricture, as the impact on quality of life from the condition may fall mostly around the time of recurrence or only present in one or two dimensions (e.g. pain, anxiety) of EQ-5D. Future research should focus on how best to capture quality of life loss during recurrence and exploring alternative measures for this type of patients using preference elicitation methods [26, 27].

When examining the cost-effectiveness over the long-term, a key uncertainty in the modelling was the choice of re-intervention. The study data showed a large proportion of patients switched to a treatment different from their previous treatment when they had a re-intervention. There is no consensus on treatment choices for re-interventions, and such choices are often influenced by many non-clinical factors such as patient choice, waiting time, and travel time [8]. However, varying the probabilities of treatment options conditional on the previous intervention in the sensitivity analyses conducted for the modelling showed that urethroplasty remained less likely to be cost-effective.

Due to the trial's follow-up period of two years, we could potentially be underestimating the costs of the urethrotomy arm, however, questions arise on how many recurrences there need to be to offset the more expensive urethroplasty and over what length of time. On the other hand, there was little evidence suggesting patients' quality of life differed significantly between the two arms, at least within the trial's follow-up period. We do not claim that cost is the only concern in the choice of treatment, but in the absence of clear evidence on the additional benefits one treatment can bring, costs may be an important factor to consider in a publicly funded health system. These issues were also extrapolated over 10 years using a Markov model, which met or exceeded internationally accepted guidelines for best practice for the conduct of such work. This analysis showed that the initial higher costs of urethroplasty were not likely to be offset by increased reintervention rates but that urethroplasty was on average more effective.

The key strength of the present study is the use of an RCT designed to detect the clinically meaningful difference in voiding symptom score. The RCT design was based on current best practice for pragmatic surgical trials and it sought to provide direct and most up to date information on costs and utilities. However, obtaining data directly from a large clinical study also has its downside. The principle limitation of the RCT was the missing data caused by trial participants being lost to follow-up; a common situation in a complex study involving several years of follow-up. We remedied this by using multiple imputation for the missing data and comparing complete case analysis with analyses using imputation. These sensitivity analyses demonstrated that the study results were robust.

Although the economic evaluation was conducted in the UK NHS, the results are generalisable to other countries with similarly public funded healthcare systems. As we have seen that there is little difference in QALYs between the two treatment options, regardless of unit costs of resources used, urethroplasty is generally more costly than urethrotomy due to the longer operating and recovery time. Therefore, the conclusions drawn for QALYs and costs would stay unchanged in other settings.

Conclusions

This paper has presented a comprehensive economic analysis of the relative efficiency of urethroplasty and urethrotomy within an RCT over 24 months and over a 10-year time horizon. Based on current practice and evidence, urethroplasty is unlikely to be cost-effective due to its higher cost. Future research should examine how the benefits of reduced recurrence by urethroplasty can be captured while finding ways to reduce its costs.

Abbreviations

OPEN: Open urethroplasty versus endoscopic urethrotomy; NHS: National Health Service; QALY: Quality adjusted life years; AUC: Area under the curve; ICER: Incremental cost-effectiveness ratio; RCT: Randomised controlled trial.

Acknowledgements

Contributors: Jing Shen, supervised by Luke Vale, led the health economic evaluation and analysis. Robert Pickard led the study, Beatriz Goulao supervised by Graeme MacLennan performed the statistical analysis, Sonya Carnell and Rebecca Forbes supported by Stephanie Currer and supervised by Jennifer Wilkinson managed the trial. John Norrie contributed to the funding application and statistical analysis plan. He also provided support to the statistical analysis team. Matt Breckons, supervised by Jing Shen, conducted a time trade off experiment reported separately. Paul Whybrow, supervised by Tim Rapley, carried out the qualitative research reported separately. Mark Forrest managed and maintained the trial database. Elaine McColl contributed to the funding application and protocol. Daniela Andrich, Anthony Mundy, James N'Dow and Stephen Payne provided clinician support to the funding application, acted as PIs at key sites. Stewart Barclay contributed a patient view to the trial, including the funding application, the protocol, and all aspects of the analysis. Jonathan Cook was involved in the design of the study and Nick Watkin co-wrote the funding application, contributed clinical insight to the trial management group. We thank the patients and health-care professionals for their participation in the study; Stewart Barclay, the patient and service user representative in the OPEN Trial Management Group; the Trial Steering committee members: Roger Kockelburg (chairperson), John Matthews, Alan McNeil, Howard Kynaston and Neil Campling; Data Monitoring Committee members: Gordon Murray (chairperson), Richard Martin and Thomas Pinkney. We also thank the following people who worked on the trial: Matthew Jackson, Research Fellow; Gladys McPherson, Data Manager; Lee Munro, Trial Manager; Rachel Stephenson, Trial Manager; Sue Tremble, Trial Manager; Robbie Brown, Trial Manager; Mark Deverill, Health Economist; Amy Collins, Project Secretary; Lavinia Miceli, Project Secretary; and Ann Payne, Project Secretary. Members of the Open Trial Group responsible for recruitment and who acted as principle investigators for their centres were: Trevor Dorkin, Freeman Hospital, Newcastle; Nick Watkin, St George's Hospital, London; Anthony Mundy, University College London Hospitals NHS Foundation Trust, London; Paul Anderson, Russells Hall Hospital, Dudley; Suzie Venn, Queen Alexandra Hospital, Portsmouth; Ian Eardley, St James's University Hospital, Leeds; Mr David Dickerson, Weston General Hospital, Weston-super-Mare; Nikesh Thiruchelvam, Addenbrooke's Hospital, Cambridge; Richard Inman and Chris Chapple, Royal Hallamshire Hospital, Sheffield; Andrew Baird, Aintree University Hospital NHS Foundation Trust, Liverpool; Andrew Sinclair, Stepping Hill Hospital, Stockport; Rajeshwar Krishnanm, Kent and Canterbury Hospital, Canterbury; Rowland Rees, University Hospital Southampton NHS Foundation Trust, Southampton; James N'dow, Aberdeen Royal Infirmary, Aberdeen; Bruce Montgomery, Frimley Park Hospital, Camberley; Michael Swinn, East Surrey Hospital, Redhill; Alastair Henderson and John Donohue, Maidstone Hospital, Maidstone; Suzie Venn, St Richard's Hospital, Chichester; Robert Mason, Torbay Hospital, Torquay; Sanjeev Madaan, Darent Valley Hospital, Kent; Mustafa Hilmy, York Hospital, York; Vivienne Kirchin, Sunderland Royal Infirmary, Sunderland; Kim Davenport, Cheltenham General Hospital, Cheltenham; John McGrath, Exeter Hospital, Exeter; Tim Porter, Yeovil District Hospital, Yeovil; Ruaraidh MacDonagh and Amerdip Birring, Musgrove Park Hospital, Taunton; Ramachandran Ravi, Basildon University Hospital; Jawad Husain, Royal Albert Edward Infirmary, Wigan; Maj Shabbir, Guy's Hospital, London; Omer Baldo, Airedale General Hospital, Keighley; Sadhanshu Chitale, Whittington Hospital, London; Mary Garthwaite, James Cook University Hospital, Middlesbrough; Shalom Srirangam, Royal Blackburn Hospital, Blackburn; Liaqat Chowoo, Bedford Hospital, Bedford; Tina Rashid, Charing Cross Hospital, London; Rob Skyrme; Jon Featherstone, Princess of Wales Hospital, Bridgend; Ammar Alhasso, Edinburgh; and Oleg Tatarov, Cardiff. We thank the following trusts for offering participant identification centre support: Basingstoke and Northamptonshire NHS Foundation Trust; Royal Liverpool and Broadgreen University Hospitals NHS Trust; Chelsea and Westminster NHS Foundation Trust; and Wirral University Teaching Hospital NHS Foundation Trust. We thank the following Trusts for offering PIC support: Basingstoke and Northamptonshire NHS Foundation Trust; Royal Liverpool and Broadgreen University Hospitals NHS Trust; Chelsea and Westminster NHS Foundation Trust; Wirral University Teaching Hospitals NHS Foundation Trust.

Authors' contributions

JS conduced the analysis, drafted the manuscript and approved the final draft; LV and NW drafted the manuscript and approved the final draft; BG, PW, SP critically reviewed the manuscript and approved the final draft.

Guidelines and regulations

The study was conducted in line with all relevant guidelines and regulations for the conduct of a randomised controlled trial. The underlying study design was approved by the funder (UK NIHR HTA programme) in the original funding application. The detailed study protocol was approved by the Trial Steering Committee (comprising an independent clinician who acted as chairperson, two further independent clinicians, an independent statistician, a lay representative and the Chief Investigator). In addition the economic evaluation reported in this paper complied with the CHEERS checklist for the reporting of an economic evaluation.

Informed consent

Study participants were consented at individual participating site following the procedure set out in the trail protocol. Trial information was provided and potential participants were given at least 48 h to consider participation in the study. Following review, at a mutually convenient time, those men who wanted to take part, who fulfilled the entry criteria and who understood the rationale and conduct of the trial, provided informed consent witnessed by research staff at site with delegated approval to do so. The right to refuse to participate without giving reasons was respected.

Competing interests

All authors declare no competing interests.

Author details

[1]Population Health Sciences Institute, Newcastle University, Newcastle upon Tyne, UK. [2]Health Services Research Unit, University of Aberdeen, Aberdeen, UK. [3]Hull York Medical School, University of Hull, Hull, UK. [4]Central Manchester Hospitals NHS Foundation Trust, Manchester, UK. [5]Department of Urology, St George's University of London, London, UK.

References

1. Buckley JC, Heyns C, Gilling P, Carney J. SIU/ICUD consultation on urethral strictures: dilation, internal urethrotomy, and stenting of male anterior urethral strictures. Urology. 2014;83(Suppl. 3):18–22. https://doi.org/10.1016/j.urology.2013.08.075.
2. Pansadoro V, Emiliozzi P. Internal urethrotomy in the management of anterior urethral strictures: long-term follow up. J Urol. 1996;156:73–5.
3. Jackson MJ, Sciberras J, Mangera A, et al. Defining a patient-reported outcome measure for urethral stricture surgery. Eur Urol. 2011;60:60–8. https://doi.org/10.1016/j.eururo.2011.03.003.
4. Meeks JJ, Erickson BA, Granieri MA, Gonzalez CM. Stricture recurrence after urethroplasty: a systematic review. J Urol. 2009;182:1266–70. https://doi.org/10.1016/j.juro.2009.06.027.
5. Chapple C, Andrich D, Atala A, et al. SIU/ICUD consultation on urethral strictures: the management of anterior urethral stricture disease using substitution urethroplasty. Urology. 2014;83(Suppl. 3):31–47. https://doi.org/10.1016/j.urology.2013.09.012.
6. Stephenson R, Carnell S, Johnson N, et al. Open urethroplasty versus endoscopic urethrotomy—clarifying the management of men with recurrent urethral stricture (the OPEN trial): study protocol for a randomized controlled trial. Trials. 2015;16:600.
7. Wessells H, Angermeier KW, Elliott S, et al. Male urethral stricture: American urological association guideline. J Urol. 2017;197:182–90.
8. Whybrow P, Pickard R, Hrisos S, Rapley T. Equipoise across the patient population: optimising recruitment to a randomised controlled trial. Trials. 2017;18(1):140.
9. Goulao B, Carnell S, Shen J, et al. Surgical treatment for recurrent bulbar urethral stricture: A randomised open label superiority trial of open urethroplasty versus endoscopic urethrotomy (The OPEN Trial). European Urology. E-pub ahead of print-4 Jul 2020
10. Briggs A, Sculpher M. An introduction to Markov modelling for economic evaluation. Pharmacoeconomics. 1998;13:397–409.
11. Consumer price index 2018, Office of National Statistics, UK.
12. Guide to methods of technology appraisal, National Institute for Health and Care Excellence, London, 2013.
13. Briggs A, Claxton K, Sculpher M. Decision modelling for health economic evaluation. Oxford: Oxford University Press; 2006.
14. Royston P. Multiple imputation of missing values. Stata J. 2004;4:227–41.
15. Brouwer W, Rutten E, Koopmanschap M. Costing in economic evaluations. In: Drummond M, McGuire A, editors. Economic evaluation in health care: merging theory and practice. Oxford: Oxford University Press; 2001.
16. Curtis LA. Unit Costs of Health and Social Care 2017. Personal Social Services Research Unit, University of Kent, Canterbury; 2017. https://doi.org/10.22024/UniKent/01.02/65559.
17. ISD Scotland. Theatre Services. 2018. www.isdscotland.org/Health-Topics/Finance/Costs/ Detailed-Tables/Theatres.asp. Accessed 9 May 2018.
18. NHS Dictionary of Medicines and Devices. 2017.
19. Devlin NJ, Shah KK, Feng Y, Mulhern B, van Hout B. Valuing health-related quality of life: an EQ-5D-5L value set for England. Health Econ. 2018;2018:7–22.
20. Matthews JN, Altman DG, Campbell MJ, Royston P. Analysis of serial measurements in medical research. BMJ. 1990;300(6719):230–5.
21. Fiebig DG. Seemingly unrelated regression. In: Baltagi BH, editor. A companion to theoretical econometrics. Malden: Blackwell Publishing Ltd.; 2003. p. 101–21.
22. MacDonald S, Haddad D, Choi A, Colaco M, Terlecki R. Anterior urethroplasty has transitioned to an outpatient procedure without serious rise in complications: data from the national surgical quality improvement program. Urology. 2017;102:225–8.
23. Poelaert F, Oosterlinck W, Spinoit A-F, Lumen N. Duration of urethral catheterization after urethroplasty: how long is enough? Italian J Urol Nephrol. 2017;69:372–6.
24. Belsante MJ, Zhao LC, Hudak SJ, Lotan Y, Morey AF. Cost-effectiveness of risk stratified follow up after urethral reconstruction: a decision analysis. J Urol. 2013;190:1292–7.
25. Pickard R, Goulao B, Carnell S, Shen J, MacLennan G, Norrie J, et al. Open urethroplasty versus endoscopic urethrotomy for recurrent urethral stricture in men: the OPEN RCT. Health Technol Assess. 2020;24(61):1–110. https://doi.org/10.3310/hta24610.
26. Shen J, Hill S, Mott D, Breckons M, Vale L, Pickard R. Conducting a time trade-off study alongside a clinical trial: a case study and recommendations. PharmacoEconomics-Open. 2019;3(1):5–20.
27. Shen J, Breckons M, Vale L, Pickard R. Using time trade-off methods to elicit short-term utilities associated with treatments for bulbar urethral stricture. PharmacoEconomics-Open. 2019;3(4):551–8.

11

Clinical significance and risk factors of urethrovesical anastomotic urinary leakage following robot-assisted radical prostatectomy

Shigenori Kakutani[1,2†], Yuta Takeshima[3†], Yuta Yamada[2*], Tetsuya Fujimura[4], Shoichi Nagamoto[5], Yutaka Enomoto[5], Yuji Hakozaki[2], Naoki Kimura[2], Taro Teshima[2], Yoshiyuki Akiyama[2], Yusuke Sato[2], Taketo Kawai[2], Daisuke Yamada[2] and Haruki Kume[2]

Abstract

Background: There has been a limited number of reports on the significance and risk factors of urethrovesical anastomotic urinary leakage (AUL) following robot-assisted radical prostatectomy (RARP). We aimed to analyze the clinical significance of AUL and evaluated its risk factors.

Methods: We conducted a multi-institutional study to review patients with prostate cancer undergoing RARP in three centers (The University of Tokyo Hospital, Mitsui Memorial Hospital, and Chiba Tokushukai Hospital). "Positive AUL" was defined as urinary extravasation at the anastomosis detected by post-operative cystogram and was further categorized into minor or major AUL. Univariate and multivariate analyses were performed to identify predictors of AUL. Postoperative continence rates and time to achieve continence were also analyzed.

Results: A total of 942 patients underwent RARP for prostate cancer in 3 centers. Of these patients, a cystogram after the RARP procedure was not performed in 26 patients leaving 916 patients for the final analysis. AUL was observed in 56 patients (6.1%); 34 patients (3.7%) with minor AUL and 22 patients (2.4%) with major AUL. Patients with major AUL exhibited a significantly longer time to achieve continence than those without major AUL. Multivariate analysis demonstrated that longer console time ($\geq$ 184 min) was significantly associated with overall AUL, and higher body mass index ($\geq$ 25 g/kg^2) was a significant predictor of both major and overall AUL.

Conclusions: The presence of major AUL was associated with the achievement of urinary continence, suggesting clinical relevance of its diagnosis by postoperative cystogram. A selective cystogram has been proposed for high-risk cases. Furthermore, identification of the risk factors of AUL will lead to optimal application.

Keywords: Anastomotic urinary leakage, Urethrovesical anastomosis, Urinary incontinence, Robot-assisted radical prostatectomy, RARP

Background

Robot-assisted radical prostatectomy (RARP) has become the most utilized treatment modality for localized prostate cancer in the past two decades [1, 2]. The improved vision of pelvic anatomy and the dexterity of robot-assisted surgical arms provided by RARP have allowed

*Correspondence: yyamada2029@gmail.com
†Shigenori Kakutani and Yuta Takeshima have contributed equally to this work
[2] Department of Urology, Graduate School of Medicine, The University of Tokyo, 7-3-1 Hongo, Bunkyo-Ku, Tokyo 113-8655, Japan

more precise and watertight urethrovesical anastomosis (UVA). A correlation between surgeon experience and quality of anastomosis has been reported, suggesting its utility as a benchmark of surgical skill for RARP [3]. This, in turn, has naturally led many to suggest that the improved quality of anastomosis resulted in reducing the incidence of urethrovesical anastomotic urinary leakage (AUL) following RARP as an advantage over conventional open retropubic radical prostatectomy (RRP) [4, 5]. However, there is presently little evidence to corroborate this, perhaps owing to a low number of events as in one study detecting no difference in AUL incidence between RRP and RARP (2.9% vs. 3.2%, *P* value = 0.49) [6]. In fact, we found that there is a lack of consensus on the importance of AUL in general, concerning its effect on the postoperative outcome, and its risk factors. A major factor contributing to this is that postoperative cystograms to detect AUL are not routinely taken at many centers around the world, leading to a significant variation in the definition of AUL, with some groups using findings of postoperative cystogram and others using confirmation of urine in the drain [7]. In 2008, Williams et al. proposed a systematic definition of AUL detected by cystogram and clarified its classification depending on severity and necessity of intervention, for objective quantification of AUL in future studies [8]. In this study, we conducted a routine postoperative cystogram following RARP and utilized this classification of cystographic findings to examine AUL objectively. Recognizing the factors associated with AUL is clinically important, since it may avert routine cystogram and provide beneficial information to surgeons for determination on patient selection regarding post-operative cystogram. To our knowledge, there is only one study that had presented statistically significant factors of AUL by performing a multivariate analysis in patients undergoing RARP [9]. Moreover, this is the first multi-institutional study to investigate the effect of AUL after RARP and its risk factors.

Methods

Patient population

The study was approved by the ethical committee of The University of Tokyo Hospital (ID: 2020039NI), the ethical committee of Mitsui Memorial hospital (ID: 2020C30), and the committee of Chiba Tokushukai Hospital (ID: 184). All clinical data were prospectively collected in a customized database and retrospectively analyzed. RARP was performed by multiple surgeons using da Vinci®Si or Xi Surgical Systems (Intuitive Surgical, Sunnydale, CA, USA) by a transperitoneal approach in 671 patients from Nov 2011 to May 2019 at The University of Tokyo Hospital, in 164 patients on the Si System from May 2017 to May 2019 at Chiba Tokushukai Hospital, and in 107 patients on the Xi System from Nov 2017 to May 2019 at Mitsui Memorial Hospital. Patients with non-metastatic prostate cancer with or without neoadjuvant hormonal therapy were treated with RARP. Contraindication of RARP included a history of rectal surgery or the presence of severe comorbidities.

Surgical technique

RARP was performed and carried out in the same fashion in all 3 centers as previously described; UVA was completed after Rocco's posterior rhabdosphincter reconstruction by a continuous running closure using two 3/0 absorbable monofilaments tied end-to-end [10, 11]. The integrity of UVA was routinely checked by an intraoperative flush test using 50–150 mL saline through the catheter. An additional suture was performed when needed to attain watertight anastomosis. A Foley catheter was placed into the bladder and the balloon was filled with 10 mL of water.

Post-surgical examination

At 6–8 days after RARP, a cystogram of anteroposterior and oblique view was taken before removal of the urethral catheter by instilling 40–120 mL of saline-diluted iodinated contrast medium into the bladder. Positive AUL was defined as the 'presence of urinary extravasation determined by cystogram.' In the absence of AUL, we removed the urethral catheter immediately or the next morning. Positive AUL was reviewed and subclassified into two categories; minor AUL within 6 cm of the UVA, in accordance with 'grade 1 urethrovesical leak,' and major AUL beyond 6 cm from the UVA, in accordance with 'grades 2 and 3 urethrovesical leaks' [8]. In patients with minor AUL, the catheter was removed within a day after the cystogram. In patients with major AUL, the catheter was placed in situ until leakage was either undetectable on a repeat cystogram or recovered to minor AUL. Time to recovery of the urinary continence was calculated from the removal of the urethral catheter.

Statistical evaluation

The collected clinical data were analyzed by using JMP Pro 15.1 software (SAS Institute, Cary, NC, USA). Valuables such as age, body mass index (BMI), initial PSA value, prostate volume, console time, blood loss volume, surgeon experience ($\geq$20, 40, or 100 cases), cavernous nerve preservation status, and pathological findings (pGS$\geq$8, pT3$\geq$, positive surgical margin) were collected. Univariate and multivariate analyses using logistic regression analysis were performed to identify factors predicting AUL. Parameters that were significantly associated with AUL in the univariate analysis and known factors based on the previous reports were included in the multivariate analyses [12]. Kaplan–Meier curves were drawn, and the Wilcoxon test was used to analyze the time to recovery of continence (≤ one pad per day) after successful removal of the catheter. Cut-off values were basically determined by the median values of each parameter, except for BMI and prostate weight which were rounded to a clinically useful number. All tests were two-sided and a P value of < 0.05 was regarded as statistically significant.

Results

Patient characteristics and perioperative status are shown in Table 1. A total of 942 patients underwent RARP procedure for prostate cancer in 3 centers (The University of Tokyo Hospital, Chiba Tokushukai Hospital, and Mitsui Memorial Hospital). The records of cystogram after RARP procedure was not available in 26 patients. A total of 916 patients were investigated for the final analysis. The number of patients included in this study was 645 patients for The University of Tokyo Hospital, 164 for Chiba Tokushukai Hospital, and 107 for Mitsui Memorial Hospital. 860 patients (93.9%) and 56 patients (6.1%) had negative and positive AUL, respectively. Of the patients with positive AUL, 34 (60.7%) were classified as minor AUL and 22 (39.3%) as major AUL. The median duration of catheterization was 7 days (IQR 6–8).

Time to recovery of continence (≤ 1 pad/day) was significantly longer in patients with major AUL than those without major AUL (Fig. 1).

In the univariate analysis, BMI (≥ 25 kg/m^2) and console time (≥ 184 min) were significantly associated with overall AUL (Table 2; $P = 0.03$ and $P = 0.04$, respectively). In the multivariate analysis, console time remained as the significant predictor of overall AUL. A similar analysis was conducted for major AUL (Table 3). In the univariate analysis, BMI (≥ 25 kg/m^2) and console time (≥ 184 min.) were associated with major AUL (Table 3; $P < 0.01$ and $P = 0.04$, respectively). There was a tendency of observing more major and overall AUL in patients with prostate weight > 40 g (Tables 2, 3; $P = 0.08$, $P = 0.006$, respectively). In the multivariate analysis, BMI remained a significant predictor of major AUL. There was no significant association between surgeon experience and overall/major AUL.

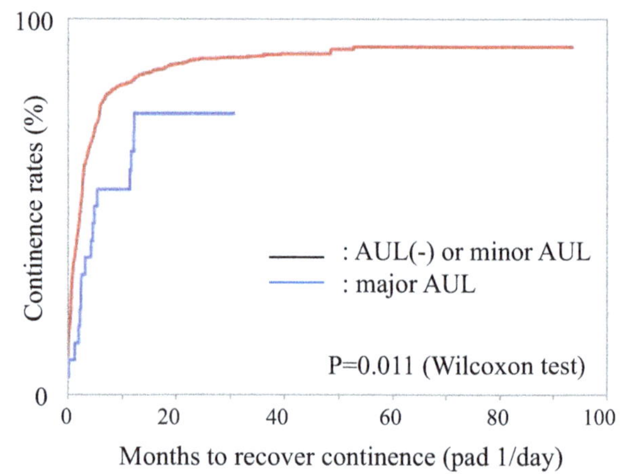

Fig. 1 Months to recover continence in patients with or without major anastomotic urinary leakage. Kaplan–Meier method analysis revealed that there was a significant delay in days to recover continence less than one pad per day in patients with major AUL

Table 1 Patients demographics

	Leakage (+)			Leakage (−)	Total
	Minor	Major	Minor + major		
Anastomotic urinary leakage after RARP					
Number of patients (%)	34 (3.7)	22 (2.4)	56 (6.1)	860 (93.9)	916
Age, (years)	68.5 (64–72)	65 (58–70)	68 (63–72)	68 (64–73)	68 (64–73)
BMI (kg/m^2)	24.1 (22.2–26.5)	25.6 (24.4–28.1)	24.9 (22.9–26.7)	23.8 (21.9–25.6)	23.9 (22–25.6)
PSA (ng/mL)	8.8 (6.2–12.6)	8.3 (5.9–15.3)	8.5 (6.2–12.9)	7.6 (5.5–11.0)	7.6 (5.6–11.1)
Operation duration (min)	279 (203–341)	295 (232–379)	289 (215–349)	240 (195–283)	241 (196–287)
Console duration (min)	212.5 (155–266)	233 (168–322)	221.5 (164–271)	183 (143–221)	184 (145–226)
Prostate weight (g)	43.1 (34–70)	50.5 (40–74)	46.5 (38–72)	40.5 (32–52)	41 (32–53)
Blood loss volume (mL)	300 (100–725)	352 (174–666)	326 (150–700)	221 (100–442)	230 (100–450)
pGS ≥ 8 (%)	29.4	22.7	26.8	28.2	29.8
pT stage ≥ 3 (%)	23.5	40.9	30.4	30.6	30.6
PSM (%)	17.6	18.2	17.9	21.3	21.7

Median values are shown (interquartile range)

RARP, robot-assisted radical prostatectomy; BMI, body mass index; PSA, prostate specific antigen; pGS, pathological Gleason score; PSM, positive surgical margin

Table 2 Univariate and multivariate analysis to predict overall anastomotic urinary leakage (AUL)

Variable	Cutoff	Univariate		Multivariate	
		Odds ratio (95%CI)	*P* value	Odds ratio (95%CI)	*P* value
Age, years	≥ 68 versus < 68	0.89 (0.52–1.54)	0.78		
BMI, kg/m^2	≥ 25 versus < 25	2.02 (1.17–3.48)	0.01*	1.80 (1.03–3.12)	0.03*
iPSA, ng/mL	≥ 7.6 versus < 7.6	1.43 (0.82–2.48)	0.22		
Diabetes	With versus without	0.19 (0.04–0.80)	0.01*		
COPD	With versus without	0.45 (0.10–1.91)	0.42		
IHD	With versus without	1.55 (0.53–4.51)	0.34		
Abdominal surgery	With versus without	1.04 (0.56–1.92)	0.87		
Surgeon volume, cases	≥ 20 versus < 20	0.95 (0.55–1.66)	0.88		
	≥ 40 versus < 40	0.84 (0.48–1.49)	0.67		
	≥ 100 versus < 100	0.66 (0.27–1.57)	0.44		
Nerve sparing	With versus without	0.92 (0.52–1.64)	0.88		
Duration of console, min	≥ 184 versus < 184	2.00 (1.13–3.54)	0.01*	1.84 (1.03–3.28)	0.03*
Prostate weight, g	≥ 40 versus < 40	1.80 (0.99–3.27)	0.05	1.69 (0.93–3.09)	0.08
Blood, mL	≥ 230 versus < 230	1.26 (0.73–2.17)	0.41		
pGS ≥ 8	≥ versus <	0.86 (0.46–1.58)	0.76		
pT3	≥ versus <	0.98 (0.54–1.77)	1.00		
PSM	With versus without	0.80 (0.39–1.62)	0.61		

BMI, body mass index; COPD, chronic obstructive pulmonary disease; IHD, ischemic heart disease; PSA, prostate specific antigen; pGS, pathological Gleason score; PSM, positive surgical margin

Statistical significance is shown as * for $P < 0.05$

Table 3 Univariate and multivariate analysis to predict major anastomotic urinary leakage (AUL)

Variable	Cutoff	Univariate		Multivariate	
		Odds ratio (95%CI)	*P* value	Odds ratio (95%CI)	*P* value
Age, years	≥ 68 versus < 68	0.64 (0.27–1.50)	0.38		
BMI, kg/m^2	≥ 25 versus < 25	4.30 (1.73–10.66)	< 0.01**	3.62 (1.44–9.09)	0.01*
iPSA, ng/mL	≥ 7.6 versus < 7.6	1.42 (0.60–3.36)	0.51		
Diabetes	With versus without	0.26 (0.03–1.95)	0.23		
COPD	With versus without	0	0.39		
IHD	With versus without	1.99 (0.45–8.83)	0.29		
Abdominal surgery	With versus without	0.44 (0.12–1.51)	0.22		
Surgeon volume, cases	≥ 20 versus < 20	0.96 (0.40–2.28)	1.00		
	≥ 40 versus < 40	0.44 (0.16–1.22)	0.12		
	≥ 100 versus < 100	0.88 (0.25–3.03)	1.00		
Nerve sparing	With versus without	1.03 (0.43–2.50)	1.00		
Duration of console, min	≥ 184 versus < 184	2.69 (1.04–6.94)	0.04*	2.23 (0.85–5.85)	0.09
Prostate weight, g	≥ 40 versus < 40	3.20 (1.07–9.56)	0.02*	2.47 (0.95–6.43)	0.06
Blood, mL	≥ 230 versus < 230	1.46 (0.61–3.46)	0.39		
pGS ≥ 8	≥ versus <	0.69 (0.25–1.90)	0.63		
pT3	≥ versus <	1.58 (0.67–3.76)	0.34		
PSM	With versus without	0.82 (0.27–2.47)	1.00		

BMI, body mass index; COPD, chronic obstructive pulmonary disease; IHD, ischemic heart disease; PSA, prostate specific antigen; pGS, pathological Gleason score; PSM, positive surgical margin

Statistical significance is shown as * for $P < 0.05$ and ** for $P < 0.01$

Discussion

AUL has been reported to occur in 0.3–15.4% of patients after RARP [12]. In our study, the incidence of AUL detected by cytogram was 6.1%, which was compatible with other reports. However, the incidence of AUL varies greatly with parameters such as postoperative date, as demonstrated in a study that showed decreasing rates of AUL incidence with a lapse of time after RRP [13]. Although the timing of postoperative cystograms from past studies range from 3–18 days and requires standardization [14–16], we set the timing of cystogram at POD 6–8, which appears to be consistent with many of the previous reports [3, 5, 8, 9, 17].

We examined post-operative continence rates and found that time to recovery of continence was negatively affected by the presence of major AUL on cystogram. This result was in line with past reports that also found an association between AUL and post-operative continence [5, 18]. This leads us to believe that major AUL is of clinical importance and that examination of factors contributing to its incidence would be beneficial in predicting postoperative outcomes.

The predictive factors of AUL have been examined in multiple previous studies. Some factors presented were obesity/BMI, ischemic heart disease, urinary tract infection, excessive blood loss, surgeon experience, eversion of the bladder mucosa, prostate size, previous prostatic surgery, or details regarding surgical technique (bladder neck eversion, posterior reconstruction, etc.) [4, 9, 19–22]. In the univariate analysis of the present study, longer console time, larger prostate weight, and higher BMI was associated with AUL. Furthermore, in the multivariate analysis, longer console time and higher BMI were significant factors of overall AUL and higher BMI was a significant factor of major AUL.

Obesity may create difficulties in accessing the vesicourethral anastomosis site or to decrease visibility. Some reports state that this only applies to RRP, while others assert that obesity also affects outcomes of RARP negatively [21, 23]. Excessive bleeding may cause natural ischemia in the bladder or urethral tissue. They also lead to impairment of visibility, making precise suture placement difficult. Unavoidable suture for maintaining hemostasis may cause further ischemia. Past studies have also reported that the postoperative bleeding was a predictor of AUL and that this was likely the result of para-anastomotic hematoma delaying the healing of UVA [17, 24]. Tillier et al. asserted that men with larger prostate size and preoperative voiding problems were predictive of major leakage in RARP due to bladder neck reconstruction and the alignment of the bladder and urethra [9]. It is obvious that the larger the prostate, the longer the distance between the bladder neck and urethra after excision of the prostate, resulting in a more challenging UVA. Console time was not mentioned in any previous study, yet it remained a predictive factor in multivariate analysis for overall AUL in our study. We surmised that console time may have been a manifestation of the level of difficulty in conducting the surgery, and in some cases the difficulty of UVA.

The above observations seem to show that difficulty in conducting the anastomosis may be a predictor of AUL. Although based on one surgeon's subjective assessment, Gnanapragasam et al. reported that a 'difficult anastomosis' was indeed an independent predictor of AUL [20]. There is also evidence that the quality of anastomosis was associated with surgeon experience [3]. We hypothesized that surgeon experience may be related to AUL and included surgeon experience as a factor, but we did not identify any association with the surgeon volume and AUL in our cohort. This may partly be due to the unique mentoring system we implemented, in which RARP was divided into sections, each with a designated time limit and blood loss criteria, and an experienced surgeon replaced an inexperienced surgeon for the remainder of the section upon exceeding the designated time or blood loss [10, 25].

A postoperative cystogram is considered a valuable diagnostic tool to detect urinary extravasation after RARP. However, it is not performed routinely at many centers around the world. Guru et al. reported that removal of catheter on postoperative days 8–10 without performing cystogram may not lead to complications in patients with RARP [26]. Although this prospective study was low-powered and consisted of only eighty patients recruited at a single institution, the fact remains that the fairly small percentage of men who develop complications relating to AUL may not be enough to justify the cost and manpower incurred by a routine cytogram for all patients with RARP. One prospective study consisting of 230 patients at a single institution indicated that selective cystogram is preferable in cases with bladder neck resection or a history of transurethral resection of the prostate [27]. Tillier et al. similarly suggested that selective cystogram in cases with larger prostate and with preoperative voiding problems may prevent early urinary retention and alleviate voiding complaints [9]. Based on these reports, a selective cystogram may be more beneficial than a routine cystogram. Prospective randomized studies under further standardization of cystogram protocols are required to better support this idea.

There are several limitations to discuss. First, this study was not a prospective randomized study, and further investigation is needed to confirm our assertion. Second, although our study analyzed the findings of a postoperative cystogram according to the criteria as defined by

Williams et al., the degree of AUL would be influenced by the amount and speed of contrast instilled into the bladder, and hence cannot be said to completely adhere to the original report [8]. Third, we may underestimate the relationship between the surgical skill and the incidence of AUL since we only examined the total console time and not the actual time to complete UVA.

Conclusion

In conclusion, we objectively examined the results of a routine cystogram after RARP and found that major AUL was associated with a longer time to recovery of continence. BMI was identified as the predictor of overall and major AUL and may be taken into consideration when performing selective cystograms after RARP.

Abbreviations

AUL: Anastomotic urinary leakage; BMI: Body mass index; GS: Gleason score; UVA: Urethrovesical anastomosis; LRP: Laparoscopic radical prostatectomy; PSA: Prostate specific antigen; PSM: Positive surgical margin; RARP: Robot-assisted radical prostatectomy; RRP: Retropubic radical prostatectomy.

Acknowledgements

The authors would like to thank K. Kawabe (former Professor of the Department of Urology, The University of Tokyo) and T. Kitamura (Honorary Professor of the Department of Urology, The University of Tokyo), for referring many of the patients included in the study.

Authors' contributions

SK and YT contributed equally to this work. YY contributed to the study conception and designed the study. SK, YT, and YY wrote the manuscript. YH, TT, NK, YS, YA, TK, DY, TF, and YY collected the data at the University of Tokyo Hospital. SK, SN, YE constructed the database in the Mitsui Memorial Hospital. YY and SK constructed the database in Chiba Tokushukai Hospital. YY and SK contributed to integrating the database and analyzing the data. HK assisted in all process of this study. All authors read and approved the final manuscript.

Competing interests

The authors declare that they have no competing interests.

Author details

[1]Department of Urology, Chiba Tokushukai Hospital, Chiba, Japan. [2]Department of Urology, Graduate School of Medicine, The University of Tokyo, 7-3-1 Hongo, Bunkyo-Ku, Tokyo 113-8655, Japan. [3]Division of Innovative Cancer Therapy, Advanced Research Center, The Institute of Medical Science, The University of Tokyo, Minato-Ku, Tokyo, Japan. [4]Department of Urology, Jichi Medical University, Tochigi, Japan. [5]Department of Urology, Mitsui Memorial Hospital, Tokyo, Japan.

References

1. Du Y, Long Q, Guan B, Mu L, Tian J, Jiang Y, Bai X, Wu D. Robot-assisted radical prostatectomy is more beneficial for prostate cancer patients: a system review and meta-analysis. Med Sci Monit. 2018;24:272–87. https://doi.org/10.12659/msm.907092.
2. Basiri A, de la Rosette JJ, Tabatabaei S, Woo HH, Laguna MP, Shemshaki H. Comparison of retropubic, laparoscopic and robotic radical prostatectomy: who is the winner? World J Urol. 2018;36:609–21. https://doi.org/10.1007/s00345-018-2174-1.
3. Moro FD, Beltrami P, Zattoni F. Can anastomotic urinary leakage in robotic prostatectomy be considered as a marker of surgical skill? Cent Eur J Urol. 2017;71:21–5. https://doi.org/10.5173/ceju.2018.1587.
4. Webb DR, Sethi K, Gee K. An analysis of the causes of bladder neck contracture after open and robot-assisted laparoscopic radical prostatectomy. BJU Int. 2009;103:957–63. https://doi.org/10.1111/j.1464-410X.2008.08278.x
5. Patil N, Krane L, Javed K, Williams T, Bhandari M, Menon M. Evaluating and grading cystographic leakage: correlation with clinical outcomes in patients undergoing robotic prostatectomy. BJU Int. 2009;103:1108–10. https://doi.org/10.1111/j.1464-410X.2008.08168.x.
6. Jacobsen A, Berg KD, Iversen P, Brasso K, Røder MA. Anastomotic complications after robot-assisted laparoscopic and open radical prostatectomy. Scand J Urol. 2016;50:274–9. https://doi.org/10.3109/21681805.2016.1145735.
7. Rebuck DA, Haywood S, McDermott K, Perry KT, Nadler RB. What is the long-term relevance of clinically detected postoperative anastomotic urine leakage after robotic-assisted laparoscopic prostatectomy? BJU Int. 2011;108:733–8. https://doi.org/10.1111/j.1464-410X.2010.09939.x.
8. Williams TR, Longoria OJ, Asselmeier S, Menon M. Incidence and imaging appearance of urethrovesical anastomotic urinary leaks following da Vinci robotic prostatectomy. Abdom Imaging. 2008;33:367–70. https://doi.org/10.1007/s00261-007-9247-8.
9. Tillier C, Van Muilekom HAM, Bloos-van der Hulst J, Grivas N, Van der Poel HG. Vesico-urethral anastomosis (VUA) evaluation of short- and long-term outcome after robot-assisted laparoscopic radical prostatectomy (RARP): selective cystogram to improve outcome. J Robot Surg. 2017;11:441–6.
10. Fujimura T, Menon M, Fukuhara H, Kume H, Suzuki M, Yamada Y, Niimi A, Nakagawa T, Igawa Y, Homma Y. Validation of an educational program balancing surgeon training and surgical quality control during robot-assisted radical prostatectomy. Int J Urol. 2016;23:160–6. https://doi.org/10.1111/iju.12993.
11. Kakutani S, Asamoto M, Araki F, Chen YN, Shinokawa M, Okagami Y, Ohata T, Taguchi S, Yamada Y, Takeshima Y, Kume H, Yamada Y, Aihara M, Ito N, Fukuhara H. Prospective evaluation of visual function in patients with ocular diseases after robot-assisted laparoscopic prostatectomy. Int J Urol. 2020;27:307–12. https://doi.org/10.1111/iju.14183.
12. Tyritzis SI, Katafigiotis I, Constantinides CA. All you need to know about urethrovesical anastomotic urinary leakage following radical prostatectomy. J Urol. 2012;188:369–76. https://doi.org/10.1016/j.juro.2012.03.126.
13. Dalton DP, Schaeffer AJ, Garnett JE, Grayhack JT. Radiographic assessment of the vesicourethral anastomosis directing early decatheterization following nerve-sparing radical retropubic prostatectomy. J Urol. 1989;141:79–81. https://doi.org/10.1016/s0022-5347(17)40595-7.
14. Schatzl G, Madersbacher S, Hofbauer J, Pycha A, Reiter WJ, Svolba G, Marberger M. The impact of urinary extravasation after radical retropubic prostatectomy on urinary incontinence and anastomotic strictures. Eur Urol. 1999;36:187–90. https://doi.org/10.1159/000067995.
15. Menon M, Hemal AK, Tewari A, Shrivastava A, Bhandari A. The technique of apical dissection of the prostate and urethrovesical anastomosis in robotic radical prostatectomy. BJU Int. 2004;93:715–9. https://doi.org/10.1111/j.1464-410X.2003.04748.x.
16. Gratzke C, Dovey Z, Novara G, Geurts N, De Groote R, Schatteman P, de Naeyer G, Gandaglia G, Mottrie A. Early catheter removal after robot-assisted radical prostatectomy: surgical technique and outcomes for the aalst technique (ECaRemA Study). Eur Urol. 2016;69:917–23. https://doi.org/10.1016/j.eururo.2015.09.052.
17. Fenig DM, Slova D, Lepor H. Postoperative blood loss predicts the development of urinary extravasation on cystogram following radical retropubic prostatectomy. J Urol. 2006;175:146–50. https://doi.org/10.1016/S0022-5347(05)00051-0.
18. Ha YS, Bak DJ, Chung JW, Lee JN, Kwon SY, Choi SH, Kwon TG. Kim THPost-operative cystographic findings as an independent predictor of urinary incontinence three months after radical prostatectomy. Minerva Urol Nephrol. 2017;69:278–84.
19. Ramsden AR, Chodak GW. Can leakage at the vesico-urethral anastomosis be predicted after radical retropubic prostatectomy? BJU Int. 2004;93:503–6. https://doi.org/10.1111/j.1464-410x.2003.04668.x.
20. Gnanapragasam VJ, Baker P, Naisby GP, Chadwick D. Identification and validation of risk factors for vesicourethral leaks following radical retropubic prostatectomy. Int J Urol. 2005;12:948–52. https://doi.org/10.1111/j.1442-2042.2005.01166.x.

21. Sandhu JS, Gotto GT, Herran LA, Scardino PT, Eastham JA, Rabbani F. Age, obesity, medical comorbidities and surgical technique are predictive of symptomatic anastomotic strictures after contemporary radical prostatectomy. J Urol. 2011;185:2148–52. https://doi.org/10.1016/j.juro.2011.02.003.
22. Coelho RF, Chauhan S, Orvieto MA, Sivaraman A, Palmer KJ, Coughlin G, Patel VR. Influence of modified posterior reconstruction of the rhabdosphincter on early recovery of continence and anastomotic leakage rates after robot-assisted radical prostatectomy. Eur Urol. 2011;59:72–80. https://doi.org/10.1016/j.eururo.2010.08.025.
23. Herman MP, Raman JD, Dong S, Samadi D, Scherr DS. Increasing body mass index negatively impacts outcomes following robotic radical prostatectomy. JSLS. 2007;11(4):438–42.
24. O'Malley RL, Telegrafi S, Laze J, Lepor H. Para-anastomotic haematoma volume predicts the presence of anastomotic extravasation after radical retropubic prostatectomy. BJU Int. 2010;105:34–6. https://doi.org/10.1111/j.1464-410X.2009.08709.x.
25. Yamada Y, Teshima T, Fujimura T, Sato Y, Nakamura M, Niimi A, Kimura N, Kakutani S, Kawai T, Yamada D, Suzuki M, Kume H. Comparison of perioperative outcomes in elderly (age ≧ 75 years) versus younger men undergoing robot-assisted radical prostatectomy. PLoS ONE. 2020;15:e0234113. https://doi.org/10.1371/journal.pone.0234113.
26. Guru KA, Seereiter PJ, Sfakianos JP, Hutson AD, Mohler JL. Is a cystogram necessary after robot-assisted radical prostatectomy? Urol Oncol. 2007;25:465–7. https://doi.org/10.1016/j.urolonc.2007.01.014.
27. Yadav R, Bansal S, Gupta NP. Selective indication for check cystogram before catheter removal following robot assisted radical prostatectomy. Indian J Urol. 2016;32:120–3. https://doi.org/10.4103/0970-1591.174776.

12

Crossing vessels with suspension versus transposition in laparoscopic pyeloplasty of patients with ureteropelvic junction obstruction

Jun Liu[1,2†], Jingjun Zhang[3†], Weinan Chen[1,2], Liulin Xiong[1,2], Xiaobo Huang[1,2] and Xiongjun Ye[1,2*]

Abstract

Purpose: To compare the effects of two different methods of laparoscopic pyeloplasty for the treatment of crossing vessels.

Methods: From January 2016 to August 2019, 33 patients with ureteropelvic junction obstruction (UPJO) underwent laparoscopic pyeloplasty at our center, including 21 men and 12 women, ranging from 14 to 66 years of age. There were 20 and 13 cases on the left and right sides, respectively. Patients underwent laparoscopic pyeloplasty (Anderson-Hynes operation). During the operation, either a Hem-o-lok clip suspension or transposition was used to treat the crossing vessels. The double-J stent was removed 8 weeks after the operation. The clinical data of patients were collected and follow-ups were regularly performed after the operation.

Results: All the crossing vessels were successfully preserved, and none of them were severed during the operation. The average operation time was 210.6 ± 58.9 min in this group and the average time to manage the crossing vessel was 8.0 ± 3.5 min, 5.9 ± 1.4 min in the suspension group, and 11.7 ± 3.0 min in the transposition group. The dilation of the affected side was 4.8 ± 1.5 cm before operation and 1.2 ± 1.3 cm 3 months after operation. The difference was statistically significant ($P < 0.05$). Follow-up to February 2020 showed no significant changes in the kidney size in all patients and hydronephrosis was relieved.

Conclusion: For UPJO patients with crossing vessel compression, the method of Hem-o-lok suspension or vascular transposition can be used to relieve crossing vascular compression and improve the success of pyeloplasty.

Keywords: Laparoscopic pyeloplasty, Crossing vessel, Ureteropelvic junction obstruction, Hydronephrosis

Introduction

Ureteropelvic junction obstruction (UPJO) is a common cause of hydronephrosis and renal dysfunction. There are several causes of UPJO, such as intraureteral stenosis, ureteral dynamic dysfunction, and ectopic vascular compression. Among them, UPJO caused by crossing vessel compression accounts for 10–28.1% of adult primary UPJO [1, 2]. Ectopic renal artery, also known as crossing vessels, refers to an extra artery of the kidney, usually entering the kidney without the renal hilum, and often is accompanied by veins. Crossing vessels usually enter the lower pole of the kidney through the ventral side of the ureteropelvic junction, where mechanical compression or traction occurs, resulting in obstruction and deformation

*Correspondence: yexiongjun@bjmu.edu.cn
†Jun Liu and Jingjun Zhang contributed equally to this work
[1] Urology and Lithotripsy Center, Peking University People's Hospital, Peking University, 133 Fuchengmen Inner Street, Xicheng District, Beijing 100034, People's Republic of China

of the local ureter, poor drainage of urine, and hydronephrosis [3]. The treatment of crossing vessels has always been controversial in clinical practice [4, 5] as these vessels can provide a part of the blood supply to the kidney; complete disconnection of the crossing vessels will cause loss of part of the renal function. Therefore, preserving the crossing vessels would mean protecting the integrity of the renal function. Several methods can be used to treat UPJO, including open pyeloplasty (OP), endoscopic pyelotomy (EP), laparoscopy (LP) and robot assisted pyeloplasty (RP). The success rate of RP is the highest, the complication of LP is lower than that of OP, the success rate of EP is relatively low, but the operation time is the shortest of all surgical methods [6]. In clinical work, the management of crossing vessels has always been a difficult challenge in laparoscopic pyeloplasty (LP).

From January 2016 to August 2019, 33 cases of UPJO with crossing vessel compression operated at Peking University People's Hospital were retrospectively analyzed to explore the treatment of crossing vessels in the LP.

Data and methods

General clinical data

From January 2016 to August 2019, 147 LP cases were completed in our hospital, including 33 cases (21 men; 12 women) of UPJO with ectopic renal vascular compression. All cases were selected continuously at the same time period. There were no patients with second pyeloplasty. The robot platform was not available and the OP was not performed. The average age was 32 years, ranging from to 14–66 years of age. There were 20 and 13 cases on the left and right sides, respectively. None of the patients had a history of ureter or kidney operation. The main symptoms were hypochondriac pain, increased RBC count in urine, and urinary tract infection. All patients were diagnosed with UPJO by abdominal ultrasound, CT tomography urography (CTU) and/or diuretic renal dynamic imaging before surgery. The indication of operation was based on clinical symptoms (such as recurrent hypochondriac pain and urinary tract infection), imaging examination results, and obvious obstruction of diuretic renal dynamic imaging [7]. The degree of hydronephrosis was classified based on the ultrasonographic grading of hydrophysis [8]. According to the legislation of the ethics committee, we obtained the moral declaration from the ethics committee and all patients signed the preoperative informed consent.

Operation method

General anesthesia was administered in all patients in the 70° lateral decubitus position. The skin was incised approximately at 2 cm from the umbilicus of the affected side, and pneumo-peritoneum was established by puncture using the Veress needle. Additionally, trocar (10 mm in the left hand and 12 mm in the right hand) was placed under the costal margin of the middle clavicle and the anterior superior iliac spine. When the affected side was on the right, a 5 mm trocar was placed under the xiphoid process to lift the liver.

The process began with the opening of the lateral peritoneum on the lateral side of the colon and the colon was pushed to the inner and lower parts. When lifting the dilated anterior wall of the renal pelvis, the energetic knife was carefully used to dissect and fully expose the anterior and posterior walls of the renal pelvis and the upper ureter. The crossing vessels on the ventral side of the dilated renal pelvis must be found and carefully dissociated to prevent damage to the crossing vessels.

Generally, according to the location and direction of the crossing vessels, the following two surgical methods are used. (1) Suspension with Hem-o-lok clips (Weck Surgical Instruments, Research Triangle Park, NC, USA) (21 cases in suspension group, Fig. 1): When the crossing vessel is close to the hilum (above the level of the

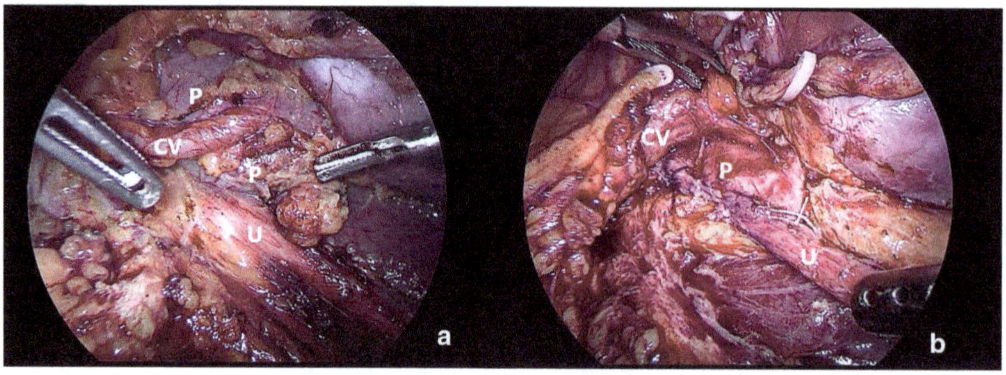

Fig. 1 Crossing vessel suspension, **a** before LP, **b** after LP

midline of the lower pole of the kidney) and in a tortuous shape, 2–3 Hem-o-lok clips can be used to clamp the fibrous connective tissue on the surface of the crossing vessel and then fix it on the perirenal fat sac above the hilum. Subsequently, the ureteropelvic junction (UPJ) could be exposed clear manner. Attention must be paid not to damage the crossing vessel during clamping. (2) Transposition of the crossing vessel (12 cases in transposition group, Fig. 2): When the crossing vessel is at the level of the lower pole of the kidney (below the level of the middle line of the lower pole of the kidney), transposition of the crossing vessel is feasible due to the lower position and the greater tension of the crossing vessel. First, the inferior pole of the kidney is exposed with an energetic knife, the lower pole of the kidney is picked up, and the crossing vessels are carefully dissociated, in order to be completely separated from the UPJ. After the ureteropelvic junction was dismembered, the crossing vessel was transferred to the dorsal side of the anastomosis and fixed on the fascia of the psoas major muscle above the anastomosis with suture to prevent the compression from forming again.

Subsequently, the, conventional dismembered laparoscopic pyeloplasty was performed, the pelvic and ureteral posterior walls were anastomosed first with 4–0 Vicryl (Johnson & Johnson Inc, New Brunswick, NJ), a 6F double-J stent was inserted, and the ureter was sutured intermittently. In the anterior wall, the redundant pelvis was closed with continuous suture by 4–0 Vicryl, a drainage tube was placed, the lateral peritoneum was closed, and the operation was completed.

Data collection and follow-up

The patient's medical records, including the operation time, time required to manage the vessels during the operation, estimated blood loss during the operation, drainage tube removal time after the operation, hospital stay time, and postoperative complications were collected. Due to the economic factors and China's medical insurance policy, not all patients can afford the cost of diuretic renal dynamic imaging. Therefore, the success criteria of these patients are complete clinical relief of abdominal pain and improvement of hydronephrosis by B-ultrasound. If the patient's pain is not relieved or B ultrasound still indicates that hydronephrosis is not improved, it means that the surgery failed. During surgery, all patients underwent insertion of double J stent, which was removed approximately 8 weeks after the surgery. The improvement of the hydronephrosis before and 3 months after the operation was evaluated by abdominal B-ultrasound. All patients were followed up for more than 6 months, and changes in renal size were recorded before and 6 months after the operation.

Statistical analysis

SPSS (version 13.0) software (SPSS, Inc., Chicago, IL) was used for data analysis. Student' s t-test was used to compare the numerical variables; Fisher's exact test was used to compare the classified variables. P values < 0.05 were considered statistically significant.

Results

All of the patients underwent successful preservation of the crossing vessels and none of them were severed during the operation. There were 5 cases of mild hydronephrosis, 15 cases of moderate hydronephrosis, and 13 cases of severe hydronephrosis (Table 1). In this group, 24 patients were confirmed to have crossing vessel compression by preoperative imaging diagnosis, and an additional 9 patients were found to have crossing vessels during the operation. Among them, 29 cases exhibited heterotopic arteries and 4 cases were accompanied by heterotopic arteries and veins. The average operation time was 210.6 ± 58.9 min in the whole

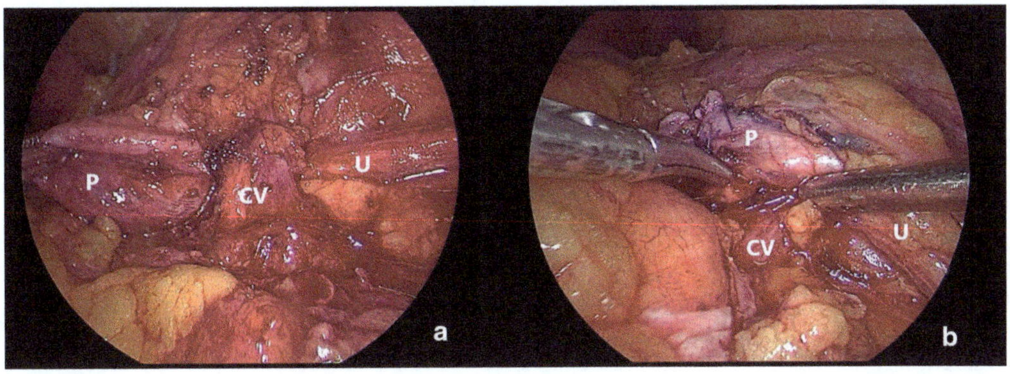

Fig. 2 Crossing vessel transposition, **a** before LP, **b** after LP

Table 1 Characteristics of patients and degree of hydronephrosis

Items	Suspension team (n = 21)	Transposition team (n = 12)	Total (n = 33)	*P* value
Age (years), $\bar{x} \pm s$	33.5 ± 13.4	31.9 ± 11.1	32.9 ± 12.2	0.513
Male/Female, n	14/7	7/5	21/12	0.222
Side (left/right), n	12/9	8/4	20/13	0.281
Degree of hydronephrosis				
Mild, n (%)	3 (14.3)	2 (16.7)	5 (15.2)	0.29
Moderate, n (%)	9 (42.9)	6 (50.0)	15 (45.5)	
Severe, n (%)	9 (42.9)	4 (33.3)	13 (39.4)	

group, 203.8 ± 61.8 min in the suspension group, and 222.5 ± 56.8 min in the transposition group. The mean treatment time of crossing vessels was 8.0 ± 3.5 min, that of suspension group was 5.9 ± 1.4 min, and that of the transposition group was 11.7 ± 3.0 min. The average volume of blood loss was 55.8 ± 25.6 mL. The average time of drainage tube removal was 4.6 ± 2.0 days and the average hospital stay was 11.4 ± 3.0 days (Table 2). In the transposition group, 1 patient exhibited slight urinary leakage and the drainage tube remained until the 9th day after the operation. The pathology of the stenosis of UPJ in all patients was chronic inflammation.

The hydronephrosis before and 3 months after the surgery were compared using abdominal B ultrasound as the standard to evaluate the effectiveness of the operation. There was a significant difference ($P < 0.05$) observed in the entire group, wherein the average hydronephrosis was 4.8 ± 1.5 cm before the operation and 1.2 ± 1.3 cm 3 months after the operation. Among them, the average hydronephrosis of the suspension group was 1.8 ± 1.0 cm 3 months after the operation, and that of the transposition group was 2.0 ± 1.8 cm 3 months after the operation. There was no significant difference in the degree of pyelocele between the two groups ($P = 0.269$).

The changes in renal length before and 6 months after the operation were compared by abdominal B-ultrasound as an indirect index to evaluate whether the crossing vessels were effectively preserved. There was no significant difference between the two groups ($P > 0.05$). All patients were followed up until February 2020, with an average follow-up of 17 months, ranging from 6 to 28 months. The size of the kidneys in all patients had no significant change compared with that before operation and hydronephrosis was relieved.

Discussion

Crossing vessel compression is one of the common causes of UPJO, mostly related to congenital development. UPJO caused by crossing vessel compression accounts for 10–28.1% of adult primary UPJO [1, 2]. The majority of the symptoms were pain or discomfort on the affected side of the waist and some patients were treated for hydronephrosis upon routine physical examination. Ectopic renal vessels (also known as renal vagal vessels) are mainly divided into ectopic renal arteries and ectopic renal veins (ectopic arteries are more common), which are usually located on the ventral side of the ureteropelvic

Table 2 Pre-operative-, intra-operative-, postoperative-, and follow-up- data of the two groups

Items	Suspension team (n = 21)	Transposition team (n = 12)	Total (n = 33)	*P* value
Operative time/min	203.8 ± 61.8	222.5 ± 56.8	210.6 ± 58.9	0.798
Crossing vascular management time/min	5.9 ± 1.4	11.7 ± 3.0	8.0 ± 3.5	0.004
Blood loss/ml	45.2 ± 36.0	74.2 ± 85.3	55.8 ± 58.4	0.182
Drainage time/d	4.3 ± 1.2	4.8 ± 2.4	4.6 ± 2.0	0.495
Hospitalization time /d	11.3 ± 2.1	11.4 ± 3.7	11.4 ± 3.0	0.967
Pre-operative hydronephrosis/cm	5.0 ± 1.6	4.6 ± 1.6	4.8 ± 1.5	0.487
Post-operative hydronephrosis/cm	1.8 ± 1.0	2.0 ± 1.8	1.2 ± 1.3*	0.269
Pre-operative length of kidney/cm	11.5 ± 1.3	11.4 ± 1.2	11.4 ± 1.8	0.720
Post-operative length of kidney/cm	11.2 ± 1.1	11.7 ± 1.3	11.5 ± 1.2#	0.291

*Compared with preoperative hydronephrosis ($P < 0.05$), #Compared with preoperative renal length, $P > 0.05$

junction and do not enter the kidney through the renal hilum. Additionally, some of them directly enter the lower pole of the kidney, with an incidence of about 6.3% [1].

There are different surgical methods for the treatment of crossing vessels. Hellström et al. [9] proposed an operation method for a vascular hitch (Hellström operation) as early as 1949, which is considered the classic operation to deal with UPJO caused by crossing vessel compression. At present, Pesce et al. [10, 11] is known to still recommend the Hellström operation by laparoscopy for UPJO with crossing vessels. It is presumed that the operation is relatively simple; on the other hand, it can decide whether to further perform pyeloplasty according to the severity of the obstruction. Also, the advantage of LP is that it can obtain better esthetic outcome (the smaller scar) than that of OP [12]. Zhang [13] reported that eight cases of UPJO with crossing vessels underwent Hellström operation by retroperitoneal laparoscopy, all of which were successful. Based on fully dissecting the crossing vessels in the upper ureter and obstruction, the crossing vessels were embedded with 4–0 absorbable sutures and fixed on the anterior wall of the renal pelvis. This operation method ensured the blood supply to the kidney and completely resolved the problem of external compression of the ureteropelvic junction. Notably, indications need to be strictly observed.

Other authors have used the method of vascular transposition to deal with UPJO with crossing vessels. Boylu et al. [14] reported that 48 cases of UPJO with crossing vessels underwent laparoscopic pyeloplasty with robot assistance, of which 18 cases were successfully transposed. According to the author's opinion, it is necessary to judge whether crossing vessels cause actual compression to the pelvic canal according to the condition during the operation. Villemagne found that furosemide challenge test is a feasible method to determine whether there is UPJO during operation [15].

Pesce [10] arrived at a conclusion regarding the method of how to judge whether a crossing vessel is the direct cause of UPJO. He observed the effective peristalsis of UPJ and the rapid passage of urine from the renal pelvis by a diuretic test in 111 patients during the operation and judged whether to perform the Hellström operation. The report stated that the success rate of this method is 98% and only one patient received suspension of operation with a poor effect. It is worth noting that crossing vascular compression is not the only factor that causes UPJO. It is equally important to resect the obstructed part of the UPJ and reconstruct the junction. In most cases, ureteral stenosis or decreased peristalsis function occurs in the compression segment. Even if the external compression is relieved, dynamic obstruction still occurs in the ureter. The data from Ellerkamp's study showed that there was no significant difference in the pathological characteristics of ureteral smooth muscle fibrosis, muscle hypertrophy, and inflammation between the UPJO patients with and without vascular compression.

Taken together, we suggest that the treatment of crossing vessels should be determined according to the position and direction of the ectopic vessels. In short, when the crossing vessels are close to the renal hilus (above the level of the lower pole midline of the kidney), the method of blood vessel suspension can be adopted (Fig. 1). When the crossing vessels are at the level of the lower pole of the kidney (below the level of the lower pole midline of the kidney), the method of crossing vessel transposition can be adopted (Fig. 2).

The average time of the crossing vessels management was 5.9 ± 1.4 min in the suspension group and 11.7 ± 3.0 min in the transposition group ($P < 0.05$). This is because the crossing vessels in the transposition group directly enter the lower pole of the kidney and the vessels are relatively short; therefore, they need to be completely free from the root of the lower pole of the kidney to the starting part. Subsequently, they should be fixed on the fascia of the psoas major muscle above the anastomosis with suture.

The obvious limitation of our study is the small number of patients. Furthermore, we know that there are several factors that can affect the final outcome of pyeloplasty: methods, approaches, techniques, as well as the manner of suturing and stenting. In addition, retrospective studies inevitably lead to case selection bias. In order to reduce the bias of the two groups of patients, only the patients who underwent laparoscopic pyeloplasty by the same surgeon were chosen.

In conclusion, the method of Hem-o-lok clips suspension or vascular transposition can be used to relieve the crossing vascular compression for UPJO patients with crossing vessel compression at the same time of pyeloplasty, according to the location and direction of the ectopic vascular, so as to further improve the success rate of pyeloplasty. It is simple and reliable to use Hem-o-lok clips to suspend ectopic blood vessels, which has a certain value in clinical applications.

Abbreviations

UPJ: Ureteropelvic junction; UPJO: Ureteropelvic junction obstruction; LP: Laparoscopic pyeloplasty; CT: Computed tomography; CTU: Computed tomography urography.

Acknowledgements

Not applicable.

Authors' contributions

J.L and JJ.Z: project development, data analysis, manuscript writing. XJ.Y: project development, manuscript editing, operation performance. WN.C:

project development, data collection. LL.X and XB.H: project development, manuscript editing. All authors read and approved the final manuscript.

Competing interest

Jun Liu: No competing financial interests exist. Jingjun Zhang: No competing financial interests exist. Weinan Chen: No competing financial interests exist. Liulin Xiong: No competing financial interests exist. Xiaobo Huang: No competing financial interests exist. Xiongjun Ye: No competing financial interests exist.

Author details

[1]Urology and Lithotripsy Center, Peking University People's Hospital, Peking University, 133 Fuchengmen Inner Street, Xicheng District, Beijing 100034, People's Republic of China. [2]Peking University Applied Lithotripsy Institute, Peking University, Beijing 100034, China. [3]Department of Urology, Peking University BinHai Hospital (Fifth Tianjin Central Hospital), Tianjin 300450, China.

References

1. Ellerkamp V, Kurth RR, Schmid E, et al. Differences between intrinsic and extrinsic ureteropelvic junction obstruction related to crossing vessels: histology and functional analyses. World J Urol. 2016;34(4):577–83.
2. Zhang X, Li HZ, Wang SG, et al. Retroperitoneal laparoscopic dismembered pyeloplasty: experience with 50 cases. Urology. 2005;66:514–7.
3. Szavay P, Heyne-Pietschmann M, Zundel SM. Uretero-pelvic junction obstruction due to crossing pole vessel: contra vascular hitch. Aktuelle Urol. 2020;51(2):121–6.
4. Polok M, Toczewski K, Borselle D, Apoznański W, Jędrzejuk D, Patkowski D. Hydronephrosis in children caused by lower pole crossing vessels-how to choose the proper method of treatment? Front Pediatr. 2019;7:83.
5. Chiarenza SF, Bleve C, Caione P, et al. Minimally invasive treatment of pediatric extrinsic ureteropelvic junction obstruction by crossing polar vessels: is vascular hitching a definitive solution? Report of a multicenter survey. J Laparoendosc Adv Surg Tech A. 2017;27(9):965–71.
6. Uhlig A, Uhlig J, Trojan L, et al. Surgical approaches for treatment of ureteropelvic junction obstruction—a systematic review and network meta-analysis. BMC Urol. 2019;19(1):112.
7. Hashim H, Christopher RJ. Ureteropelvic junction obstruction. Eur Urol Suppl. 2012;11:25–32.
8. Ellenbogen P, Scheible F, Talner L, et al. Sensitivity of gray scale ultrasound in detecting urinary tract obstruction. AJR Am J Roentgenol. 1978;130(4):731–3.
9. Hellström J, Giertz G, Lindblom K. Pathogenesis and treatment of hydronephrosis. J Belge Urol. 1951;20(1):1–6.
10. Pesce C, Campobasso P, Costa L, Battaglino F, Musi L. Ureterovascular hydronephrosis in children: is pyeloplasty always necessary? Eur Urol. 1999;36(1):71–4.
11. Sakoda A, Cherian A, Mushtaq I. Laparoscopic transposition of lower pole crossing vessels ('vascular hitch') in pure extrinsic pelvi-ureteric junction (PUJ) obstruction in children. BJU Int. 2011;108(8):1364–8.
12. Masieri L, Sforza S, Cini C, et al. Minilaparoscopic versus open pyeloplasty in children less than 1 year. J Laparoendosc Adv Surg Tech A. 2019;29(7):970–5.
13. Zhang X, Xu K, Fu B, et al. The retroperitoneal laparoscopic Hellström technique for pelvi-ureteric junction obstruction from a crossing vessel. BJU Int. 2007;100(6):1335–8.
14. Boylu U, Oommen M, Lee BR, et al. Ureteropelvic junction obstruction secondary to crossing vessels-to transpose or not? Robot Exp J Urol. 2009;181(4):1751–5.
15. Villemagne T, Fourcade L, Camby C, et al. Long-term results with the laparoscopic transposition of renal lower pole crossing vessels. J Pediatr Urol. 2015;11(4):174.e1-174.e1747.

13

Effect of pre-operative internal obturator muscle mass index in MRI on biochemical recurrence of prostate cancer patients after radical prostatectomy

Won Tae Kim[1,2], Ho Won Kang[1,2], Sung Pil Seo[2], Yong-June Kim[1,2], Sang Cheol Lee[1,2], Wun-Jae Kim[1,2], Bum Sang Cho[3], Yun Sok Ha[4], Tae Gyun Kwon[4], Jinsung Park[5], Seung Chol Park[6], Young Beom Jeong[7], Taek Won Kang[8], Sung-Woo Park[9] and Seok Joong Yun[1,2*]

Abstract

Background: Recent reports show that the pre-operative or post-operative skeletal mass index (sarcopenia) affects survival rates for various cancers; however, the link between prostate cancer survival and sarcopenia is unclear. Therefore, this study examined the effect of the pre-operative internal obturator muscle (IOM) mass index on biochemical recurrence (BCR) of prostate cancer (PCa) patients who underwent radical prostatectomy.

Methods: In total, 222 patients, who underwent open, laparoscopic, or robot-assisted radical prostatectomy at seven centers in 2011 and were followed up for 5 years, were enrolled. BCR was examined in the context of pre-operative IOM mass index and BMI.

Results: The mean age of the patients was 67.82 ± 6.23 years, and the mean pre-operative prostate-specific antigen (PSA) level was 11.61 ± 13.22 ng/ml. There was no significant difference in baseline characteristics between the low and high IOM mass index groups ($p > 0.05$). Age, pre-op PSA level, ECE, and T-stage were associated with BCR ($p = 0.049$, $p < 0.001$, $p = 0.001$, $p = 0.004$, respectively). BMI, prostate volume, Gleason score, resection margin, N-stage, M-stage and IOM mass index was not associated with BCR ($p > 0.05$).

Conclusions: Pre-operative IOM mass index was not associated with BCR; however, long-term follow-up is necessary to evaluate cancer-specific and overall survival of PCa patients.

Keywords: Prostatic neoplasms, Sarcopenia, Internal obturator muscle, Recurrence

Background

Prostate cancer (PCa) is the most common cancer in men worldwide [1]. The incidence of PCa in Asia is among the lowest in the world [1]. However, the incidence in the Republic (Rep.) of Korea is increasing rapidly [2]. PCa mortality rates have fallen in high-resource countries, but have increased or remain stable in low-resource countries [1]. PCa-associated mortality in the Rep. of Korea is increasing along with incidence [2].

Sarcopenia is a condition characterized by progressive and generalized loss of muscle mass and strength [3]. Sarcopenia predicts drug toxicity and time-to-tumor progression in patients undergoing chemotherapy [4]. The impact of sarcopenia in cancer patients has been studied,

*Correspondence: sjyun@chungbuk.ac.kr
[1] Department of Urology, College of Medicine, Chungbuk National University, 62, Kaeshin-dong, Heungduk-ku, Cheongju, Chungbuk 361-711, South Korea

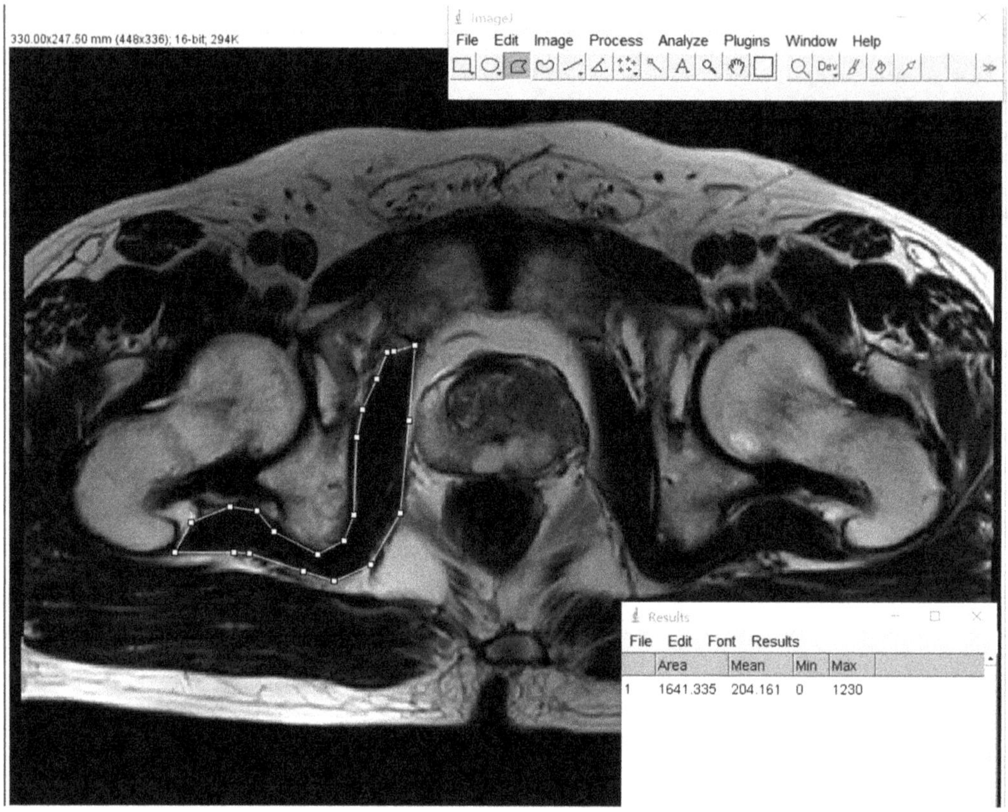

Fig. 1 The measuring methods of internal obturator muscle width in the pelvis MRI for IOM mass index

and data suggest that sarcopenia is independently associated with post-operative outcome following resection of colorectal cancer, hepatocellular carcinoma, pancreatic cancer, and bladder cancer [5–8]. In addition, sarcopenia is a prognostic marker for disease recurrence and mortality in patients with urologic cancers [8–11].

Radical prostatectomy (RP) is the gold standard treatment for localized PCa. RP is often the treatment of choice for younger and less morbid patients. A previous report suggests that sarcopenia is associated with non-cancer-related death in PCa patients undergoing radiotherapy [12]. Conversely, Mason et al. report that sarcopenia is not independently associated with perioperative complications or oncologic outcomes after RP [13]. Therefore, there is a lack of evidence supporting an association between sarcopenia and oncologic outcomes in PCa. Generally, sarcopenia, skeletal mass index (SMI) was defined as the cross-sectional area of the rectus abdominis; internal, external, and transverse obliques; psoas; quadratus lumborum; and erector spinae muscles from L3 down. Most surgeon performed MRI imaging work-up for prostatectomy. However, preoperative CT imaging is the option and surgeon's preference. Unfortunately, cross sectional area of whole muscle from L3 down level cannot be taken in the MRI imaging. Internal obturator muscle (IOM) is the only measurable muscle in the pelvis MRI axial cut. Additionally, there was no study between pre-operative IOM mass index and oncologic outcomes in PCa. Therefore, we investigated the effect of pre-operative IOM mass index on biochemical recurrence (BCR) in Korean patients after RP.

Methods

Study population and data collection

In total, 222 PCa patients, who underwent open, laparoscopic, or robot-assisted RP at seven academic centers in 2011 and were followed up for 5 years, were enrolled. All patients had histologically confirmed primary adenocarcinoma of the prostate, and all had undergone pre-operative MRI within 3 months of surgery. Patients were excluded if they had previously received androgen deprivation therapy (ADT) or radiotherapy (RT). In addition, patients undergoing testosterone replacement

Table 1 Baseline characteristics of all patients and according to the Internal obturator muscle (IOM) mass Index

Parameters	Overall	According to the IOM mass index		
		Low IOM	High IOM	*p*-value
Number	222	111	111	
Age (years)	67.82 ± 6.23	68.55 ± 6.11	67.10 ± 6.29	0.083
IOM (mm²/cm²)	11.23 ± 2.22			
BMI (kg/m²)	24.46 ± 2.86	24.17 ± 2.86	24.74 ± 2.85	0.136
Pre-op PSA (ng/mL)	11.61 ± 13.22	11.12 ± 12.29	12.11 ± 14.12	0.579
Prostate volume (cc)	34.58 ± 14.13	35.56 ± 15.68	33.57 ± 12.33	0.313
Type of operation				0.200
RRP	163 (73.4)	77 (69.4)	86 (77.5)	
LRP	1 (0.5)	0	1 (0.9)	
RARP	58 (26.1)	34 (30.6)	24 (21.6)	
Gleason score				0.441
≤ 6	59 (26.6)	24 (21.6)	35 (26.6)	
7	145 (65.3)	78 (70.3)	67 (65.3)	
8	8 (3.6)	4 (3.6)	4 (3.6)	
9	10 (4.5)	5 (4.5)	5 (4.5)	
T-stage				0.717
T2a	28 (12.6)	14 (12.6)	14 (12.6)	
T2b	38 (17.1)	19 (17.1)	19 (17.1)	
T2c	119 (53.6)	56 (50.5)	63 (56.8)	
T3a	21 (9.5)	13 (11.7)	8 (7.2)	
T3b	16 (7.2)	9 (8.1)	7 (6.3)	
N-stage				0.155
0	267 (97.1)	111 (100)	109 (98.2)	
1	8 (2.9)	0 (0.0)	2 (1.8)	
cM stage				0.316
0	221 (99.5)	110 (99.1)	111 (100)	
1	1 (0.5)	1 (0.9)	0 (0.0)	
BCR				0.871
0	173 (77.9)	87 (78.4)	86 (77.5)	
1	49 (22.1)	24 (21.6)	25 (22.5)	

BMI, body mass index; pre-op PSA, pre-operative prostate-specific antigen; RRP, radical retropubic prostatectomy; LRP, laparoscopic radical prostatectomy; RARP, robot-assisted radical prostatectomy; BCR, biochemical recurrence

Table 2 Comparison of clinical and pathological parameters according to body mass index

Parameter	≤ Normal	Overweight	Obese	*p*-value
Number	63	73	86	
Age (years)	68.57 ± 6.06	68.07 ± 6.85	67.07 ± 5.76	0.321
IOM (mm²/cm²)	10.84 ± 2.18	11.13 ± 2.02	11.59 ± 2.37	0.115
BMI (kg/m²)	21.11 ± 1.45	24.06 ± 0.51	27.25 ± 1.79	< 0.001
Pre-op PSA (ng/mL)	13.97 ± 17.97	11.01 ± 10.93	10.40 ± 10.57	0.237
Prostate volume (cc)	32.54 ± 12.95	33.01 ± 14.39	37.54 ± 14.42	0.062
Type of operation				0.291
RRP	48 (76.2)	58 (79.5)	57 (66.3)	
LRP	0 (0.0)	0 (0.0)	1 (1.2)	
RARP	15 (23.8)	15 (20.5)	28 (32.6)	
Gleason score				0.165
≤ 6	14 (22.2)	20 (27.4)	25 (29.1)	
7	43 (68.3)	49 (67.1)	53 (61.6)	
8	5 (7.9)	1 (1.4)	2 (2.3)	
9	1 (1.6)	3 (4.1)	6 (7.0)	
T-stage				0.220
T2a	7 (11.1)	14 (19.2)	7 (8.1)	
T2b	7 (11.1)	13 (17.8)	18 (20.9)	
T2c	37 (58.7)	37 (50.7)	45 (52.3)	
T3a	5 (7.9)	5 (6.8)	11 (12.8)	
T3b	7 (11.1)	4 (5.5)	5 (5.8)	
N-stage				0.524
0	62 (98.4)	72 (98.6)	86 (100)	
1	1 (1.6)	1 (1.4)	0 (0.0)	
cM stage				0.282
0	62 (98.4)	73 (100)	86 (100.0)	
1	1 (1.6)	0 (0.0)	0 (0.0)	
BCR				0.521
0	46 (73.0)	59 (80.8)	68 (79.1)	
1	17 (27.0)	14 (19.2)	18 (20.9)	

IOM, Internal obturator muscle mass index; BMI, body mass index; pre-op PSA, pre-operative prostate-specific antigen; RRP, radical retropubic prostatectomy; LRP, laparoscopic radical prostatectomy; RARP, robot-assisted radical prostatectomy; BCR, biochemical recurrence

therapy or taking medications that affect muscle mass were excluded.

Clinical and pathologic data included age, height, body weight, prostate-specific antigen (PSA) levels, prostate volume, pathologic T-, N-, and M-stage, receipt of adjuvant RT or ADT, and follow-up duration. BCR after RP was defined as a post-operative PSA level > 0.2 ng/mL. Patients undergoing adjuvant ADT or RT after RP were excluded in the BCR group. IOM mass index was measured by dividing the mean internal obturator muscle area (calculated from MRI) by height (squared). All internal obturator muscle area measurements were performed by a single radiologist using ImageJ (https://imagej.nih.gov/ij/) at the level of symphysis pubis (Cho, BS, Fig. 1). Median value of IOM mass index was used to determine the cutoff value between high and low IOM mass index. Using this median value (11.47708194 cm^2/m^2), patients were classified into high or low IOM mass index group. BMI group were divided into 3 groups according to Korean BMI criteria (normal < 23 kg/m^2; 23 kg/m^2 ≤ overweight < 25 kg/m^2; 25 kg/m^2 ≤ obese).

Table 3 Cox proportional hazards model analysis of biochemical recurrence

Parameter	HR	95% CI	*p*-value
Age (years)	0.945	0.892–1.000	0.049
IOM (mm^2/cm^2) (low vs. high)	0.891	0.462–1.719	0.731
BMI (kg/m^2)			0.142
≤Normal	–		
Overweight	0.880	0.379–2.042	
Obesity	0.455	0.195–1.063	
Pre-op PSA (ng/ml)	1.064	1.045–1.083	<0.001
Prostate volume (cc)	1.016	0.990–1.042	0.226
Gleason score			0.364
≤6	–		
7	1.263	0.478–3.340	
8	1.473	0.317–6.844	
9	3.064	0.798–11.760	
ECE (no vs. yes)	5.551	2.011–15.322	0.001
Resection margin (– vs. +)	1.040	0.479–2.262	0.920
T-stage			0.004
T2a	–		
T2b	13.260	2.218–79.262	
T2c	3.157	0.609–16.373	
T3a	1.564	0.177–13.785	
T3b	4.830	0.700–33.326	
N-stage (no involvement vs. LN involvement)	0.300	0.028–3.202	0.319
M-stage (no meta vs. meta)	0.000	0.000–	0.985

IOM, internal obturator muscle mass index; BMI, body mass index; pre-op PSA, pre-operative prostate-specific antigen; ECE, extracapsular extension; LN, lymph node

Statistical analysis

IOM mass index was divided into two groups according to a median cut-off value. BMI was divided to three groups according to Korean BMI criteria [14]. The baseline characteristics of the patients with a low IOM mass index and a high IOM mass index were compared using an independent t-test and the Chi-square test as appropriate. Comparisons of clinical and pathological parameters according to BMI were made using ANOVA and the Chi-square test as appropriate. The association between BCR and pre-operative IOM mass index or BMI values were examined using a Cox proportional hazards model and a Kaplan–Meier survival analysis. Statistical analyses were performed using the Statistical Package for Social Sciences, version 25 software (SPSS, Inc., Chicago, IL, USA). A p-value <0.05 was considered statistically significant.

Results

Baseline characteristics of the study population according to IOM mass index

The baseline characteristics of all the patients are shown in Table 1. The mean age was 67.82 ± 6.23 years, and the mean pre-operative PSA level was 11.61 ± 13.22 ng/mL. There was no significant difference in baseline characteristics between the low IOM mass index and high IOM mass index groups ($p > 0.05$).

Comparison of clinical and pathological parameters according to BMI

As shown in Table 2, there was no significant difference in clinical and pathological parameters according to BMI ($p > 0.05$).

Cox proportional hazards model analysis of biochemical recurrence

Age, pre-op PSA, ECE, and T-stage was associated with BCR ($p = 0.049$, $p < 0.001$, $p = 0.001$, $p = 0.004$, respectively). However, there was no association between BCR and BMI, prostate volume, Gleason score, resection margin, N-stage, or M-stage ($p > 0.05$; Table 3). In particular, IOM mass index was not associated with BCR ($p > 0.05$; Fig. 2).

Discussion

The results of the present study suggest that IOM mass index is not associated with BCR after RP in Korean men. The present study is the first to show no significant association between IOM mass index and BCR in men with RP. Thus, IOM mass index may not be a prognostic marker for BCR in Korean men with localized PCa undergoing RP.

Previous studies suggest that high BMI is associated with increased risk of PCa [15, 16]. A meta-analysis by Bergstrom et al. reports a 6% increase in the risk of PCa in overweight men and a 12% increase in obese men compared with men of normal weight [16]. MacInnis et al. reported a weak positive association between BMI and risk of PCa; BMI was associated with moderate increase in the risk of advanced PCa [15].

The relationship between BMI and BCR after RP remains controversial. Freedland et al. reported that obesity among men treated with RP was associated with high-grade tumors, a trend toward increased risk of a positive surgical margin, and high BCR [17]. Magheli et al. reported that high BMI is associated with adverse pathological findings and is a strong independent predictor of BCR after RP [18]. Asmar et al. reported that both obesity and hypertension are associated with an increased risk of BCR after RP, independent of age at the

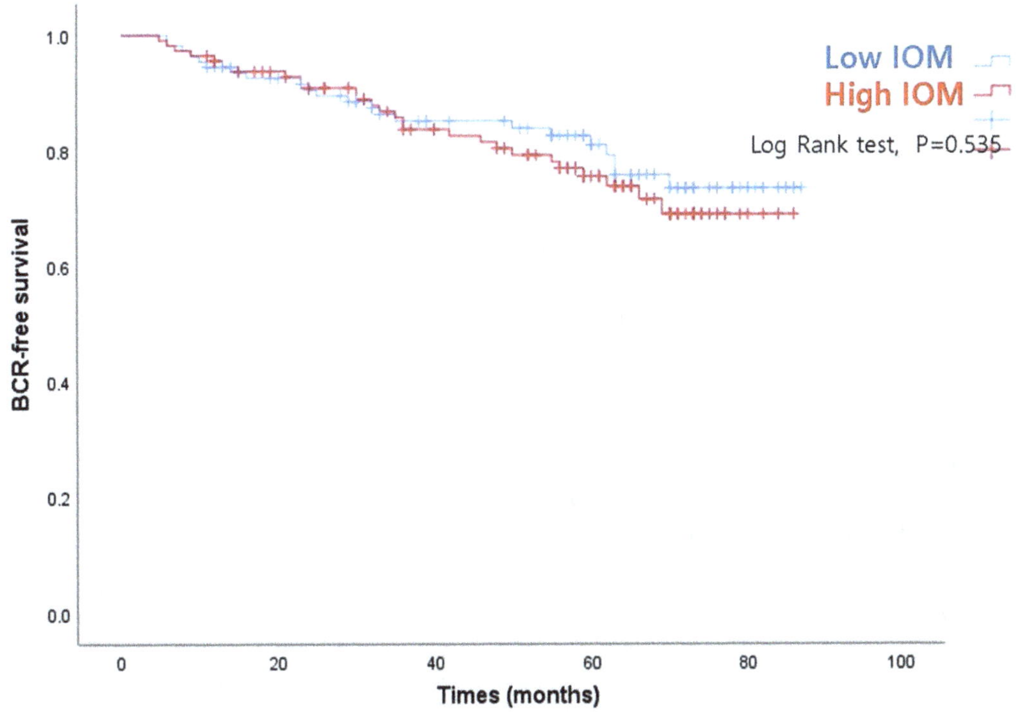

Fig. 2 Biochemical recurrence (BCR)-free survival according to internal obturator muscle (IOM) mass index status (low IOM vs. high IOM)

time of diagnosis or tumor pathological features [19]. By contrast, Tomaszewski et al. reported that obesity is not associated with adverse pathologic features, positive surgical margin, or BCR [20]. They suggested that their data provide evidence that obese men undergoing RP are not more likely to suffer PCa progression. In addition, Siddiqui et al. reported that obese patients appeared to have worse pathologic features at the time of prostatectomy; however, BMI did not appear to be an independent predictor of recurrence or survival after prostatectomy [21]. The present study found no association between BMI and BCR. Therefore, we believe that the relationship between BMI and BCR after RP remains unclear.

Sarcopenia is a process associated with normal aging; however, it is exacerbated by the hypercatabolic state and inflammatory responses caused by malignancy [22]. A systematic review by Joglekar et al. investigated the impact of sarcopenia on outcome following surgical resection of cancer and reported that sarcopenia is an independent prognostic factor for both complications and survival following surgical resection [23]. Sarcopenia is a more objective and comprehensive pre-operative risk factor that predicts all-cause survival for bladder cancer after radical cystectomy (RC) [9, 24]. With respect to PCa, several reports link sarcopenia and survival [12, 25]. Thus, sarcopenia could be used to predict non-cancer-related death in men with PCa after RT [12] and may be a poor prognostic factor for CRPC treated with chemotherapy [25]. However, the association between sarcopenia and survival after RP is very unclear. Only one study was reported that sarcopenia was not significantly associated with the risks of BCR, systemic progression, or all-cause mortality after RP [13]. This study is the first study to evaluate the association between IOM and prognosis in all cancer patients. IOM mass index is the only measurable muscle mass index in pelvic MRI. So, there was no options to select the muscle mass index in pelvic MRI. However, long-term follow-up studies are necessary to identify (or not) any association between sarcopenia or IOM mass index and survival.

We recognize that this study has several limitations. First, we only measured internal obturator muscle mass, but not SMI. In general, SMI was defined as the cross-sectional area of the rectus abdominis; internal, external, and transverse obliques; psoas; quadratus lumborum; and erector spinae muscles from L3 down. However, because this was a multi-institutional study, different authors have different protocols for pre-operative CT and MRI. Therefore, we selected only the internal obturator muscle area in the pelvis in the MRI, because of internal obturator muscle is the only measurable muscle in the pelvis MRI axial cut. So, we couldn't compared IOM mass with general SMI. Second, many patients who underwent RP at these institutions were excluded from the analysis due to differences in CT or MRI protocols. In some institutions, radiologists were not able to measure the internal obturator muscle at the same levels. Third, the follow-up period was too short to get an accurate picture of survival. In this case we did not examine cancer-specific or overall survival; studies may need follow-up data spanning more than 15 years to get an accurate picture of the association between IOM mass index and the survival of PCa patients.

Conclusions

Pre-operative IOM mass index was not associated with BCR; however, long-term (> 15 years) follow-up is necessary to better answer this still controversial question.

Acknowledgements
Not applicable.

Authors' contributions
WTK wrote the original draft and editing of the final draft. SJY contributed to the concept and project planning. YJK, SCL, WJK contributed significantly to the writing of this paper. HWK, SPS, BSC, YSH, TGK, JP, SCP, YBJ, TWK, SWP contributed to the selecting data. The authors read and approved the final mansuscript.

Competing interests
The authors declare no competing interests.

Author details
[1]Department of Urology, College of Medicine, Chungbuk National University, 62, Kaeshin-dong, Heungduk-ku, Cheongju, Chungbuk 361-711, South Korea. [2]Department of Urology, Chungbuk National University Hospital, Cheongju, South Korea. [3]Department of Radiology, College of Medicine, Chungbuk National University, Cheongju, South Korea. [4]Department of Urology, College of Medicine, Kyungpook National University, Daegu, South Korea. [5]Department of Urology, College of Medicine, Eulji University, Daejeon, South Korea. [6]Department of Urology, College of Medicine, Won Kang University, Iksan, South Korea. [7]Department of Urology, College of Medicine, Jeonbuk National University, Jeonju, South Korea. [8]Department of Urology, College of Medicine, Jeonnam National University, Kwangju, South Korea. [9]Department of Urology, College of Medicine, Pusan National University, Pusan, South Korea.

References

1. Center M, Jemal A, Lortet Tieulent J, Ward E, Ferlay J, Brawley O, et al. International variation in prostate cancer incidence and mortality rates. Eur Urol. 2012;61:1079–92.
2. Lee HY, Park S, Doo SW, Yang WJ, Song YS, Kim JH. Trends in prostate cancer prevalence and radical prostatectomy rate according to age structural changes in South Korea between 2005 and 2015. Yonsei Med J. 2019;60:257–66.
3. Cruz Jentoft AJ, Baeyens JP, Bauer JM, Boirie Y, Cederholm T, Landi F, et al. Sarcopenia: European consensus on definition and diagnosis: Report of the European Working Group on Sarcopenia in Older People. Age Ageing. 2010;39:412–23.
4. Prado CM, Baracos VE, McCargar LJ, Reiman T, Mourtzakis M, Tonkin K, et al. Sarcopenia as a determinant of chemotherapy toxicity and time to tumor progression in metastatic breast cancer patients receiving capecit abine treatment. Clin Cancer Res. 2009;15:2920–6.
5. Miyamoto Y, Baba Y, Sakamoto Y, Ohuchi M, Tokunaga R, Kurashige J, et al. Sarcopenia is a negative prognostic factor after curative resection of colorectal cancer. Ann Surg Oncol. 2015;22:2663–8.
6. Harimoto N, Shirabe K, Yamashita YI, Ikegami T, Yoshizumi T, Soejima Y, et al. Sarcopenia as a predictor of prognosis in patients following hepatectomy for hepatocellular carcinoma. Br J Surg. 2013;100:1523–30.
7. Peng P, Hyder O, Firoozmand A, Kneuertz P, Schulick RD, Huang D, et al. Impact of sarcopenia on outcomes following resection of pancreatic adenocarcinoma. J Gastrointest Surg. 2012;16:1478–86.
8. Smith AB, Deal AM, Yu H, Boyd B, Matthews J, Wallen EM, et al. Sarcopenia as a predictor of complications and survival following radical cystectomy. J Urol. 2014;191:1714–20.
9. Psutka SP, Carrasco A, Schmit GD, Moynagh MR, Boorjian SA, Frank I, et al. Sarcopenia in patients with bladder cancer undergoing radical cystectomy: impact on cancer-specific and all-cause mortality. Cancer. 2014;120:2910–8.
10. Psutka SP, Boorjian SA, Moynagh MR, Schmit GD, Frank I, Carrasco A, et al. Mortality after radical cystectomy: impact of obesity versus adiposity after adjusting for skeletal muscle wasting. J Urol. 2015;193:1507–13.
11. Psutka SP, Boorjian SA, Moynagh MR, Schmit GD, Costello BA, Thompson RH, et al. Decreased skeletal muscle mass is associated with an increased risk of mortality after radical nephrectomy for localized renal cell cancer. J Urol. 2016;195:270–6.
12. McDonald AM, Swain TA, Mayhew DL, Cardan RA, Baker CB, Harris DM, et al. CT Measures of bone mineral density and muscle mass can be used to predict noncancer death in men with prostate cancer. Radiology. 2017;282:475–83.
13. Mason RJ, Boorjian SA, Bhindi B, Rangel L, Frank I, Karnes RJ, et al. The association between sarcopenia and oncologic outcomes after radical prostatectomy. Clin Genitourin Cancer. 2018;16:e629–36.
14. Kim MK, Lee WY, Kang JH, Kim BT, Kim SM, Kim EM, et al. 2014 clinical practice guidelines for overweight and obesity in Korea. Endocrinol Metab. 2014;29:405–9.
15. MacInnis RJ, English DR. Body size and composition and prostate cancer risk: systematic review and meta-regression analysis. Cancer Causes Control. 2006;17:989–1003.
16. Bergström A, Pisani P, Tenet V, Wolk A, Adami HO. Overweight as an avoidable cause of cancer in Europe. Int J Cancer. 2001;91:421–30.
17. Freedland SJ, Aronson WJ, Kane CJ, Presti JC, Amling CL, Elashoff D, et al. Impact of obesity on biochemical control after radical prostatectomy for clinically localized prostate cancer: a report by the Shared Equal Access Regional Cancer Hospital database study group. J Clin Oncol. 2004;22:446–53.
18. Magheli A, Rais Bahrami S, Trock BJ, Humphreys EB, Partin AW, Han M, et al. Impact of body mass index on biochemical recurrence rates after radical prostatectomy: an analysis utilizing propensity score matching. Urology (Ridgewood, NJ). 2008;72:1246–51.
19. Asmar R, Beebe Dimmer JL, Korgavkar K, Keele GR, Cooney KA. Hypertension, obesity and prostate cancer biochemical recurrence after radical prostatectomy. Prostate Cancer Prostatic Dis. 2013;16:62–6.
20. Tomaszewski J, Chen Y, Bertolet M, Ristau BT, Woldemichael E, Nelson JB. Obesity is not associated with aggressive pathologic features or biochemical recurrence after radical prostatectomy. Urology (Ridgewood, NJ). 2013;81:992–6.
21. Siddiqui SA, Inman BA, Sengupta S, Slezak JM, Bergstralh EJ, Leibovich BC, et al. Obesity and survival after radical prostatectomy: A 10-year prospective cohort study. Cancer. 2006;107:521–9.
22. Prado CM, Wells JC, Smith SR, Stephan BC, Siervo M. Sarcopenic obesity: a critical appraisal of the current evidence. Clin Nutr (Edinburgh). 2012;31:583–601.
23. Joglekar S, Nau PN, Mezhir J. The impact of sarcopenia on survival and complications in surgical oncology: a review of the current literature. J Surg Oncol. 2015;112:503–9.
24. Hirasawa Y, Nakashima J, Yunaiyama D, Sugihara T, Gondo T, Nakagami Y, et al. Sarcopenia as a novel preoperative prognostic predictor for survival

in patients with bladder cancer undergoing radical cystectomy. Ann Surg Oncol. 2016;23:1048–54.

25. Ohtaka A, Aoki H, Nagata M, Kanayama M, Shimizu F, Ide H, et al. Sarcopenia is a poor prognostic factor of castration-resistant prostate cancer treated with docetaxel therapy. Prostate Int. 2019;7:9–14.

14

No staghorn calculi and none/mild hydronephrosis may be risk factors for severe bleeding complications after percutaneous nephrolithotomy

Xue Dong[1], Dongnv Wang[1], Huangqi Zhang[1], Shuzong You[1], Wenting Pan[1], Peipei Pang[4], Chaoqian Chen[2], Hongjie Hu[3*] and Wenbin Ji[1*]

Abstract

Background: To explore the risk factors for severe bleeding complications after percutaneous nephrolithotomy (PCNL) according to the modified Clavien scoring system.

Methods: We retrospectively analysed 2981 patients who received percutaneous nephrolithotomies from January 2014 to December 2020. Study inclusion criteria were PCNL and postoperative mild or severe renal haemorrhage in accordance with the modified Clavien scoring system. Mild bleeding complications included Clavien 2, while severe bleeding complications were greater than Clavien 3a. It has a good prognosis and is more likely to be underestimated and ignored in retrospective studies in bleeding complications classified by Clavien 1, so no analysis about these was conducted in this study. Clinical features, medical comorbidities and perioperative characteristics were analysed. Chi-square, independent *t* tests, Pearson's correlation, Fisher exact tests, Mann–Whitney and multivariate logistic regression were used as appropriate.

Results: Of the 2981 patients 70 (2.3%), met study inclusion criteria, consisting of 51 men and 19 women, 48 patients had severe bleeding complications. The remaining 22 patients had mild bleeding. Patients with postoperative severe bleeding complications were more likely to have no or slight degree of hydronephrosis and have no staghorn calculi on univariate analysis ($p < 0.05$). Staghorn calculi (OR, 95% CI, *p* value 0.218, 0.068–0.700, 0.010) and hydronephrosis (OR, 95% CI, *p* value 0.271, 0.083–0.887, 0.031) were independent predictors for severe bleeding via multivariate logistic regression analysis. Other factors, such as history of PCNL, multiple kidney stones, site of puncture calyx and mean corrected intraoperative haemoglobin drop were not related to postoperative severe bleedings.

Conclusions: The absence of staghorn calculi and a no or mild hydronephrosis were related to an increased risk of post-percutaneous nephrolithotomy severe bleeding complications.

Keywords: Percutaneous nephrolithotomy, Postoperative complications, Staghorn calculi, Hydronephrosis, The modified Clavien scoring, Computed tomography

Background

Percutaneous nephrolithotomy (PCNL) is the primary choice for the treatment of larger than 2 cm renal stones [1]. PCNL, which is a commonly applied operation, has a lower complication rate than open surgery.

*Correspondence: hongjiehu@zju.edu.cn; wb.j@163.com
[1] Department of Radiology, Taizhou Hospital, Zhejiang University, Taizhou 318000, Zhejiang, China
[3] Department of Radiology, School of Medicine, Sir Run Run Shaw Hospital, Zhejiang University, Hangzhou 310023, Zhejiang, China

However, severe bleeding after percutaneous nephrolithotomy is still a challenge for urologists. Different research groups have evaluated the potential impact of several clinical, radiological, and perioperative variables on postpercutaneous nephrolithotomy bleeding [2, 3].

Unfortunately, because there is no general consensus on the definition of bleeding complications [4], few published reports have applied specific bleeding complication scores to urological surgery. Surgery, including urology, has used the Clavien-Dindo classification system extensively [5, 6] due to its simplicity and usability in classifying postoperative complications [7]. Postoperative complications after urological surgery were recommended to be reported by the European Association of Urology (EAU) guidelines panel, and the Clavien-Dindo classification system was the primary choice [8]. In 2012 de la Rosette et al. found that urologists tended to have a lower rate of agreement for grading minor complications (Clavien score 1) and best agreement was identified to define severe complications (Clavien greater than 3a) [9].

Past analysis of prognostic factors showed that puncture correctness [2], blood transfusion [3], puncture via the inferior calyx, and multiple or isolated kidney stones [10] were previously reported to be independently associated with severe bleeding after PCNL. Severe postoperative bleeding complications are a challenge to urologists and patients. To the best of our knowledge, no studies have investigated the factors associated with severe bleeding complications based on the modified Clavien score. The goal of our work was to identify factors associated with severe bleeding complications after PCNL according to the modified Clavien score [9]. We determined the clinical, radiological, and perioperative features that were related to severe bleeding complications after PCNL.

Methods

Study design and patients

This retrospective research was approved by the institutional review board. The requirement to obtain patient consent was waived. The study analysed the data of 2,981 patients who received PCNL at Taizhou Enze Medical Center (Group) Taizhou Hospital from January 2014 to December 2020. Cases with missing data and no significant complications related to bleeding were excluded. Only patients with complete clinical data who underwent unenhanced abdominal computed tomography (CT) (slice thickness 5 mm) to assess renal stone information and nephrosonography to evaluate hydronephrosis preoperatively were included.

Clinical data

The information collected included demographics, clinical and perioperative characteristics and renal stone characteristics. Demographic features included age, sex, and BMI. The clinical characteristics assessed were clinical characteristics (urinary tract infections, haematuria and pain), preoperative creatinine, history of anticoagulation, medical comorbidities (hypertension, diabetes mellitus, ischaemic heart disease, chronic lung disease, cardiorespiratory diseases, and chronic kidney disease), open surgery history and a previous history of PCNL. Renal stone features included laterality, stone location, stone count, peak Hounsfield unit, and the presence of staghorn calculi. Staghorn calculi is defined any branched stone occupying more than one portion of the collecting system [11]. Hydronephrosis was graded as either none/mild or moderate/severe using the Society of Fetal Urology grading system [12, 13]. Perioperative characteristics were the calyx of access, dilatation type, operative time (OT) and corrected intraoperative haemoglobin drop. Haemoglobin levels were corrected (corrected haemoglobin drop) for any prior transfusion. One unit of packed red blood cells or whole blood transfused was defined as the equivalent of 10 g/L haemoglobin drop [14].

Bleeding complications were collected during postoperative follow-up and categorized according to the modified Clavien score. It has a lower rate of agreement for grading minor complications (Clavien score 1) [9] and a good prognosis, so no analysis about these was conducted in this study. Major bleeding complications were defined as greater than Clavien 2. Mild bleeding complications in this study were defined as Clavien 2, and severe bleeding were classified as Clavien 3a, 3b, 4a, 4b and 5. When patients had more than 1 complication, the final analysis included only the highest Clavien score (Additional file 1: Table S1). Examples of views are shown for a mild bleeding complication undergoing blood transfusion in Fig. 1 and a severe bleeding complication undergoing a superselective renal arteriogram in (Fig. 2).

Surgical technique

PCNL procedures were performed according to the local clinical guidelines and practices. After placing the patient in the lithotomy position, retrograde ureter catheterization was performed. All other procedures were completed in the prone position. The standard technique involved using ultrasound and/or fluoroscopy in obtaining percutaneous renal access. After obtaining renal access, the tract was dilated using either balloon dilation or Amplatz serial dilation before placement of an access sheath and nephroscope. Amplatz dilatation or balloon dilatation were used according to indications on the

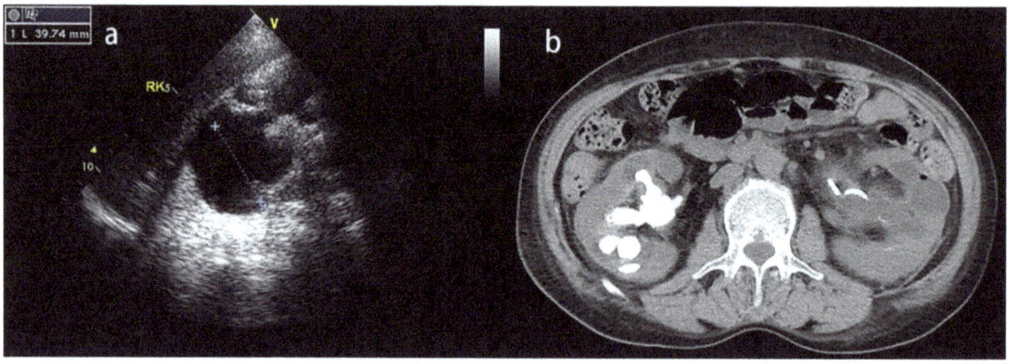

Fig. 1 Mild complication after PCNL in 57-year-old woman who underwent CT scan and nephrosonography preoperatively. **a** Sonagraphic view demonstrated anteroposterior diameter (APD) of right kidney was 39.74 mm, severe hydronephrosis. **b** CT view of staghorn calculi

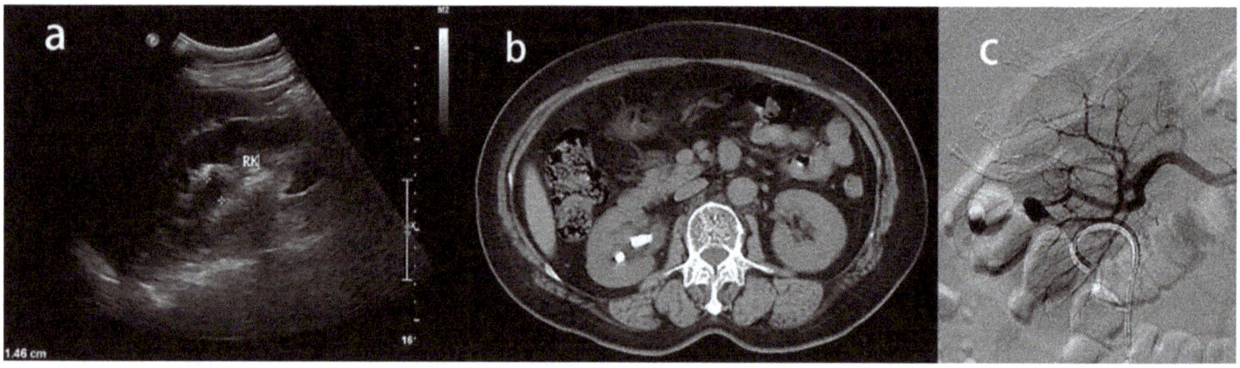

Fig. 2 Severe complication after PCNL in 56-year-old woman who underwent CT scan and nephrosonography preoperatively. **a** Sonagraphic view demonstrated anteroposterior diameter (APD) of right kidney was 14.6 mm, mild hydronephrosis. **b** CT view of no staghorn calculi. **c** Superselective renal arteriogram showed extravasation in right kidney mid segmental branches

patients. An intracorporeal lithotripsy device was then introduced through the working channel of the nephroscope and stones were broken down using a pneumatic lithotripter and/or holmium laser and then stone fragments were removed. At the end of the procedure, the system may be examined with a flexible endoscope. The procedure was considered to have been completed when all removable stones have been taken out. Internal and/or and external drain(s) were positioned according to the judgment of the surgeon.

Statistical analysis

Statistical analysis was performed with IBM SPSS (version 25; IBM, New York, USA). To evaluate significant factors for severe bleeding after PCNL, chi-square, Fisher's exact tests were used for the categorical variables. The independent *t*-test, Pearson correlation, and Mann–Whitney *U* test were used for the analysis of quantitative variables. To identify predictive factors associated with severe bleeding, multivariable logistic regression was used, and the corresponding odds ratios (ORs) and 95% confidence intervals (CIs) were determined. All p values were two-tailed, and a p value of < 0.05 was considered statistically significant.

Results

Of the 2981 patients who received PCNL, In accordance with the modified Clavien score [15], the mild bleeding group included 22 patients (22 blood transfusions), and the severe bleeding group included 48 patients (45 angioembolization, 2 multiple bladder washouts, 1 nephrectomy and ICU management). The mean ± SD age of 70 patients was 57.5 ± 13.7, and men accounted for 72.9%. The mean ± SD BMI was 22.6 ± 3.1 kg/m^2. According to our preoperative assessment, 62.9% of the cases suffered from flank pain, 7.1% of patients presented with a history of haematuria, and 92.9% had a history of previous urinary tract infections. Hypertension and chronic renal disease, accounting for 42.9% and 32.9% of the cohort, were two of the most common comorbidities. A total of

4.3% of the patients had a history of using anticoagulant medication.

A preoperative test revealed an IQR serum creatinine of 81.5 μmol/L (67.8–127.5). According to the preoperative imaging, 50.0% of patients of major bleeding had staghorn calculi. A total of 57.1% of the patient's calculi were located in the left kidney, and multiple calculi were present in 71.4% of the cases. A total of 71.4% of the patients had no hydronephrosis or only a mild degree of hydronephrosis. A total of 28.6% of the patients presented with a mid or severe degree of hydronephrosis. The pole access was used the upper calyx in 0 cases, the middle calyx in 63 cases, the lower calyx in 1 cases and multiple calyx the upper in 6 cases. The average corrected intraoperative haemoglobin drop from the pre-PCNL to the first post-PCNL day was 20.6 ± 15.2 g/dL (range 0–68). The mean OT was 108.5 ± 39.9 (range 31–236) minutes. Occurrence times of management strategy of the highest Clavien grade in final analysis were ranged from 1 to 24 days after PCNL.

Table 1 shows a comparison of the patient demographics, preoperative clinical characteristics and renal stone characteristics between mild bleeding complications and severe bleeding complications. Staghorn calculi

Table 1 Patient demographic, preoperative clinical characteristics and renal stone characteristics

No. pts (%)	Major bleeding complication	Mild bleeding complication	Severe bleeding complication	*p*
	70	22	48	
Sex (%)				
Male	51 (72.9)	14 (63.6)	37 (77.1)	0.240
Female	19 (27.1)	8 (36.4)	11 (22.9)	
Age (years, mean ± SD)	57.5 (13.7)	59.3 (13.6)	56.7 (13.8)	0.471
BMI (kg/m^2, mean ± SD)	22.6 (3.1)	21.8 (3.1)	23.0 (3.0)	0.139
Preop creatinine (μmol/L, IQR)	81.5 (67.8–127.5)	83.0 (70.5–163.8)	80.5 (67.0–124.0)	0.494
History of anticoagulation (%)	3 (4.3)	2 (9.1)	1 (2.1)	0.231
Preop clinical (%)				
Pain	44 (62.9)	12 (54.5)	32 (66.7)	0.330
Hematuria	5 (7.1)	1 (4.5)	4 (8.3)	1.000
UTIs	65 (92.9)	20 (90.9)	45 (93.8)	0.646
Preop. comborbidities (%)				
Hypertension	30 (42.9)	12 (54.5)	18 (37.5)	0.181
Diabetes mellitus	11 (15.7)	4 (19.0)	7 (14.6)	0.725
Ischemic heart disease	14 (20.0)	6 (27.3)	8 (16.7)	0.344
Chronic lung disease	6 (8.6)	2 (9.1)	4 (8.3)	1.000
Chronic kidney disease	23 (32.9)	7 (31.8)	16 (33.3)	0.900
At least 1	48 (68.6)	18 (81.8)	30 (62.5)	0.106
Open surgery history (%)	11 (15.7)	6 (27.3)	5 (10.4)	0.088
History of PCNL (%)	11 (15.7)	5 (22.7)	6 (12.5)	0.303
Calculi side (%)				
Lt	40 (57.1)	11 (50.0)	29 (60.4)	0.414
Rt	30 (42.9)	11 (50.0)	19 (39.6)	
Stone count (%)				
Single	20 (28.6)	7 (31.8)	13 (27.1)	0.684
Multiple	50 (71.4)	15 (68.2)	35 (72.9)	
Stone type (%)				
Staghorn[a]	35 (50.0)	16 (72.7)	19 (39.6)	0.010
Others	35 (50.0)	6 (27.3)	29 (60.4)	
peak Hounsfield unit (Hu, IQR)	1095.0 (735.0–1406.0)	1282.0 (723.5–1506.3)	1086.0 (710.0–1334.0)	0.425
Hydronephrosis (%)				
None or mild	50 (71.4)	12 (54.5)	38 (79.2)	0.034
Moderate or severe	20 (28.6)	10 (45.5)	10 (20.8)	

UTIs urinary tract infections, *BMI* body mass index, *IQR* interquartile range

[a] Any branched stone occupying more than one portion of the collecting system

Table 2 Perioperative characteristics

No. pts (%)	Major bleeding complication	Mild bleeding complication	Severe bleeding complication	*p*
	70	22	48	
OT (min, mean ± SD)	108.5 (39.9)	119.2 (41.7)	103.4 (38.4)	0.127
Corrected intraoperative hemoglobin drop (g/dL, mean ± SD)	20.6 (15.2)	19.8 (18.0)	20.9 (13.9)	0.785
Dilatation type (%)				
Amplatz	51 (72.9)	16 (72.7)	35 (72.9)	0.987
Balloon	19 (27.1)	6 (27.3)	13 (27.1)	
No. renal accesses (%)				
Single	64 (91.4)	20 (90.9)	44 (91.7)	1.000
Multiple	6 (8.6)	2 (9.1)	4 (8.3)	
Pole access (%)				0.697
Upper calyx	0 (0)	0 (0)	0 (0)	
Mid calyx	63 (90)	19 (86.4)	44 (91.7)	
Lowe calyx	1 (1.4)	1 (4.5)	0 (0)	0.314
Multiple calyx	6 (8.6)	2 (9.1)	4 (8.3)	

OT operative time

Table 3 Multivariate analysis of severe bleeding complication after percutaneous nephrolithotomy

	OR (95% CI)	*p*
Staghorn	0.218 (0.068–0.700)	0.010
Hydronephrosis	0.271 (0.083–0.887)	0.031

OR corresponding odds ratio, *CIs* confidence interval

Table 4 Major bleeding complications by modified Clavien score

	Clavien category	No. cases
2	Bleeding requiring blood transfusion	22
3a	Bleeding requiring multiple bladder washouts	2
3b	Bleeding managed by angioembolisation	45
4a	Bleedingrequiring ICU management	1
Total		70

($p = 0.010$) and the degree of hydronephrosis ($p = 0.034$) were significantly related to severe bleeding complications in univariate analysis. None of perioperative characteristics were significantly associated with severe bleeding complications in Table 2. Multivariate analysis showed that only the absence of staghorn stones (OR, 95% CI, *p* value 0.218, 0.068–0.700, 0.010) and none or mild degree of hydronephrosis (OR, 95% CI, *p* value 0.271, 0.083–0.887, 0.031) were a higher risk of severe bleeding in Table 3. The mild and severe bleeding complications are shown in Table 4. By the modified Clavien

Table 5 Angiographic findings in 45 patients

Angiographic findings	No. cases
Contast extravasation	26
PA	8
AVF	4
PA and AVF	2
PA and Contast extravasation	3
AVF and Contast extravasation	2

PA Pseudoaneurysm, *AVF* Arteriovenous fistula

score. 45 cases' bleeding complications were managed by angioembolization and their angiographic findings are shown in Table 5.

Discussion

PCNL plays an indispensable role in treating large kidney stones [16]. Since PCNL was popularized in 1976 [15], it has been proven to be a valid procedure for the removal of kidney stones after decades of surgical experience.

Bleeding complications after PCNL are dangerous or even life-threatening. Conservative treatment can be used to control venous haemorrhage, while arterial lesions are rare but require immediate intervention. Several studies have shown that the occurrence of blood transfusions caused by PCNL varies widely, from 1 to 5% [4, 17]. The rate of postoperative angioembolization is not high, ranging from 0 to 1.5% [18]. Due to the simple treatment methods, such as using intravenous fluid without blood transfusion, requiring a single episode of nephrostomy clamping or skin compression/pressure dressing [19], minor bleeding only poses a slight threat to patients and has a lower rate of agreement with urologists [9], and therefore cases of bleeding complications classified as Clavien 1 were not included in this research.

Several studies have identified prognostic factors for severe bleeding complications after PCNL [2, 3, 10, 20]. However, due to the absence of standardized reporting classification systems, their results are difficult to interpret and compare. Sitki et al. [3] showed that the predictors for severe bleeding complications were stone load and renal abnormalities. However, this study evaluated risk factors for post-PCNL bleeding that required embolization from blood transfusion so these cases of direct angioembolization without a blood transfusion have been ignored. Therefore, we evaluated bleeding complications in accordance with the modified Clavien scoring system, which is advised when reporting urological operation outcomes [16, 21].

Severe postoperative bleeding is a challenge to both the patient and the surgeon. Our analysis sought to identify prognostic factors for severe bleeding complications after PCNL in our hospital. In this study, we found that staghorn calculi and the degree of hydronephrosis were related to severe bleeding complications. In multivariate analysis, no staghorn calculi and none or mild hydronephrosis were significant predictors of the severe bleeding.

Staghorn stones represent 10–20% of all nephrolithiasis cases [22]. In our experience, the absence of staghorn calculi is a predictor of severe bleeding post-PCNL. Previous studies have come to inconsistent conclusions. In previous studies, the presence of staghorn stones [23, 24] was a predictor of severe postoperative bleeding. Zehri et al. reported [23] that the occurrence of staghorn stones can significantly predict severe vascular lesions after PCNL. In El-Nahas's [24] study, vascular embolization was needed in 39 of 3878 patients undergoing PCNL, and multivariate analysis found that staghorn stones were a significant risk factor. One explanation is that staghorn stones may prolong the operative time, leading to an increased chance of bleeding after surgery.

However, the conclusions of these studies were not different from the common bleeding complications reported by other studies after PCNL [17, 25, 26] and were not consistent with the results of our study. One reason for this may be that previous studies have compared outcomes in patients who underwent embolization with those who did not have any bleeding complications, while in our study, risk factors for severe bleeding were only discussed in patients with bleeding complications of greater than Clavien 2 as reported by the modified Clavien scoring system. Another reason for presence of staghorn calculi predicting mild bleeding may be that the patients formating staghorn stones without obvious symptoms leading to medical treatment indicate that the kidneys of them may have a better tolerance than these of no staghorn stones that occur less severe bleeding complication after PCNL.

In this study, mild or absence of hydronephrosis was observed to be associated with an increased risk of severe bleeding complications following PCNL. This result is consistent with the research of Lee et al. [27]: no hydronephrosis was a predictor for severe bleeding after PCNL. Similarly, Hee et al. stated that a lack of hydronephrosis was an important risk factor for transfusion in conventional PCNL [28]. Senocak et al. [13] found that the degree of hydronephrosis was significantly related to the reduction of blood loss during paediatric PCNL. Wang et al. [29] reported that no hydronephrosis occurred in patients with severe renal haemorrhage.

There are several possible explanations for the findings of our study. Patients without moderate or severe hydronephrosis may have a thicker renal parenchyma, which increases the risk of severe bleeding from puncture. Moderate and severe hydronephrosis can lead to thinning of the renal cortex and eventually ischaemia, which may be related to reduced renal blood flow. Another possible explanation is that none or mild hydronephrosis may reduce the availability of calculi and thus requiring more manipulation during the surgery, which may cause larger lesions to renal vessels and parenchyma.

In Sitki's [3] study, the risk factors were analysed for bleeding complications that required renal arterial embolization and blood transfusion, and the stone load, renal abnormalities, and the mean corrected haemoglobin drop predicted severe bleeding after PCNL. Tan et al. [10] demonstrated that severe haemorrhage after PCNL is related to lower calyx puncture and multiple kidney stones. Diabetes was a predictor of bleeding in both studies [13, 25]. In our study, factors such as BMI, hypertension, diabetes, chronic kidney disease, corrected haemoglobin drop, site of punctured calyx, and multiple stones did not have any significant correlation with severe bleeding. This suggests that these covariates may be predictors for postoperative blood loss in general but not for severe bleeding complications.

The significance of this study is that in patients who have already experienced relatively observable bleeding, those who have no staghorn stones and/or none or mild hydronephrosis preoperatively need to be managed carefully because they are more likely to have severe bleeding complications. PCNL patients with none or mild hydronephrosis may benefit from retrograde intrarenal surgery [30] with a holmium laser and may be ideal candidates for its use. The findings of this study may play a role in the surgical decision-making for patients with renal stones.

Several limitations exist in our study. First, any retrospective study may result in an underestimate of postoperative bleeding complications. However, patients with bleeding complications of greater than Clavien 2 are hardly ignored because further or invasive operations are required, which is why we focused on this group. Second, the sample size of this study was small, which had a certain impact on the results, but samples with severe bleeding are difficult to obtain. Moreover, all PCNLs in our hospital were conducted in the prone position, so these findings may not be applicable to PCNLs performed in the supine position.

Conclusions

After reviewing our experience with PCNL, we identified predictors of severe bleeding postoperatively. Absence of staghorn stones or no/mild hydronephrosis were independently associated with the high risk of severe bleeding. In patients with obvious bleeding, it is necessary to take extreme precautions for those with no staghorn stones and/or none or mild hydronephrosis such that preventive measures against severe bleeding can be taken to reduce the threat to their lives (Additional file 1).

Abbreviations

PCNL: Percutaneous nephrolithotomy; UTIs: Urinary tract infections; EAU: European Association of Urology; CT: Computed tomography; BMI: Body mass index; APD: Anteroposterior diameter; OT: Operative time; ORs: Corresponding odds ratios; CIs: Confidence intervals; ICU: Intensive Care Unit; IQR: Interquartile range.

Acknowledgements

Not applicable.

Authors' contributions

XD, WJ, DW, SY, HH Project development; XD, WP, CC Data collection or management; XD, HZ Data analysis; XD Manuscript writing; PP, XD, WP Manuscript editing. The authors read and approved the final manuscript.

Competing interests

The authors declare that they have no competing interests.

Author details

[1]Department of Radiology, Taizhou Hospital, Zhejiang University, Taizhou 318000, Zhejiang, China. [2]Department of Urology, Taizhou Hospital of Zhejiang Province, Taizhou 318000, Zhejiang, China. [3]Department of Radiology, School of Medicine, Sir Run Run Shaw Hospital, Zhejiang University, Hangzhou 310023, Zhejiang, China. [4]Department of Pharmaceuticals Diagnosis, GE Healthcare, Hangzhou, China.

References

1. Turk C, Petrik A, Sarica K, et al. EAU guidelines on interventional treatment for urolithiasis. Eur Urol. 2016;69:475–82. https://doi.org/10.1016/j.eururo.2015.07.04.
2. Kim HY, Lee KW, Lee DS. Critical causes in severe bleeding requiring angioembolization after percutaneous nephrolithotomy. BMC Urol. 2020;20(1):22.
3. Li Z, Wu A, Liu J, et al. Risk factors for hemorrhage requiring embolization after percutaneous nephrolithotomy: a meta-analysis. Transl Androl Urol. 2020;9(2):210–7.
4. Seitz C, Desai M, Häcker A, et al. Incidence, prevention, and management of complications following percutaneous nephrolitholapaxy. Eur Urol. 2012;61(1):146–58.
5. Moriarty MA, Uhlman MA, Bing MT, et al. Evaluating the safety of intraop erative instillation of intravesical chemotherapy at the time of nephroure terectomy. BMC Urol. 2015;15:45.
6. De la Rosette J, Assimos D, Desai M, et al. The Clinical Research Office of the Endourological Society Percutaneous Nephrolithotomy Global Study: indications, complications, and outcomes in 5803 patients. J Endourol. 2011;25(1):11–7.
7. Dindo D, Demartines N, Clavien PA. Classification of surgical complications: a new proposal with evaluation in a cohort of 6336 patients and results of a survey. Ann Surg. 2004;240(2):205–13.
8. Mitropoulos D, Artibarni W, Graefen M, Remzi M, Roupret M, Truss M. Reporting and grading of complications after urologic surgical procedures: an ad hoc EAU guidelines panel assessment and recommendations. Eur Urol. 2012;61(2):341–49.
9. de la Rosette JJMCH, Opondo D, Daels FPJ, et al. Categorisation of complications and validation of the Clavien score for percutaneous nephrolithotomy. Eur Urol. 2012;62(2):246–55.
10. Tan J, Chen B, He L, et al. Renal access through the inferior calyx is associated with higher risk of severe bleeding after percutaneous nephrolithotomy. Arch Med Sci. 2015;11(2):340–5.
11. Mishra S, Sabnis RB, Desai MR. Percutaneous nephrolithotomy monotherapy for staghorn: paradigm shift for "staghorn morphometry" based clinical classification. Curr Opin Urol. 2012;22(2):148–53.
12. Fernbach SK, Maizels M, Conway JJ. Ultrasound grading of hydronephrosis: introduction to the system used by the Society for Fetal Urology. Pediatr Radiol. 1993;23(6):478–80.
13. Senocak C, Ozbek R, Bozkurt OF, Unsal A. Predictive factors of bleeding among pediatric patients undergoing percutaneous nephrolithotomy. Urolithiasis. 2018;46(4):383–9.
14. Mehran R, Rao SV, Bhatt DL, et al. Standardized bleeding definitions for cardiovascular clinical trials: a consensus report from the Bleeding Academic Research Consortium. Circulation. 2011;123(23):2736–47.
15. Fernström I, Johansson B. Percutaneous pyelolithotomy: a new extraction technique. Scand J Urol Nephrol. 1976;10(3):257–9.
16. Roodneshin F, Poor Zamany Nejat Kermany M, Rostami P, Ahmadzadeh N, Gharaei B, Kamranmanesh MR. Comparison of hemodynamic stability and pain control in lateral and prone positions in patients undergoing percutaneous nephrolithotomy: a randomized controlled trial. Urol J. 2020;17(2):124–8.
17. Keoghane SR, Cetti RJ, Rogers AE, Walmsley BH. Blood transfusion, embolization and nephrectomy after percutaneous nephrolithotomy. BJU Int. 2013;111:628–32.
18. Siskin GP, Englander M, Stainken BF, Ahn J, Dowling K, Dolen EG. Embolic agents used for uterine fibroid embolization. AJR Am J Roentgenol. 2000;175:767–73.
19. Nuño de la Rosa I, Palmero JL, Miralles J, Amorós A, Ferrer MD, Esteban E. Treatment of hemorrhagic complications of percutaneous nephrolithotomy in Galdakao position. Actas Urol Esp. 2013;37:587–91.
20. Dong X, Ren Y, Han P, et al. Superselective renal artery embolization management of post-percutaneous nephrolithotomy hemorrhage and its methods. Front Surg. 2020;7:582261.
21. Opondo D, Gravas S, Joyce A, et al. Standardization of patient outcomes reporting in percutaneous nephrolithotomy. J Endourol. 2014;28(7):767–74.
22. Mohammadi Sichani M, Jafarpisheh A, Ghoreifi A. Evaluation and comparison of metabolic disorders between patients with unilateral and bilateral staghorn renal stones. Urol J. 2019;16(3):242–5.
23. Zehri AA, Biyabani SR, Siddiqui KM, Memon A. Triggers of blood transfusion in percutaneous nephrolithotomy. J Coll Phys Surg Pak JCPSP. 2011;21(3):138–41.
24. El-Nahas AR, Shokeir AA, El-Assmy AM, Mohsen T, Shoma AM, Eraky I, et al. Post-percutaneous nephrolithotomy extensive hemorrhage: a study of risk factors. J Urol. 2007;177(2):576–9.

25. Akman T, Binbay M, Sari E, Yuruk E, Tepeler A, Akcay M, et al. Factors affecting bleeding during percutaneous nephrolithotomy: single surgeon experience. J Endourol. 2011;25(2):327–33.
26. Jinga V, Dorobat B, Youssef S, et al. Transarterial embolization of renal vascular lesions after percutaneous nephrolithotomy. Chirurgia (Bucur). 2013;108(4):521–9.
27. Lee JK, Kim BS, Park YK. Predictive factors for bleeding during percutaneous nephrolithotomy. Korean J Urol. 2013;54(7):448–53.
28. Kim HY, Choe HS, Lee DS, Yoo JM, Lee SJ. Is absence of hydronephrosis a risk factor for bleeding in conventional percutaneous nephrolithotomy. Urol J. 2020;17(1):8–13.
29. Wang Y, Jiang F, Wang Y, et al. Post-percutaneous nephrolithotomy septic shock and severe hemorrhage: a study of risk factors. Urol Int. 2012;88(3):307–10.
30. Gökce Mİ, Ibiş A, Sancı A, et al. Comparison of supine and prone positions for percutaneous nephrolithotomy in treatment of staghorn stones. Urolithiasis. 2017;45(6):603–8.

15

Transvaginal natural orifice specimen extraction surgery (NOSES) in 3D laparoscopic partial or radical nephrectomy

Qinxin Zhao[1†], Dongdong Han[1,2†], Feiya Yang[1], Sujun Han[1] and Nianzeng Xing[1*]

Abstract

Background: With the development of minimally invasive technology, more and more people pay attention to aesthetics of the wound after operation. This study is aim to introduce a new surgical technique of transvaginal natural orifice specimen extraction surgery (NOSES) in 3D laparoscopic partial or radical nephrectomy and evaluate the safety, feasibility and clinical effect.

Methods: Eleven patients who underwent 3D laparoscopic partial nephrectomy (n = 7) or radical nephrectomy (n = 4) and NOSES were included in this study. The surgical procedures and techniques, especially the NOSES operation, are reported in detail. In addition, the basic clinical data, perioperative related data, perioperative complications were analyzed.

Results: All 11 patients were performed successfully without conversion to open surgery. The mean total operative time was 133 (84, 150) min. NOSES time was 15 (13, 16) min, and the postoperative hospital stay was 5 (5, 5) d. The mean visual analogue score (VAS) was 3 (2, 4) point and 1 (0, 1) point at 24 h and 48 h after operation, respectively. No patient had recurrence, metastasis and death during the follow-up period of 3 to 17 months. The median Vancouver Scar Scale (VSS) was 1 (1, 1) point. The mean of Female Sexual Function Index (FSFI) was 21.60 (20.20, 21.60), 21.80 (19.80, 21.80) respectively between preoperative and postoperative 3 months, which has no statistical difference ($P = 0.179$). There was no statistical difference in the Pelvic Floor Distress Inventory-short form 20 (PFDI-20) score between preoperative and postoperative 3 months ($P = 0.142$).

Conclusions: Transvaginal NOSES is safe and feasible in 3D laparoscopic partial or radical nephrectomy. Furthermore, it results in low incision-related pain without affecting the pelvic floor and sexual function.

Keywords: Natural orifice specimen extraction surgery (NOSES), Laparoscopy, Partial nephrectomy, Radical nephrectomy, Renal carcinoma

Background

With the development of laparoscopic technology, more and more patients are pursuing the aesthetic condition of the wound after operation. Laparoscopic radical nephrectomy is still recommended for the operation of renal cancer, and partial nephrectomy or radical nephrectomy is recommended for unilateral renal tumors with T1a–T1b

*Correspondence: xingnianzeng@126.com
†Qinxin Zhao and Dongdong Han have contributed equally and shared first author
[1] Department of Urology, National Cancer Center/National Clinical Research Center for Cancer/Cancer Hospital, Chinese Academy of Medical Sciences and Peking Union Medical College, Beijing, People's Republic of China

stage or localized tumors [1, 2]. However, the traditional laparoscopic partial nephrectomy or radical nephrectomy are still using the median incision of the lower abdomen to remove specimens, which increase the pain feeling of patients after operation, and affect the wound healing and other related complications. Nowadays natural orifice specimen extraction surgery (NOSES) has attracted wide attention. Compared with the traditional operation, the amount of bleeding, length of hospital stays, and the time of the first postoperative exhaust are significantly better than the traditional laparoscopic specimen extraction [3, 4]. But there are relatively few studies on laparoscopic partial or radical nephrectomy plus transvaginal NOSES. Therefore, since July 2019, our center has performed partial nephrectomy or radical nephrectomy and transvaginal NOSES for 11 female patients and analyzed the relevant data of the patients preoperative and postoperative, and the report is as follows.

Methods

Basic clinical data

In this study, 11 patients with renal carcinoma underwent 3D laparoscopic partial nephrectomy or radical nephrectomy and transvaginal NOSES, 7 patients (63.63%) underwent laparoscopic partial nephrectomy and transvaginal NOSES, and 4 patients (36.36%) underwent laparoscopic radical nephrectomy and transvaginal NOSES. All patients were operated on by one experienced urologist. All patients received abdominal magnetic resonance or enhanced computed tomography or abdominal ultrasonography before surgery. Perioperative period, postoperative recovery, complications and oncologic prognosis were recorded. The study was approved by Research Ethics Committee of Cancer Hospital, Chinese Academy of Medical Sciences. All the patients agreed to participate in the study and signed the informed consent. All methods were carried out in accordance with relevant guidelines and regulations.

Indications and contraindications of NOSES

Indications for surgery: a. Estimate the size of surgical specimens can be taken out from the vagina; b. Married adult female patients; c. Preoperative imaging examination indicates possible renal cancer or renal cancer patients.

Absolute contraindications for surgery: a. Unmarried and infertile women; b. Contractile scar of vagina caused by trauma or surgery; c. Patients with intravaginal infection, cervical neoplasia or carcinogenesis, gynecological pelvic inflammation and other diseases that are not cured before surgery.

Relative contraindications: a. History of pelvic or lower abdominal surgery; b. Obesity.

Preoperative preparation

Bowel preparation: use glycerol enema machine for enema in the morning before operation; vaginal preparation: use Iodophor for vaginal irrigation 3 days before operation, once a day.

Surgical methods

Preparation steps

Under general anesthesia, the patient was placed in an oblique position of 70°. After disinfection with Iodophor in vagina, a piece of iodophor gauze ball was left to maintain pneumoperitoneal pressure. Figure 1 shows the location of Trocar.

Radical nephrectomy

a. Exposure of retroperitoneal tissue: Free fascial tissue of colon and abdominal cavity with ultrasound scalpel, and expose retroperitoneal tissue (Fig. 2A). b. Free ureter: Peel off the lower part of Gerota fascia with an ultrasonic scalpel, free the ureter, clamp with Hem-o-lock clip and cut off the ureter (Fig. 2B). c. Free renal artery and vein and ligation, cutting: Free along ureter and genital vein toward proximal end, free and fully expose renal vein, reveal renal artery behind it, clip renal artery with 3 Hem-o-locks and cut it (Fig. 2C), renal veins were treated in the same way (Fig. 2D). d. Preservation of adrenal

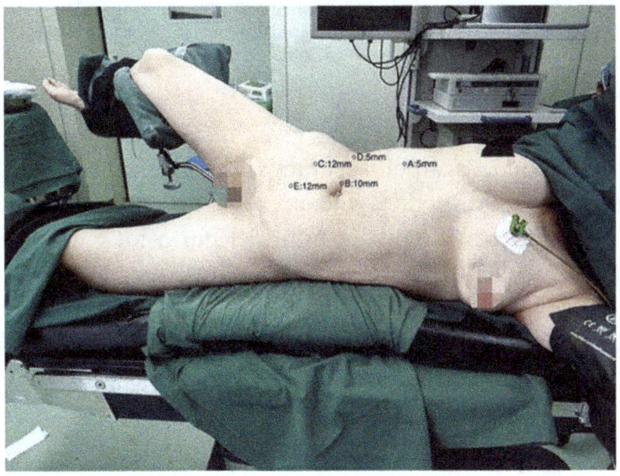

Fig. 1 The patient's position and location of trocar. The patient was placed in an oblique position of 70°. The location of trocar: A hole is located under the costal margin of the mid-clavicular line on the affected side, and 5 mm cannula is punctured into the abdominal cavity; B hole is located around the umbilicus and makes a longitudinal incision about 1 cm, and 10 mm Trocar cannula is placed into the laparoscope; C, D and E holes are located at the midpoint of the anterior superior iliac crest and umbilicus line on the affected 12 mm, 12 mm and 5 mm Trocar cannulas were placed at the horizontal intersection of axillary front line and umbilical cord for the placement of operating instruments

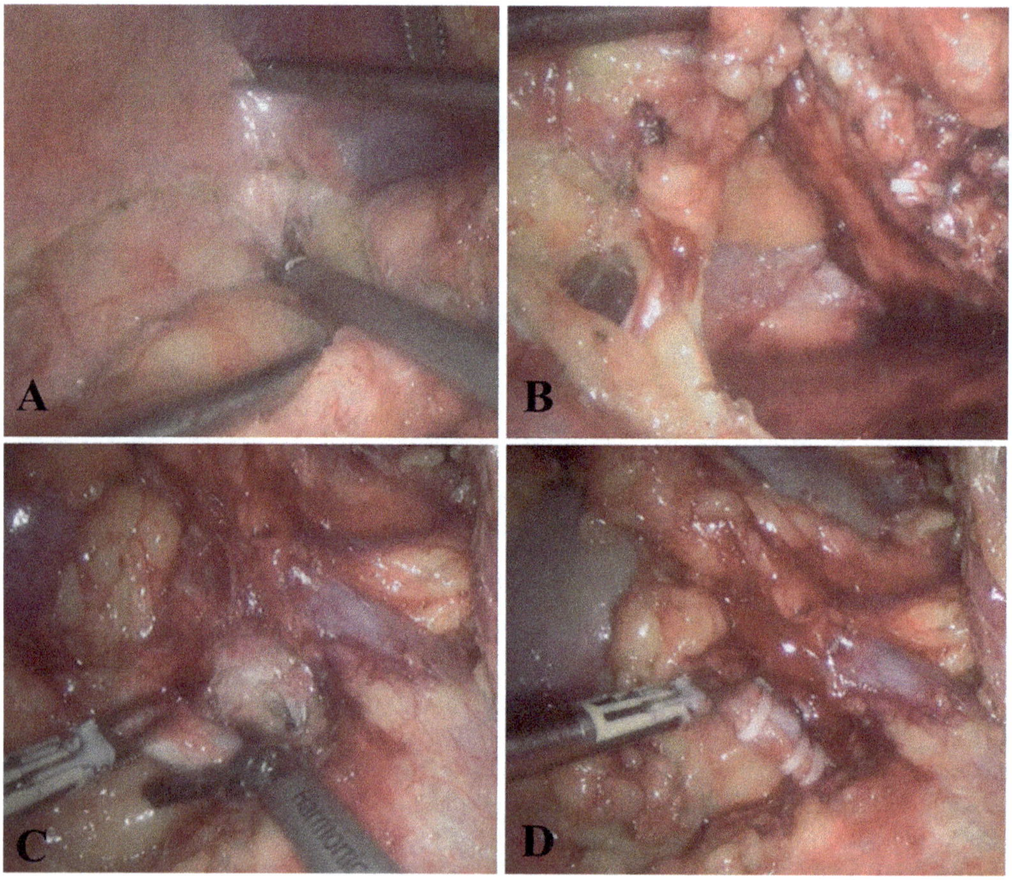

Fig. 2 Surgical procedures of laparoscopic radical nephrectomy. **A** Free fascial tissue of colon and abdominal cavity with ultrasound scalpel, and expose retroperitoneal tissue. **B** Peel off the lower part of Gerota fascia with an ultrasonic scalpel, free the ureter, clamp with Hem-o-lock clip and cut off the ureter. **C, D** Free along ureter and genital vein toward proximal end, expose renal vein, renal artery behind it, clip renal artery with 3 Hem-o-locks and cut it, renal veins were treated in the same way

gland: Peel off the anterior layer of Gerota fascia with an ultrasound scalpel, separate the perirenal fat toward the superior direction, and preserve the adrenal gland. e. Removal of kidney and tumor: Hem-o-lock was used to clamp the small blood vessels and lymphatic vessels around the renal hilum and cut them off. The kidney and tumor were completely free and removed.

Partial nephrectomy

a. Exposure of retroperitoneal tissue: Release the fascial tissue of the colon and abdominal cavity with an ultrasound scalpel, turn the hepatic or splenic flexure of the colon to the opposite side, expose the retroperitoneal tissue (Fig. 3A1-2). b. Separate the renal artery and vein: Separate the plane of the renal vein along the

(See figure on next page.)

Fig. 3 Surgical procedures of laparoscopic partial nephrectomy. a. Exposure of retroperitoneal tissue: Release the fascial tissue of the colon and abdominal cavity with an ultrasound scalpel, turn the hepatic or splenic flexure of the colon to the opposite side, expose the retroperitoneal tissue (**A1-2**). b. Separate the renal artery and vein: Separate the plane of the renal vein along the retroperitoneal and Gerota fascial space, free the renal vein, and find the renal artery behind the renal vein, free the renal artery (**B1-2**). c. Location of the tumor: Cut the perirenal fat capsule in the middle of the kidney to find the location of the tumor, free the adipose tissue around the tumor, expose the tumor at the boundary of normal kidney tissue, preserve the adipose tissue above the tumor (**C**), d. Resect the tumor: Block the main renal artery with vascular clips, and resect the tumor with scissors and aspirator 1 cm outside the edge of the tumor, together with part of normal kidney tissue (**D**). e. Hemostasis and suture: Initial hemostasis using bipolar electrocoagulation on the wound surface. The inner layer was sutured with 3-0 barbed suture, and the renal wound was sutured with 2-0 barbed coil layer, and the suture was fixed intermittently with Hem-o-lock (**E**). f. Restore blood flow and observe blood supply: Loosen the renal artery blocking clamp, observe whether the blood supply, color, elasticity of renal tissue are normal, whether there are obvious bleeding foci, and explore whether the ureter is normal, whether the urine color is normal (**F**). Protein glue can be used to plug the wound to assist hemostasis if necessary, and the perirenal fat capsule can be re-sutured

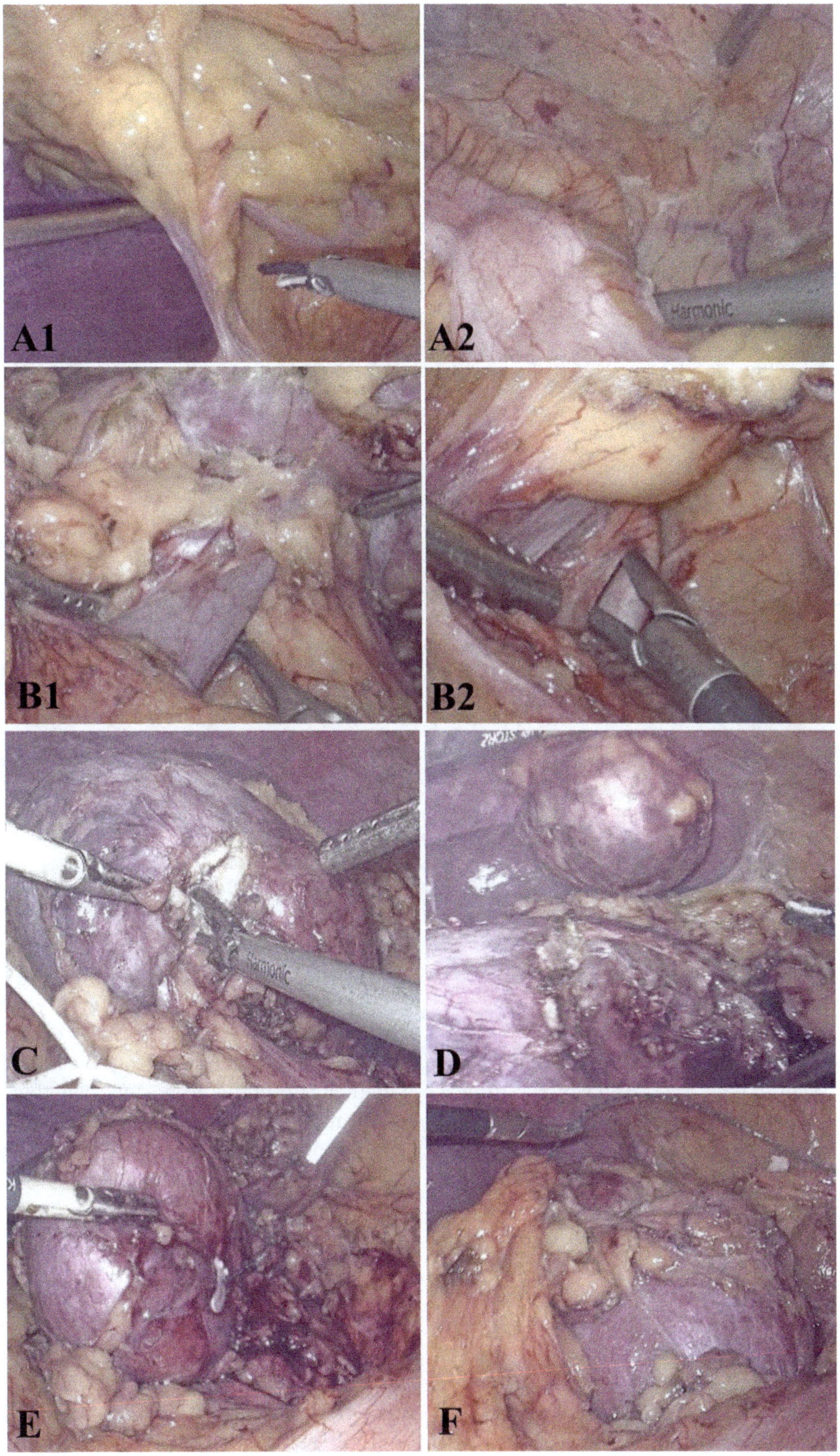

Fig. 3 (See legend on previous page.)

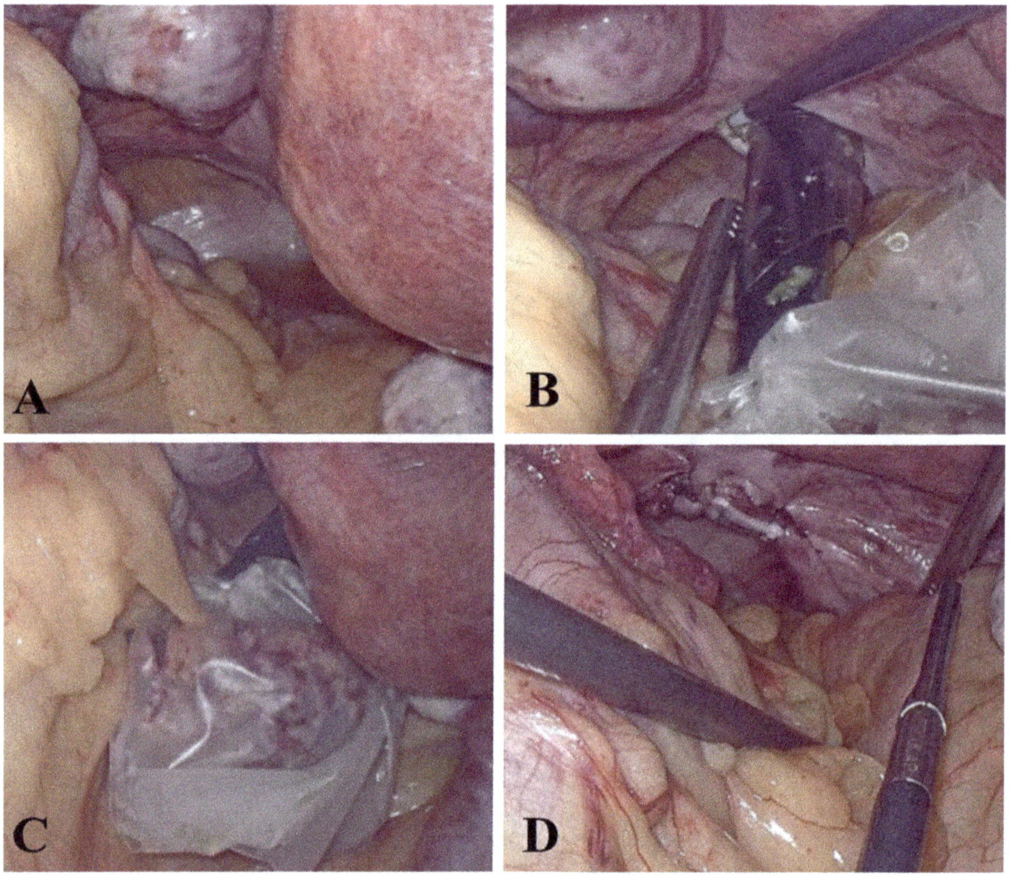

Fig. 4 Surgical procedures of laparoscopic transvaginal NOSES. The laparoscopic field of view was transferred to the pelvis, the posterior vaginal fornix was exposed (**A**), 12 mm Trocar was placed in the vagina which had been fully sterilized by gauze strips, and the posterior vaginal fornix was closely attached to the posterior vaginal fornix. The posterior vaginal fornix was transversely cut (**B**) with an electrocoagulation knife to both sides, so that the incision was about 2–3 cm long. The specimen band (**C**) was placed in the transvaginal Trocar, and the excised kidney and part of the ureter were placed into the specimen. Take out the band, hang the vagina with 2-0 barbed thread, and suture the vaginal incision and the posterior fornix exactly (**D**), and suture the lateral peritoneum with 2-0 barbed thread

retroperitoneal and Gerota fascial space, free the renal vein, and find the renal artery behind the renal vein, free the renal artery (Fig. 3B1-2). c. Location of the tumor: Cut the perirenal fat capsule in the middle of the kidney to find the location of the tumor, free the adipose tissue around the tumor, expose the tumor at the boundary of normal kidney tissue, preserve the adipose tissue above the tumor (Fig. 3C), d. Resect the tumor: Block the main renal artery with vascular clips, and resect the tumor with scissors and aspirator 1 cm outside the edge of the tumor, together with part of normal kidney tissue (Fig. 3D). e. Hemostasis and suture: Initial hemostasis using bipolar electrocoagulation on the wound surface. The inner layer was sutured with 3–0 barbed suture, and the renal wound was sutured with 2-0 barbed coil layer, and the suture was fixed intermittently with Hem-o-lock (Fig. 3E). f. Restore blood flow and observe blood supply: Loosen the renal artery blocking clamp, observe whether the blood supply, color, elasticity of renal tissue is normal, whether there are obvious bleeding foci, and explore whether the ureter is normal, whether the urine color is normal (Fig. 3F). Protein glue can be used to plug the wound to assist hemostasis if necessary, and the perirenal fat capsule can be re-sutured.

Transvaginal NOSES

The laparoscopic field of view was transferred to the pelvis, the posterior vaginal fornix was exposed (Fig. 4A), 12 mm Trocar was placed in the vagina which had been fully sterilized by gauze strips, and the posterior vaginal fornix was closely attached to the posterior vaginal fornix. The posterior vaginal fornix was transversely cut (Fig. 4B) with an electrocoagulation knife to both sides, so that the incision was about 2–3 cm long. The specimen band (Fig. 4C) was placed in the transvaginal Trocar, and the excised kidney and part of the ureter were placed into the specimen. Take out the band, hang the vagina with 2-0 barbed thread, and suture the vaginal incision and the posterior fornix exactly (Fig. 4D), and suture the lateral peritoneum with 2-0 barbed thread.

Evaluation of surgical effect

Total operation time, estimated intraoperative bleeding volume, intraoperative blood transfusion volume, postoperative creatinine value, postoperative ambulation time, recovery time to resume eating, first time to flatus, postoperative VAS score, postoperative follow-up data (including sexual function, pelvic floor function, vaginal posterior fornix and abdominal incision healing).

Statistical methods

The data was processed by IBM SPSS statistics v26.0. Continuous data were expressed by means and standard deviation and range. K-S test was used to check whether the preoperative and postoperative data conformed to normal distribution, and t test was used to verify whether the data conformed to normal distribution. Otherwise, rank sum test was used. The test result $P < 0.05$ represented statistical significance.

Results

All 11 patients were performed successfully without conversion to open surgery. The average of age was 50 (48, 61) years, the average of BMI was 21.3 (23.3, 25.0) kg/m^2. The Charlson Comorbidity Index (CCI) score was 1 (1, 2) point. The average of American Society of Anesthesiologists (ASA) score was 1 (1, 1) point (Table 1). Three patients (27.27%) had a previous history of abdominal surgery. The mean total operative time was 133 (84, 150). NOSES time was 15 (13, 16) min, and the postoperative hospital stay was 5 (5, 5) d. The time to resume eating was 1 (1, 2) d, and the time to ambulation was 1 (1, 1) d. The time to flatus was 2 (1, 2) d. The mean visual analogue score (VAS) was 3 (2, 4) point and 1 (0, 1) point at 24 h and 48 h after operation, respectively. Postoperative pathological results were clear cell carcinoma in 9 cases (81.82%), chromophobe cell carcinoma in one case (9.09%) and renal angiomyolipoma in one case (9.09%) (Table 2).

The follow-up time was 3–17 months. There were no related complications during the perioperative period. There were no complications such as abdominal distension, constipation, wound pain and so on (Table 3). For the follow-up of pelvic floor function. The mean of preoperative and postoperative 3 months Female Sexual Function Index (FSFI) was 21.60 (20.20, 21.60), 21.80 (19.80, 21.80) respectively, which has no statistical difference ($P = 0.179$). There was no statistical difference in the Pelvic Floor Distress Inventory-short form 20 (PFDI-20) score between preoperative and postoperative 3 months ($P = 0.142$). The median Vancouver Scar Scale (VSS) was 1 (1, 1) point. (Table 4). The trocar wound healed well and was close to the surrounding normal skin tissue, with almost no mark.

Table 1 Base information of all 11 patients

Variables	Data
Patient, n	11
Age [median, (IQR)], y	50 (48, 61)
BMI [median, (IQR)], kg/m^2	21.3 (23.3, 25.0)
CCI [median, (IQR)]	1 (1, 2)
ASA score, n (%)	
1	10 (90.91%)
2	1 (9.09%)
Abdominal surgery history, n (%)	3 (27.27%)
Partial nephrectomy, n (%)	7 (63.63%)
Radical nephrectomy, n (%)	4 (36.36%)

BMI body mass index, *CCI* Charlson Comorbidity Index, *ASA* American Society of Anesthesiologists

Table 2 Perioperative data of all 11 patients

Variables	Data
Postoperative hospital stays [median, (IQR)], d	5 (5, 5)
Estimated blood lose [median, (IQR)], ml	20 (10, 30)
Transfusion, n (%)	0 (0%)
Total operation time [median, (IQR)], min	133 (84, 150)
NOSES time [median, (IQR)], min	15 (13, 16)
Specimen size [median, (IQR)], cm	6 (4.5, 13)
VAS score [median, (IQR)]	
24 h	3 (2, 4)
48 h	1 (0, 1)
Final pathologic stage	
Clear cell carcinoma, n (%)	9 (81.82%)
Chromophobe cell carcinoma, n (%)	1 (9.09%)
Renal angiomyolipoma, n (%)	1 (9.09%)
T1a	5 (45.45%)
T1b	5 (45.45%)
T2	0 (0%)
T3	1 (9.09%)
T4	0 (0%)
Pathologic stage	
N0	0 (0%)
N1	0 (0%)
N2	0 (0%)
N3	0 (0%)

NOSES natural orifice specimen extraction surgery, *VAS* visual analogue scale

Table 3 Follow up data of all 11 patients

Variables	Data
Follow-up time [median, (IQR)], m	6 (4, 15)
VSS score [median, (IQR)]	1 (1, 1)
Recurrence, n (%)	0 (0%)
Metastasis, n (%)	0 (0%)
Overall survival, n%	11 (100%)

VSS Vancouver Scar Scale

Table 4 Preoperative and postoperative sexual function and pelvic floor function contrast of all 11 patients

Variables	Data		
	Preoperative at 3 months [median, (IQR)]	Postoperative at 3 months [median, (IQR)]	*P*
PFDI-20	7 (5, 8)	7 (3, 9)	0.142
FSFI	21.60 (20.20, 21.60)	21.80 (19.80, 21.80)	0.179

PFDI-20 pelvic floor distress inventory-short form 20, *FSFI* Female Sexual Function Index

Discussion

With the development of minimally invasive technology, people gradually start to pay more attention to the quality of life and wound aesthetics after surgery. It is well known that laparoscopic partial nephrectomy or radical nephrectomy is currently one of the most effective treatment modalities for renal cancer. But intraoperatively, it is not possible to avoid removing specimens from the abdominal wall incision, consequently increasing postoperative complications such as slower wound healing, increased postoperative pain, and increased infection.

In 1993. Breda et al. [5] reported that the retrieval of specimens from the vaginal natural cavity reduced the disadvantages of extended wound retrieval specimens. However, there is no complete standard and guideline reference for intraperitoneal specimen retrieval in women, so we aimed to do the above studies to explore the feasibility and efficacy of NOSES in 3D laparoscopic partial or radical nephrectomy. Several studies [6, 7] have shown that transvaginal specimen retrieval surgery achieved promising clinical results. In a meta-analysis summarizing 665 patients who underwent surgery via NOSES versus 772 via conventional laparoscopy, patients showed no significant difference in terms of postoperative recurrence rate, postoperative pain, hospital stay, time to first flatus, aesthetic outcome of the wound, and wound infection compared with conventional laparoscopy [8]. But some scholars believe that transvaginal NOSES may cause problems with tumor implantation or wound infection, one meta-analysis concluded that there was no significant difference in oncological outcomes between the NOSES group and the traditional abdominal incision group [9]. Similar results were obtained by Gao et al. [10] who showed no significant difference in 3-year overall survival and disease-free survival between the two groups. In our study, patients did not experience tumor recurrence, implant metastasis within the follow-up date, and also did not experience infection problems in their perioperative wounds, which were more desirable than those of conventional surgery.

Recently, some scholars have used the natural orifice endoscopic surgery (NOTES) in obstetrics and gynecological surgery, urological surgery, and gastrointestinal surgery [11, 12]. However, transvaginal NOTES surgery requires dedicated instruments, and the surgical difficulty is high, with a long learning curve, at present, there are still a small number of developing clinical NOTES at home and abroad, which also makes it difficult to generalize and clinical application [13–15].

The NOSES procedure can be performed without special instruments, and we developed the relevant surgical methods and precautions of transvaginal NOSES in partial nephrectomy or radical nephrectomy based on the above experience. During the operation, we placed a retractable specimen bag, put the specimen into it, and tighten one end of the bag to take the specimen out visually, which can prevent the spread and implantation of tumors. In terms of posterior vaginal vault wound, we use 2-0 barbed suture to avoid fistula and muscle damage in the wound. At the same time, NOSES should also protect the female uterus and adnexa, although the malleability of the female vagina is better, to prevent patients from postoperative pelvic floor dysfunction. We do not recommend NOSES surgery in patients with bulky tumors or already existing metastases. In our study, no patient had vaginal prolapse, labored urination and suffered oncological recurrence. In addition, patients were satisfied with wound healing during the postoperative follow-up time. Most studies [16, 17] have shown that patients do not experience impaired sexual function after transvaginal fornix incision specimen retrieval, and the sexual function of surgical patients, which was consistent with our findings.

Conclusions

To sum up, transvaginal NOSES is safe and feasible in 3D laparoscopic partial or radical nephrectomy. Furthermore, it results in low incision-related pain without affecting the pelvic floor and sexual function. However, the number of cases is small, and multicenter randomized controlled trials with more cases are needed to further evaluate and verify this conclusion.

Abbreviations

NOSES: Nature orifice specimen extraction surgery; VAS: Visual analogue score; VSS: Vancouver Scar Scale; FSFI: Female Sexual Function Index; PFDI-20: Pelvic Floor Distress Inventory-short form 20; BMI: Body mass index; CCI: Charlson Comorbidity Index; ASA: American Society of Anesthesiologists; NOTES: Natural orifice endoscopic surgery.

Acknowledgements

Not applicable.

Authors' contributions

QXZ: Manuscript writing, data collection and management, and manuscript editing. DDH: Data collection and management, data analysis, and manuscript writing. FYY: Data collection and management. SJH: Data analysis and management. NZX: Project development, and manuscript editing. All authors read and approved the final manuscript.

Competing interests

The authors declare that they have no competing interests.

Author details

[1]Department of Urology, National Cancer Center/National Clinical Research Center for Cancer/Cancer Hospital, Chinese Academy of Medical Sciences and Peking Union Medical College, Beijing, People's Republic of China.
[2]Department of Urology, Beijing Chaoyang Hospital, Capital Medical University, Beijing, People's Republic of China.

References

1. Motzer RJ, Jonasch E, Boyle S, et al. NCCN guidelines insights: kidney cancer, version 1.2021. J Natl Compr Canc Netw. 2020;18(9):1160–70.
2. Hsieh JJ, Purdue MP, Signoretti S, et al. Renal cell carcinoma. Nat Rev Dis Primers. 2017;3:17009–28.
3. Wolthuis AM, Overstraeten ADBV, D'Hoore A. Laparoscopic naturalorifice specimen extraction-colectomy: a systematic review. World J Gastroenterol. 2014;20(36):12981–92.
4. Wolthuis AM, Fieuws S, Van Den Bosch A, et al. Randomized clinical trial of laparoscopic colectomy with or without natural-orifice specimen extraction. Br J Surg. 2015;102(6):630–7.
5. Breda G, Silvestre P, Giunta A, et al. Laparoscopic nephrectomy with vaginal delivery of the intact kidney. Eur Urol. 1993;24(1):116–7.
6. Palanivelu C, Rangarajan M, Jategaonkar PA, et al. An innovative technique for colorectal specimen retrieval: a new era of "natural orifice specimen extraction" (NOSE). Dis Colon Rectum. 2008;51(7):1120–4.
7. Efetov SK, Tulina IA, Kim VD, et al. Natural orifice specimen extraction (NOSE) surgery with rectal eversion and total extra-abdominal resection. Tech Coloproctol. 2019;23(9):899–902.
8. Lin J, Lin S, Chen Z, et al. Meta-analysis of natural orifice specimen extraction versus conventional laparoscopy for colorectal cancer. Langenbecks Arch Surg. 2020;406:283–99.
9. Wolthuis AM, de Buck van Overstraeten A, D'Hoore A. Laparoscopic natural orifice specimen extraction-colectomy: a systematic review. World J Gastroenterol. 2014;20(36):12981–92.
10. Gao G, Chen L, Luo R, et al. Short- and long-term outcomes for transvaginal specimen extraction versus minilaparotomy after robotic anterior resection for colorectal cancer: a mono-institution retrospective study. World J Surg Oncol. 2020;18(1):190.
11. KaoukJH HGP, Goel RK, et al. Pure natural orifice translumenal endoscopic surgery (NOTES) transvaginal nephrectomy. Eur Urol. 2010;57:723–6.
12. Zou X, et al. Natural orifice transluminal endoscopic surgery in urology: the Chinese experience. Asian J Urol. 2020;7(1):1–9.
13. Zou X, Zhang G, Yuan Y, et al. Pure transvaginal natural orifice translumenal endoscopic surgery for renal cyst decortication: report of initial five cases. Int J Urol. 2014;21(1):64–8.
14. Xue Y, Zou X, Zhang G, et al. Transvaginal natural orifice transluminal endoscopic nephrectomy in a series of 63 cases: stepwise transition from hybrid to pure NOTES. Eur Urol. 2015;68(2):302–10.
15. Bazzi WM, Stroup SP, Cohen SA, et al. Comparison of transrectal and transvaginal hybrid natural orifice transluminal endoscopic surgery partial nephrectomy in the porcine model. Urology. 2013;82(1):84–9.
16. Letticè S, Sener TE, Lucan VC, et al. Hybrid transvaginal NOTES nephrectomy: postoperative sexual outcomes. A three-center matched study. Urology. 2017;99:131–5.
17. Linke GR, Luz S, Janczak J, et al. Evaluation of sexual function in sexually active women 1 year after transvaginal NOTES: a prospective cohort study of 106 patients. Langenbecks Arch Surg. 2013;398:139–45.

16

Minimally invasive management versus open surgery in the treatment of penetrating bladder injuries

John Culhane[1*], Johar Raza Syed[1] and Sameer Siddiqui[2]

Abstract

Background: While blunt extra-peritoneal bladder injury is typically treated non-operatively or with minimally invasive management, the treatment for penetrating bladder injury is generally open surgery. We identify a group of patients with penetrating bladder injury who were treated with minimally invasive management and compare the results with those who underwent traditional open surgical treatment.

Methods: This retrospective cohort study analyzes penetrating bladder injuries from a single trauma center from 2012 through 2019, and from the National Trauma Data Bank for 2016 and 2017. Mortality, complications, and length of stay were compared for minimally invasive management versus open surgery. We used Chi square to test significance for categorical variables, Mann–Whitney U test for ordinal variables, and T-test for continuous variables. Multivariate analysis was performed with multiple logistic, ordinal, and linear regression.

Results: Local: 117 (0.63%) had a bladder injury; 30 (25.6%) were penetrating. 6 (20.0%) were successfully treated with minimally invasive management with no complication versus 24 complications in 11 patients (45.8%) for open surgery ($p = 0.047$). Open surgical management was not a significant independent predictor of mortality or hospital length of stay. National Trauma Data Bank: 5330 (0.27%) had a bladder injury; 963 (19.5%) were penetrating. 97 (10.1%) were treated with minimally invasive management. The minimally invasive management group had 12 complications in 5 patients (4.9%) versus 280 complications in 169 patients (19.7%) for open surgery ($p = < 0.001$). Open surgery was a significant independent predictor of complications (OR 1.57, $p = 0.003$) and longer hospital length of stay ($B = 5.31$, $p < 0.001$).

Conclusions: Most penetrating bladder injury requires open surgery, however a small proportion can safely be managed with minimally invasive management. Minimally invasive management is associated with lower total complications and shorter hospital length of stay in select patients.

Keywords: Penetrating, Bladder, Trauma, Minimally invasive

Introduction

Selective non-operative or minimally invasive management (MIM) has become standard of care for blunt extraperitoneal bladder injury, however MIM for penetrating bladder injury remains controversial. MIM can reduce the morbidity of large open incisions and potentially

*Correspondence: john.culhane@health.slu.edu
[1] Department of Trauma, Saint Louis University, 1008 Spring Ave, Saint Louis, MO 63110, USA

decrease recovery time, but this must be balanced against the risk of delayed diagnosis and treatment which could lead to peritonitis, abscess, and other complications. There is disagreement among major guidelines regarding penetrating mechanism as an absolute indication for open exploration and repair.

The latest American Association for the Surgery of Trauma (AAST) urologic trauma guidelines recommend selective MIM of extraperitoneal bladder injury for both blunt and penetrating trauma [1]. European Urologic Association (EUA) guidelines recommend operative treatment of all penetrating bladder injury [2], and American Urologic Association (AUA) guidelines do not distinguish treatment based on mechanism [3]. The individual studies that form the basis of the guidelines include very little penetrating trauma. Often the mechanism is not specified, or blunt and penetrating cases are grouped together. We present a retrospective cohort study of exclusively penetrating injuries in which MIM was implemented. Our local study is supplemented by a review of the National Trauma Data Bank (NTDB). Our hypothesis is that MIM can be performed safely for a carefully selected subset of penetrating bladder injuries. We believe that ours is the first study focused specifically on MIM of penetrating bladder injury.

Materials and methods

Study design and population

This is a retrospective cohort study that compares outcomes of patients who underwent open surgical versus minimally invasive management of penetrating bladder trauma. Local patients were treated at a level I trauma center with a prospectively maintained trauma database. After internal review board approval, penetrating bladder injuries between 2012 and 2019 were queried. We defined MIM as observation, prolonged bladder drainage, or use of endoscopic procedures such as cystoscopy. We excluded both open and laparoscopic bladder repair. Any patient who was coded for open peritoneal inspection or any other procedure that is normally done via an open trans-peritoneal approach was placed into the open group.

Patients were chosen for MIM based on hemodynamic stability, lack of peritonitis, and no intraperitoneal contrast extravasation on CT cystogram. Patients with other indications for open pelvic surgery such as orthopedic procedures, vascular repair, and repair of full thickness rectal perforation would also undergo open bladder repair.

The NTDB is a registry of trauma data from multiple US trauma centers. The years 2016 and 2017 were chosen because these are the first years which use ICD10 coding, which is necessary to classify diagnoses and procedures with adequate precision for this study. NTDB and local patients were analyzed separately rather than pooling the cases because differences in reporting could introduce bias, and because access to the charts provides more detail for the local cohort.

Data collection and statistical analysis

Chi square was used to test for significance for categorical variables. Mann–Whitney U test was used to test for significance for ordinal variables. T-test and Mann–Whitney U test were used to test for significance for continuous variables based on the sample size and distribution. Multivariate analysis was performed with multiple logistic regression for binary categorical outcome, multiple ordinal regression for ordinal outcome, and multiple linear regression for continuous outcome. The independent variables for the regressions are open surgery, age, gender, race, comorbidity index, trauma injury severity score (TRISS), university versus non-university hospital, verification level of trauma center, firearm injury, and grade of bladder injury according to the AAST Trauma Organ Injury Scale (OIS).

A comorbidity index was created by assigning a point to major comorbid conditions and totaling them into a single numerical score. We compared patients who had no open surgery (minimally invasive management—MIM), with those who had an open urologic procedure or other open peritoneal surgery. We chose these groups to examine whether it was safe to omit open exploration for both diagnosis and treatment. The MIM group would be most likely to suffer the consequences of missed or undertreated injury, and to show the benefits of less invasive treatment.

All statistical analysis was conducted with SPSS Statistics, version 26.0 (IBM Corp., Armonk, N.Y., USA).

Results

Patient characteristics

There were 18,506 trauma patients treated at our level I trauma center during the years 2012 through 2019. 1,961,104 NTDB patients were analyzed for the years 2016 and 2017. For the local group, 117 (0.63%) had a bladder injury. 30 (25.6%) of the injuries were penetrating. Discharge disposition is missing for one patient. The other 29 all survived to discharge. The injury was due to a firearm for all patients. For the NTDB group, 5330 (0.27%) had a bladder injury. 1042 (19.5%) of the injuries were penetrating. We eliminated 71 patients who died or were transferred within 24 h because they may not have undergone bladder surgery due to short survival or hospital stay. This leaves 963 to analyze. The mechanisms of injury were: 911 (94.7%) firearms, 48 (5.0%) sharp objects, 3 (0.3%) lawn mower, 1 (0.1%) nail gun. Baseline characteristics for bladder injury patients are reported in Table 1.

Type of surgery

For the local patients, 6 (20.0%) were treated without an open bladder repair or inspection. All injuries were extraperitoneal. Three were AAST grade I, consisting of 3 bladder hematomas, 2 of which were associated with proximal urethral injuries which were treated endoscopically. Three were grade II, consisting of extraperitoneal injuries with contained extravasation of contrast. All were treated with drainage only. None failed non-operative management.

For the NTDB, 866 (89.9%) patients had surgical bladder repair or other open peritoneal surgery. Presumably, the bladder was inspected during open surgery, although

Table 1 Baseline characteristics of penetrating bladder injury patients

Characteristics	MIM	Open
Local data		
Sex—Female	3 (50.0%)	2 (8.3%)
Race—White	2 (33.3%)	4 (16.7%)
Chest Injury AIS > 2	0 (0.0%)	2 (8.3%)
Abdominal Injury AIS > 2	0 (0.0%)	14(58.3%)
Extremity Injury AIS > 2	4 (66.7%)	17(70.8%)
Rectal Injury	0(0%)	5(16.7%)
Pelvic Fracture	1(16.7%)	5(16.7%)
Abdomino-Pelvic Vascular Injury	0(0%)	7(23.3%)
Age	33.3	31
BMI	28.4	27.5

	MIM		Open	
	Mean	Median	Mean	Median
Injury severity Score	11.2	13	17.5	18
TRISS	0.98		0.95	
Comorbidity Index	0.67	1	1.4	1

Characteristics	MIM	Open
NTDB data		
Sex—Female	12 11.7%)	74 (8.6%)
Race—White	37(35.9%)	227(26.4%)
Head Injury AIS > 2	1 (1.0%)	12 (1.4%)
Chest Injury AIS > 2	4 (3.9%)	71 (8.3%)
Abdominal Injury AIS > 2	33(32.0%)	602(70.0%)
Extremity Injury AIS > 2	37(35.9%)	308(35.8%)
Rectal Injury	6(6.2%)	216(24.9%)
Pelvic Fracture	47(48.4%)	368(42.5%)
Abdomino-Pelvic vascular injury	6(6.2%)	114(13.2%)
University Hospital	61(59.2%)	516(60.0%)
Level 1 Designation	46(44.7%)	420(48.8%)
Firearm Injury	90(87.4%)	821(95.5%)
Age	32	29.9
BMI	27.5	27.1

	MIM		Open	
	Mean	Median	Mean	Median
Injury severity Score	12.1	12	15.5	14
TRISS	0.97		0.94	
Comorbidity index	0.19	0	0.21	0

it is not always recorded. 97 (10.1%) did not have any open urologic procedure, surgical bladder repair or open peritoneal surgery. This comprises the MIM group. Mechanisms of injury in this group consist of 89 GSW, 10 sharp objects, 1 nail gun, and 2 lawn mowers.

Of the 97 MIM patients, 43 had 65 minimally invasive urologic procedures, 32 of which were drainage. 75 (7.8%) of penetrating bladder injury patients did not have open peritoneal surgery or any urologic procedure other than drainage. Urologic injury in this group was treated with drainage and observation only.

The NTDB recorded the location of the injury for 54 of the patients. 51 of these were classified as extraperitoneal. Exceptions were 2 patients who had an organ injury scale Grade IV injury. A 27 year old male had laparoscopic inspection and drainage of the peritoneal cavity but no repair. An 18 y/o male went to the floor from the ED. He was ultimately discharged to court/law enforcement. A fourteen year old male had a Grade V injury. He had laparoscopic inspection of the peritoneal cavity and drainage of the bladder, but no repair. He survived to discharge home.

Outcomes and complications

Univariate analysis

The local MIM group had no complications versus 24 complications in 11 patients (45.8%) for open surgery: $p=0.047$. Average length of stay (LOS) was 5.5 days for MIM versus 15.1 days for open surgery ($p=0.03$). The NTDB MIM group had 12 complications in 5 patients (4.9%) versus 280 complications in 169 patients (19.7%) for open surgery ($p= <0.001$). Average LOS was 6.1 days for MIM versus 12.9 days for open surgery ($p=0.01$). This represents significantly decreased overall complications and average LOS with MIM for both the local and NTDB groups. Intensive Care Unit (ICU) LOS was not significantly different for either group.

Multivariate analysis

For the local group multiple linear regression showed that open surgery was a significant predictor of increased LOS: B=9.72 (1.10 to 18.33) $p= <0.029$, meaning that open surgery predicted a 9.72 day average increase in LOS. Other independent predictors were TRISS and severe chest injury. Open surgery was not an independent predictor of ICU LOS or complications. Since no local patients died, multivariate analysis was not conducted for mortality.

For the NTDB group, multiple logistic regression showed that age and TRISS, but not open surgery were significant independent predictors of mortality. Multivariate ordinal regression showed that open surgery was associated with 1.57 (0.544 to 2.60) unit increase in the log odds of being in a group with a higher number of complications ($p=0.003$). Other independent predictors of increased complications include age, TRISS, and number of comorbidities. Multivariate linear regression showed that open surgery predicted a 5.31 day increase in LOS (2.45 to 8.16, $p<0.001$). Open surgery did not predict increased ICU LOS.

Discussion

MIM has become standard for many blunt injuries, but acceptance has been slower for penetrating trauma. As with trauma in general, there has been a shift to MIM for urologic trauma, including bladder injuries. Not all bladder injuries are appropriate for MIM. Major guidelines agree that surgeons should repair all intraperitoneal bladder injuries, both blunt and penetrating [2–6]. Hemodynamically unstable patients and patients with other hollow viscus injuries are not candidates for MIM [6]. For extraperitoneal injury, operative repair is recommended if the patient is already undergoing pelvic surgery for another injury such as exploratory laparotomy or orthopedic repair of the pelvis [2, 3]. Complicated injuries involving the ureteral orifice or trigone may require surgery to prevent future incontinence [4].

These restrictions leave hemodynamically stable patients with extraperitoneal injuries and no other indication for pelvic surgery as potential candidates for MIM. Most studies of MIM of bladder injury are in the blunt setting, where it has become the standard of care, however there is disagreement among urologic trauma guidelines regarding whether the blunt bladder injury paradigm applies to penetrating bladder injury (PBI) as well. Some advocate a mandatory surgical approach. A 2004 consensus statement by Gomez et al. and the 2005 European Urologic Association (EUA) guidelines recommend surgical exploration of all PBI [7, 8]. In a 2015 review of lower urinary tract injuries by the EUA trauma guidelines panel, Lumen et al. strongly recommended that all PBI should undergo emergency exploration with bladder repair [2]. Stein published a narrative review and update on 2014 AUA guidelines based on personal experience. The author's conclusion was that penetrating injuries should be explored and treated primarily [9]. Phillips published a review in 2017 which listed penetrating mechanism as an indication for open surgery, citing the AUA university core curriculum [10].

In contrast, in a 2019 statement, AAST urologic trauma guidelines recommend MIM of extraperitoneal bladder injury for both blunt and penetrating trauma [1]. Other guidelines do not explicitly state whether the recommendation applies to both blunt and penetrating injury. In the 2004 Eastern Association trauma guidelines for genitourinary trauma for all mechanisms, Holevar reported that catheter drainage shows results equal to surgical repair [6]. The latest AUA guidelines recommend MIM with drainage for extraperitoneal bladder injury without mention of injury mechanism [3]. Bryk published a 2013 review of urologic trauma guidelines. The recommendation after synthesizing all guidelines was that MIM of extraperitoneal injuries is acceptable without specifying the mechanism of injury [11].

Evidence for MIM of bladder injury consists mainly of retrospective reviews which contain few cases of penetrating injury. In some studies, the mechanism is not specified. If there are any penetrating injuries, they are grouped together with blunt [12–16]. There are few examples in the literature focused on PBI. Zaid et al. published a narrative review of penetrating urologic injury. The authors stated that PBI can be managed non-operatively, but the reference provided [7], another review, states that operative exploration and repair is the standard approach [17].

Limitations

As with any large multi-center database, the NTDB has inherent limitations with respect to granularity and coding accuracy [18]. The choice of MIM tends to select patients with less severe injuries, which could account for the shorter LOS and lower complication rate in the univariate analysis. We included the TRISS and AAST grade of bladder injury in the multivariate analyses to adjust for severity of injury, but subtle biases could remain. All injuries managed with MIM in the local group and the vast majority of those with location recorded in the NTDB group were extraperitoneal. We believe that the most conservative policy is to restrict MIM to extraperitoneal injuries. Our population includes mainly firearm lesions. Results could differ for populations with different injury patterns.

In summary, reports of MIM of PBI in the literature are rare, making it difficult to generate consistent treatment guidelines. For the small number of cases reported, the practice appears safe. Our report adds 6 cases from our institution and 97 cases from the NTDB to the total. All local patients were managed successfully without complication. Total complications were significantly lower for both local and NTDB cohorts and LOS was lower for the NTDB cohort, thus in our study, the practice appears safe as well.

Conclusion

Minimally invasive management of penetrating bladder injury remains controversial. Our analysis describes successful minimally invasive management of PBI, but it is important to bear in mind that this only applies to a narrow subset of patients. We propose the following criteria for MIM of PBI: hemodynamically stable patients with no other indication for pelvic surgery, extraperitoneal location, and partial thickness injury or well contained extraperitoneal contrast extravasation (AAST Grades I and II). Our results are largely based on firearm lesions, therefore outcome may differ for other mechanisms.

Patients meeting these criteria may be managed without any open exploration or any other open urologic procedure. MIM of PBI may involve minimally invasive percutaneous or endoscopic techniques, but some injuries may be managed with observation only, omitting urologic procedures of any kind. MIM of PBI is not associated with increased mortality or increase of any specific reported complication. MIM is associated with significantly fewer total complications and is an independent predictor of decreased hospital LOS. We believe that these results indicate that for a minority of PBI patients, observation and if necessary, endoscopic urologic procedures represent a safe treatment option.

Abbreviations

MIM: Minimally invasive management; NTDB: National trauma data bank; AAST: American association for the surgery of trauma; OIS: Organ injury scale; AUA: American Urologic Association; EUA: European Urologic Association; ICU: Intensive care unit; LOS: Length of stay; ISS: Injury severity score; TRISS: Trauma injury severity score; GSW: Gunshot Wound.

Acknowledgements

None.

Authors' contributions

JC and JS gathered, analyzed and interpreted the patient data regarding the treatment groups and outcomes. SS participated in gathering and analyzing the data and interpreting its clinical significance. All authors read and approved the final manuscript.

Competing interests

The authors declare no competing interests.

Author details

[1]Department of Trauma, Saint Louis University, 1008 Spring Ave, Saint Louis, MO 63110, USA. [2]Department of Urology, Saint Louis University, 1008 Spring Ave, Saint Louis, MO 63110, USA.

References

1. Coccolini F, et al. WSES-AAST. Expert panel kidney and uro-trauma: WSES-AAST guidelines. World J Emerg Surg. 2019;14:54.
2. Lumen N, Kuehhas FE, Djakovic N, et al. Review of the current management of lower urinary tract injuries by the EAU Trauma Guidelines Panel. Eur Urol. 2015;67(5):925–9.
3. Morey AF, Broghammer JA, Hollowell CMP, et al. Urotrauma guideline 2020: AUA guideline. J Urol. 2021;205(1):30–5.
4. Mahat Y, Leong JY, Chung PH. A contemporary review of adult bladder trauma. J Int Violence Res. 2019;11(2):101–6.
5. Como JJ, Bokhari F, Chiu WC, et al. Practice management guidelines for selective nonoperative management of penetrating abdominal trauma. J Trauma. 2010;68(3):721–33.
6. Holevar M, et al. Genitourinary trauma, Management of. https://www.east.org (2004)

7. Gomez RG, Ceballos L, Coburn M, et al. Consensus statement on bladder injuries. BJU Int. 2004;94(1):27–32.
8. Lynch TH, Martínez-Piñeiro L, Plas E, et al. EAU guidelines on urological trauma. Eur Urol. 2005;47(1):1–15.
9. Stein DM, Santucci RA. Current Opinion in Urology. 2015; 25(4), 323–30.
10. Phillips B, Holzmer S, Turco L, et al. Trauma to the bladder and ureter: a review of diagnosis, management, and prognosis. Eur J Trauma Emerg Surg. 2017;43(6):763–73.
11. Bryk DJ, Zhao LC. Guideline of guidelines: a review of urological trauma guidelines. BJU Int. 2016;117(2):226–34.
12. Hsieh CH, Chen RJ, Fang JF, et al. Diagnosis and management of bladder injury by trauma surgeons. Am J Surg. 2002;184(2):143–7.
13. Madiba TE, Haffejee AA. Causes and outcome of bladder injuries in Durban. East Afr Med J. 1999;76(12):676–9.
14. Robards VL, Haglund RV, Lubin EN, et al. Treatment of rupture of the bladder. J Urol. 1976;116:178–9.
15. Urry RJ, Clarke DL, Bruce JL, et al. The incidence, spectrum and outcomes of traumatic bladder injuries within the Pietermaritzburg Metropolitan Trauma Service. Injury. 2016;47(5):1057–63.
16. Anderson RE, et al. Current Management of Extraperitoneal Bladder Injuries: Results from the Multi-Institutional Genito-Urinary Trauma Study (MiGUTS). J Urol. 2020;204(3):538–44.
17. Zaid UB, Bayne DB, Harris CR, et al. Penetrating trauma to the ureter, bladder, and urethra. Curr Trauma Rep. 2015;1(2):119–24.
18. Haws BE, et al. Misclassification of pelvic ring injuries in the national trauma data bank. J Orthop Trauma. 2015. PMID: 25866941

17

Metal stent for the ureteral stricture after surgery and/or radiation treatment for malignancy

Wei Wang[†], Xiaoshuai Gao[†], Jixiang Chen[†], Zhenghuan Liu, Liao Peng and Xin Wei[*]

Abstract

Background: To assess the efficacy and safety of self-expanding metal ureteral stent for the stricture following surgery and/or radiation for malignancy.

Methods: We performed 36 metal ureteral stent insertion procedures (32 patients) between May 2019 and June 2020. The main inclusion criterion was the patients with ureteral stricture due to surgery and/or radiation treatment for malignancy. The diagnosis of stricture was ascertained by history and radiographic imaging. The etiologies underlying the strictures were: surgery and/or radiation therapy for cervical and rectal cancer, surgery for ovarian cancer. The primary outcome was the stent patency rate, and the secondary outcomes were the postoperative complications and glomerular filtration rate (GFR). Stent patency was defined as stent in situ without evident migration, unanticipated stent exchange or recurrent ureteral obstruction. Cost analysis was calculated from stent cost, anesthesia cost and operating room fee.

Results: The pre-metallic stent GFR was 22.53 ± 6.55 mL/min/1.73 m^2. Eight patients were on double-J stents before insertion of metallic stents. The total annual cost of per patient in our study was $10,600.2 US dollars (range $9394.4–$33,527.4 US dollars). During a median follow-up time of 16 months (range 8–21 months), 27 cases (31 sides, 84%) remained stent patency. Twelve patients died from their primary malignancy carrying a patency stent. Stent migration was observed in 4 patients within 10 months after insertion. Ectopic stents were endoscopically removed and replaced successfully. Three stents were occluded, and no encrustation was seen in our study. Three and four patients had postoperative fever and gross hematuria, respectively. Infection was observed in 2 cases, mandating antibiotics therapy. In addition, postoperative volume of hydronephrosis postoperatively was significantly reduced compared with preoperation (54.18 ± 15.42 vs 23.92 ± 8.3, $P = 0.019$). However, no statistically significant differences regarding GFR, creatinine levels, blood urea nitrogen and hemoglobin existed between preoperation and last follow-up.

Conclusions: The current study demonstrated that metal ureteral stent is effective and safe in the treatment of stricture following surgery and/or radiation therapy for malignant cancer. Patients hydronephrosis could be improved by the stent placement.

Keywords: Metal stent, Ureteral stricture, Iatrogenic

*Correspondence: weixinscu@scu.edu.cn
[†]Wei Wang, Xiaoshuai Gao and Jixiang Chen contributed equally to this work and should be considered as co-first author
Department of Urology, Institute of Urology, West China Hospital, Sichuan University, No. 37 Guo Xue Xiang, Chengdu, Sichuan 610041, People's Republic of China

Introduction

It is reported that nearly 75% of all ureteral strictures were caused by Iatrogenic injury and radiation treatment [1]. If left untreated, prolonged obstruction and narrowing of ureter can lead to hydronephrosis, decreased renal function, renal failure and even loss of a renal unit. Timely removal of obstruction is the golden principle for treating ureteral strictures. Currently, there are several therapeutic options available, including open surgery, laparoscopic or robotic reconstruction surgery, endoscopic ureterotomy, nephrostomy and stent insertion. For patients who developed ureteral stricture after surgery and/or radiation treatment for malignancy, it is more difficult to conduct open surgery again due to the formation of intra-abdominal adhesion in this scenario. Nephrostomy and double-J stent insertion are commonly used in these patients, but they are associated with high complication rates and require frequent replacement with increased medical cost [2–4]. Moreover, double-J stent is prone to occlude because of extrinsic compression [5].

Allium® ureteral stent is a self-expanding, large caliber stent. It consists of a super-elastic nickel-titanium alloy to provide long-term direct wall support. One retrospective study had determined the role of Allium stent in the treatment of malignant ureteral stricture [6]. However, they failed to assess the change of hydronephrosis and renal function before and after stent placement procedure, and they did not present cost analysis in their study [6]. Therefore, we presented our experience with the Allium® ureteral stent in the treatment of stricture following surgery and/or radiation treatment for malignancy. We evaluated the stent patency rate and complications during a median follow-up time of 16 months, the hydronephrosis and glomerular filtration rate (GFR) improvement after stent placement was also assessed. Moreover, cost analysis of Allium stent was performed for the first time.

Method

This prospective clinical trial was approved by the Ethics Approval Committee of West China Hospital, and the registered number was 2019-009. The current study was conducted according to the international ethical recommendations stated in the Declaration of Helsinki and its later amendments or comparable ethical standards [7]. All participants were informed of the risks and benefits of stent placement. The inclusion criterion was that the patients with ureteral stricture due to surgery and/or radiation treatment for malignancy. The diagnosis of stricture was ascertained by history and radiographic imaging. We performed 36 Allium® ureteral stent placement procedures (32 patients) between May 2019 and June 2020. All procedures were conducted or supervised by a single consultant endourologist. All stent placement procedures stuck with the same technique as detailed below. The primary endpoint was the patency rate of the Allium® ureteral stent, while the secondary outcomes were the postoperative complications and GFR. Stent patency was defined as stent in situ without evident migration, unanticipated stent exchange or recurrent ureteral obstruction (increasing hydronephrosis and associated deterioration of renal function). The volume of hydronephrosis was evaluated according to the meridian measured by computed tomography (CT): hydronephrosis volume = length * width * depth * 0.523 [8, 9]. The GFR was evaluated by Single-Photon Emission Computed Tomography (SPECT). Postoperative complications were graded based on the Clavien-Dindo classification [10]. Cost analysis was calculated from stent cost, anesthesia cost and operating room fee.

Technique

The Allium ureteral stent has two calibers (24F and 30F) and two lengths (10 cm and 12 cm). The main body has a high radial force with softer end segments (Fig. 1). In all patients, the procedure was conducted in the lithotomy position under general anesthesia with a prophylactic antibiotic used. After rigid cystoscopy, a hydrophilic guidewire was inserted under fluoroscopic guidance to the renal pelvis. For patients who were not possible to pass a guidewire, a small channel was incised with holmium laser (1.1 to 1.3 j, 30 Hz) under the fluoroscopy and ureteroscope guidance. The ureters were contrasted anterogradely through the nephrostomy tube or retrogradely via ureteroscope under X-ray guidance to show the location and length of ureteral stenosis. Subsequently, a guide wire was introduced and a ureteral balloon dilator (21 F) was utilized to pass over the site of stenosis and inflated to 25 atm (2.53 MPa) for 3 min. Afterwards, Allium stent (10 or 12 cm, 24F or 30F) was introduced into the stricture segment and identified by fluoroscopic image. The operative time was the interval between insertion of cystoscope and the completion of stent placement. Length of hospital stay was defined as

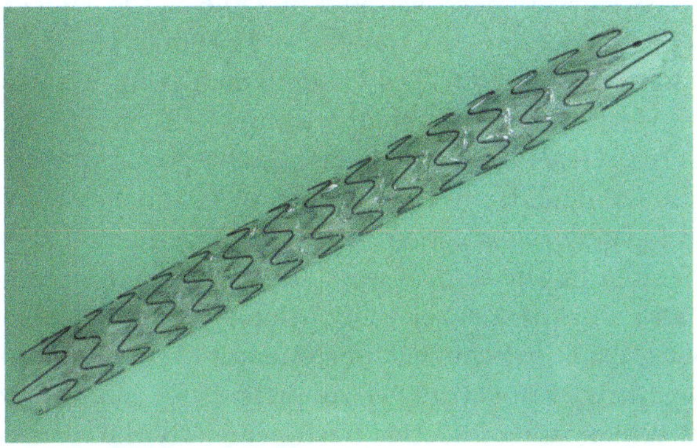

Fig. 1 The Allium ureteral stent

the duration passed from the operative day to the hospital discharge day.

Follow-up

Kidney, ureter, bladder (KUB) X-ray was conducted 1 day after stent insertion to determine the position of the stent. CT imaging and SPECT were conducted in all patients 1 month after stent insertion. Then CT scan, creatinine measurement, urine cultures, urinalysis and serum biochemistry were carried out every 3 months in the stable patients.

Statistical analysis

Continuous variables were presented with mean ± SD (standard deviation) or median (range) based on normal or non-normal distribution. Categorical variables were summarized with a count and percentage. A paired analysis (Student's t-test or Wilcoxon signed rank test) was conducted with the volume of hydronephrosis, creatinine levels, blood urea nitrogen (BUN), GFR and hemoglobin (Hb) between preoperation and the last follow-up. SPSS v. 24 software (SPSS Inc. IBM Corp, Somers, NY, USA) were utilized to conduct statistical analysis. All tests were two-sided, and a p value of < 0.05 was deemed statistically significant.

Results

From May 2019 until June 2020, we enrolled 32 patients (36 ureteral strictures) into the study. 11 patients suffered ureteral stricture following surgery and 6 patients suffered stricture following surgery and radiation therapy combined for cervical cancer.

Additionally, 4 patients suffered ureteral stricture following surgery and 6 patients suffered stricture following surgery and radiation therapy combined for rectal cancer. Five patients had stricture following surgery for ovarian cancer. The median length of ureteral stricture was 10.8 cm (range 3–17 cm) (Table 1).

All stents were inserted successfully and positioned correctly in the 36 ureters. The procedure-related characteristics were demonstrated in Table 2. The total cost of per patient in our study was $10,600.2 US dollars (range $9394.4–$33,527.4 US dollars). During a median follow-up time of 16 months (range 8–21 months), 27 cases (31 sides, 84%) remained stent patency. Twelve patients died from their primary malignancy carrying a patency stent. Three stents occluded and 4 stents migrated in our study. Two stents occluded due to the obstruction of urinary blood clots. Three (9.3%) and four (12.5%) patients had postoperative fever and gross hematuria, respectively. Two patients (6.2%) suffered the urinary tract infection postoperatively. The patients were managed by antibiotics treatment. Stent migration (3, 4, 6, and 10 months after the procedure) occurred in 4 (12.5%) ureters (one into the bladder, two into renal pelvis, and one within ureter). Primary stricture site of

Table 1 Patient demographics

Variable	US
Number of patients	32
Age, years, median (range)	46.8 (35–66)
Gender, male/female, n	7/25
BMI, kg/m^2	22.9 ± 1.35
Etiology of stricture, n	
Surgery/radiation therapy for cervical cancer	17
Surgery/radiation therapy for rectal cancer	10
Surgery for ovarian cancer	5
Stricture side, n	
Unilateral	28
Bilateral	4
Stricture site, n	
Upper ureter	7
Middle ureter	4
Lower ureter	25
Length of US, cm, median (range)	10.8 (3–17)
Urinary infection before placement, n	5/32
Previous treatment, n	
Nephrostomy ≥ 1	2/32
PS ≥ 2	8/32
Endoincision ≥ 1	0/32
Balloon dilation ≥ 1	5/32

US, ureteral stricture; BMI, body mass index; PS, polymeric double-J stent

Table 2 Procedure-related characteristics and follow-up

Variable	US (n = 32)
Operative time, min, median (range)	75 (40–125)
Length of hospital stay, days, median (range)	7 (4–17)
Total cost, $, median (range)	10,600.2 (9394.4–33,527.4)
Stent cost, $, median (range)	7558 (7377–7992)
Anesthesia cost, $	270
Operating room fees, $	2200
Follow up, months, median (range)	16 (8–21)
Stent patency, n (%)	27 (84)
Postoperative complications, n (%)	
Clavien Dindo grade I	
Gross hematuria	4 (12.5)
Fever	3 (9.3)
Clavien Dindo grade II	
Infection needed antibiotics	2 (6.2)
Clavien Dindo grade III–IV	
Stent migration	4 (12.5)
Stent encrustation	0

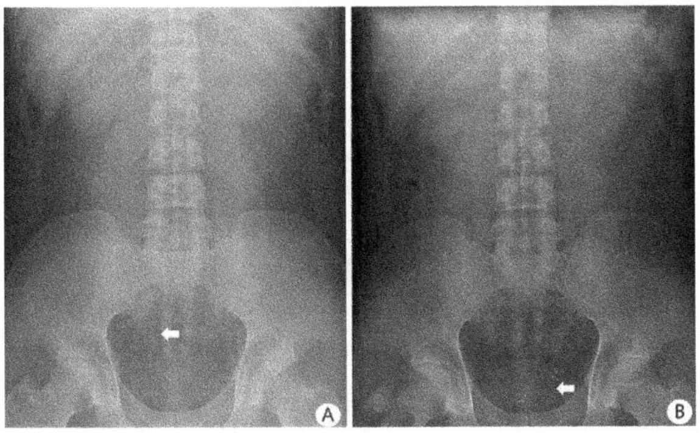

Fig. 2 KUB radiography of stent displacement in patient with lower ureteral stricture 1 day and 6 months after insertion: **A** KUB radiography showing the normal position of stent 1 day after insertion; **B** KUB radiography demonstrating the stent migration into the bladder 6 months after placement

Table 3 Difference between preoperation and last follow-up

Factors	Preoperation	Last follow-up	*p* value
Volume of hydronephrosis/cm^3	54.18±15.42	23.92±8.3	0.019
Creatinine levels/(μmol/L)	103.45±31.86	90.1±30.96	0.082
BUN/(μmol/L)	6.77±1.98	5.76±1.57	0.134
Norm GFR of affected kidney/(mL/min/1.73 m^2)	22.53±6.55	25.1±13.1	0.33
Uptake of affected kidney (%)	30.9±6.26	34.3±8.69	0.161
Hb/(g/L)	113.2±28.5	117.8±22.9	0.14

BUN, blood urea nitrogen; GFR, glomerular filtration rate; Hb, hemoglobin

ectopic stents includes 2 cases of upper, 1 case of middle and 1 case of the lower ureter. The median length of ureteral stricture of 4 patients who suffered stent migration was 5.4 cm (range 3.9–7.9 cm). As shown in Fig. 2, the stent migrated into the bladder 6 months after stent placement. Ectopic stents were endoscopically removed and a new Allium® ureteral stent was reinserted successfully. In all four patients, no clinical symptoms of fever or infections were observed, and computed tomography revealed no aggravated hydronephrosis. There were no patients experienced stent encrustation in our study (Table 2).

The volume of hydronephrosis postoperatively was significantly reduced compared with preoperation (54.18±15.42 vs 23.92±8.3, $P=0.019$). There was no statistically significant difference regarding GFR (22.53±6.55 vs 25.1±13.1, $P=0.33$), creatinine levels (103.45±31.86 vs 90.1±30.96, $P=0.082$), BUN (6.77±1.98 vs 5.76±1.57, 0.134) and Hb (113.2±28.5 vs 117.8±22.9, $P=0.14$) between preoperation and last follow-up (Table 3).

Discussion

This is the largest study evaluating the efficacy and safety of Allium ureteral stent in the management of ureteral stricture following surgery and/or radiation therapy for malignancy. The current study showed that Allium ureteral stent patency rate was 84% during a median observation time of 16 months. Twelve patients died from their primary malignancy carrying a patency stent. The placement of Allium stent significantly decreased average volume of hydronephrosis from preoperative 54.18 cm^3 to postoperative 23.92 cm^3 ($P=0.019$). Three stents occluded and 4 cases of stent migrated. No encrustation was observed in our series. Three (9.3%) and four (12.5%) patients had postoperative fever and gross hematuria, respectively. Infection was observed in 2 cases (6.2%), mandating antibiotics therapy. Additionally, the total cost of per patient in our study was $10,600.2 US dollars (range $9394.4–$33,527.4 US dollars). Therefore, our study demonstrated that Allium ureteral stent is effective and safe in the treatment of ureteral stricture following surgery and/or radiation therapy for malignant cancer.

It is reported that nearly 75% of all ureteral strictures were caused by iatrogenic injury and radiation treatment [1]. Ureter is prone to be injured during gynecologic and general surgery as it is proximal to anatomical position of ovaries, cervix, colon and rectum [11]. In addition, the delicate blood supply of ureter renders it less likely to self-repair after injury. Common mechanisms of iatrogenic surgery are direct injury (crushing, squeezing, transection, suture ligation and coagulation) and indirect injury (devascularization, energy induced and generation of free oxygen radicals) [12]. Iatrogenic ureteral stricture is more likely to be induced in the lower third of ureter than the middle and upper third [13, 14]. Nearly 70% of stricture located in the lower third ureter in our study, which is consistent with the previous report [13, 14].

The Allium ureteral stent is a fully covered, self-expanding, large caliber metal stent. The stent is made of super elastic nickel-titanium alloy, which maintain lumen patency via providing long-term direct wall support. The stent patency rate was 84% during a median observation time of 16 months in our study, which is slightly lower compared with previous study [15]. Zhong et al. reported a success rate of 87.5% with the use of Allium ureteral stent in the treatment of ureteral stricture after kidney transplantation [15]. However, the mean length of ureteral stricture was 2.5 cm in their series. Moskovitz et al. reported that a total success rate of 95% with the insertion of Allium ureteral stent for a median indwelling time of 17 months [6]. The patients who underwent stent exchange and had a secondary luminal patency were also considered as successful [6]. In contrast, unanticipated stent exchange was regarded as stent failure in our study.

The distinct success definition might account for our slightly lower stent patency rate.

The covered biocompatible, biostable polymer makes Allium ureteral stent a nonpermeable tube to avoid tissue ingrowth and early encrustation. In our study, no cases of stent encrustation were observed, which might be attributed to the specific unraveling materials of stents. Similarly, previous study published by Moskovitz and colleagues did not observe encrustation with the placement of Allium ureteral stent [6]. Stent migration is a relatively rare but significant postoperative complication. Polymer double-J stent provides self-retaining capability because of J-shaped design at two extremities which anchor the stent in the renal pelvis and the bladder. Compared with traditional double-J stent, Allium stent has a large caliber and strong supporting force. In our series, stent migration occurred in 4 out of 36 (12.5%) placements, which is slightly lower than the previous report of 14.2% [6]. In two patients, the stent migrated into the renal pelvis, while the other two stents migrated into bladder and within ureter, respectively. Primary stricture site of ectopic stents includes 2 cases of upper, 1 case of middle and 1 case of the lower ureter. Three patients with stent migration had engaged in bending, lifting heavy objects and running. Consequently, we speculated that the displacement of stents might be related to ureteral peristalsis and physical activity of patients. Ectopic stents were endoscopically removed and a new Allium ureteral stent was reinserted successfully. In all four patients, no clinical symptoms of fever or infections were observed, and CT scan revealed no aggravated hydronephrosis.

The volume of hydronephrosis is significantly decreased from preoperative 54.18 cm^3 to postoperative 23.92 cm^3 after stent insertion ($P=0.019$), demonstrating that the Allium stent was effective for relieving hydronephrosis and function protection. Similarly, Dong et al. reported that the average width of the renal pelvis significantly reduced from 2.65 to 1.34 cm after stent placement procedure [16], which supports our results. The stent patency rate was 84% during a median observation time of 16 months in our analysis, and the cost of Allium stent was based on the annual procedure. Cost for single Allium ureteral stent is between $7377 to $7992 US dollars, and the anesthesia and operating room fee were $270 and $2200 US dollars. Therefore, the median total cost was $10,600.2 US dollars (range $9394.4–$33,527.4 US dollars) in our analysis. In contrast, annual cost for double-J stents was extrapolated on the basis of stent exchange made every 3 to 6 months. The cost for single polymer stent insertion is between $2255 and $3125 US dollars, and the extrapolated annual cost for polymer stent would then be $9648 to $13,128 US dollars [17], which is comparable to the annual cost for Allium stent. The annual charge for Resonance metal stent was $9469.5 US dollars [18], this analysis was conducted based on Resonance stent exchange only once a year. Additionally, the annual cost for another thermo-expandable nickel-titanium alloy ureteral stent, Memokath 051, was calculated at $7841 US dollars [19], which is slightly lower than Allium stent. However, 17% of re-operation rate for Memokath 051 stent migration and/or occlusion might negate the cost savings potential in patients [19]. Two patients had an average total cost more than $30,000 US dollars. Both of them had bilateral ureteral stricture and two Allium stents were inserted during the procedure. Our results demonstrated a stent median life surpassing 1 year in the majority of patients. Longer stent life results in less frequent stent exchange, decreased patients' discomfort and improved quality of life.

Polymeric double-J stent is an appealing first choice for managing ureteral stricture. Moreover, no special facilities are required and all urologists are familiar with this common procedure. However, application of polymeric stent can be plagued with an approximately 20% failure rate [20] and complications such as urinary tract infection, encrustation and obstruction [21]. The Resonance metallic stent has a tightly coiled wire structure and is made of Ni-Co-Cr-M alloy. Several retrospective studies have been conducted with a 65–78% stent patency rates at various duration of follow-up [22–24]. Notably, the effectiveness of Resonance in alleviating ureteral obstruction was not observed in children, and pediatric patients needed further treatment to relieve the obstruction [25]. In addition, a number of studies have reported the efficacy of Memokath 051 metal-mesh ureteral stent. Agrawal et al. prospectively collected data on patients who had a Memokath 051 stent insertion [26]. 14 patients (19%) needed re-insertion during a mean follow-up of 7.1 months [26]. They also identified chronic kidney disease, diabetes and ureteropelvic junction strictures as predictive factors for migration and the need for re-insertion. Another study published by Maan et al. evaluated stent-related symptoms between double-J stent and the Memokath 051 [27]. They found that the Memokath group significantly outperformed the double-J stent group regarding general health, pain and urinary symptom index. However, this conclusion should be drawn cautiously because of retrospective biases of study. In addition to single ureteral stent insertion, it is possible to place 2 stents side-by-side (Tandem ureteral stents). Tandem ureteral stents improve the urine flow through providing additional scaffolding to withstand the compressive forces. In addition, the use of 2 ipsilateral stents increases the stiffness and reduces kinking [28]. Vogt el al. switched to tandem stents after obstruction of the stiffest stent in less than 6 months [29]. They performed 18 tandem ureteral stent insertion and found 2 cases (11.1%) experienced stent failure, which might be predictive for a decrease in survival [29, 30]. Active clinical and ultrasound are also needed in patients with tandem stents to evaluate renal function.

The current study had several limitations. Firstly, we could not compare the efficacy and safety between Allium ureteral stent and polymer double-J stent. Secondly, stent-related symptoms were not assessed by questionnaire in the current study. However, this is the largest study evaluating treatment outcomes of Allium ureteral stent in the ureteral stricture following surgery and/or radiation therapy for malignancy. We also performed the cost analysis of Allium ureteral stent in the management of stricture for the first time.

Conclusions

In summary, the current study demonstrated that Allium ureteral stent is effective and safe for patients with stricture following surgery and/or radiation therapy for malignancy. The stent could maintain a high patency rate and low complication rate for a long period of time. Moreover, patients' hydronephrosis could be improved by the stent placement.

Abbreviations
KUB: Kidney, ureter, bladder; SD: Standard deviation; BUN: Blood urea nitrogen; GFR: Glomerular filtration rate; Hb: Hemoglobin.

Acknowledgements
Not applicable.

Authors' contributions
WW collected the data, analyzed the data and prepared the manuscript. XSG collected the data. JXC analyzed the data and prepared a manuscript. ZHL analyzed the data and prepared a manuscript. LP prepared a statistical analysis and tables and figures. XW collected the data, analyzed the data and prepared a manuscript. All authors have read and approved the final manuscript.

Competing interests
The authors declared that they had no competing interest related to this work.

References

1. Abboudi H, Ahmed K, Royle J, Khan MS, Dasgupta P, N'Dow J. Ureteric injury: a challenging condition to diagnose and manage. Nat Rev Urol. 2013;10(2):108–15.
2. De S, Autorino R, Kim FJ, Zargar H, Laydner H, Balsamo R, Torricelli FC, Di Palma C, Molina WR, Monga M, et al. Percutaneous nephrolithotomy versus retrograde intrarenal surgery: a systematic review and meta-analysis. Eur Urol. 2015;67(1):125–37.
3. Fernández-Cacho LM, Ayesa-Arriola R. Quality of life, pain and anxiety in patients with nephrostomy tubes. Rev Lat Am Enfermagem. 2019;27:e3191.
4. Lange D, Bidnur S, Hoag N, Chew BH. Ureteral stent-associated complications–where we are and where we are going. Nat Rev Urol. 2015;12(1):17–25.
5. Chung SY, Stein RJ, Landsittel D, Davies BJ, Cuellar DC, Hrebinko RL, Tarin T, Averch TD. 15-year experience with the management of extrinsic ureteral obstruction with indwelling ureteral stents. J Urol. 2004;172(2):592–5.
6. Moskovitz B, Halachmi S, Nativ O. A new self-expanding, large-caliber ureteral stent: results of a multicenter experience. J Endourol. 2012;26(11):1523–7.
7. World Medical Association Declaration of Helsinki. ethical principles for medical research involving human subjects. JAMA. 2013;310(20):2191–4.
8. Gao X, Chen J, Wang W, Peng L, Di X, Xiao K, Li H, Wei X. Step-by-step technique for the endoscopic treatment of ureteric stricture. BJU Int 2021
9. Leung VY, Rasalkar DD, Liu JX, Sreedhar B, Yeung CK, Chu WC. Dynamic ultrasound study on urinary bladder in infants with antenatally detected fetal hydronephrosis. Pediatr Res. 2010;67(4):440–3.
10. Clavien PA, Barkun J, de Oliveira ML, Vauthey JN, Dindo D, Schulick RD, de Santibañes E, Pekolj J, Slankamenac K, Bassi C, et al. The Clavien-Dindo classification of surgical complications: five-year experience. Ann Surg. 2009;250(2):187–96.
11. Delacroix SE Jr, Winters JC. Urinary tract injures: recognition and management. Clin Colon Rectal Surg. 2010;23(2):104–12.
12. Cichoń W, Maciukiewicz P. Iatrogenic ureteral injury in adults–diagnosis and treatment. Przegl Lek. 2014;71(12):700–2.
13. Vorobev V, Beloborodov V, Golub I, Frolov A, Kelchevskaya E, Tsoktoev D, Maksikova T. Urinary system iatrogenic injuries: problem review. Urol Int. 2021;105:460–9.
14. Lobo N, Kulkarni M, Hughes S, Nair R, Khan MS, Thurairaja R. Urologic complications following pelvic radiotherapy. Urology. 2018;122:1–9.
15. Zhong Q, Song T, Zeng J, Lin T, Fan Y, Wei X. Initial experiment of self-expanding metal ureteral stent in recurrent ureteral stenosis after kidney transplantation. Am J Transplant. 2020;21:1983–4.
16. Dong WM, Wang MR, Hu H, Wang Q, Xu KX, Xu T. [Initial clinical experience and follow-up outcomes of treatment for ureteroileal anastomotic stricture with Allium coated metal ureteral stent]. Beijing Da Xue Xue Bao Yi Xue Ban. 2020;52(4):637–41.
17. Baumgarten AS, Hakky TS, Carrion RE, Lockhart JL, Spiess PE. A single-institution experience with metallic ureteral stents: a cost-effective method of managing deficiencies in ureteral drainage. Int Braz J Urol. 2014;40(2):225–31.
18. Taylor ER, Benson AD, Schwartz BF. Cost analysis of metallic ureteral stents with 12 months of follow-up. J Endourol. 2012;26(7):917–21.
19. Papatsoris AG, Buchholz N. A novel thermo-expandable ureteral metal stent for the minimally invasive management of ureteral strictures. J Endourol. 2010;24(3):487–91.
20. Ganatra AM, Loughlin KR. The management of malignant ureteral obstruction treated with ureteral stents. J Urol. 2005;174(6):2125–8.
21. Rosenberg BH, Bianco FJ Jr, Wood DP Jr, Triest JA. Stent-change therapy in advanced malignancies with ureteral obstruction. J Endourol. 2005;19(1):63–7.
22. Nagele U, Kuczyk MA, Horstmann M, Hennenlotter J, Sievert KD, Schilling D, Walcher U, Stenzl A, Anastasiadis AG. Initial clinical experience with full-length metal ureteral stents for obstructive ureteral stenosis. World J Urol. 2008;26(3):257–62.
23. Wah TM, Irving HC, Cartledge J. Initial experience with the resonance metallic stent for antegrade ureteric stenting. Cardiovasc Intervent Radiol. 2007;30(4):705–10.
24. Wang HJ, Lee TY, Luo HL, Chen CH, Shen YC, Chuang YC, Chiang PH. Application of resonance metallic stents for ureteral obstruction. BJU Int. 2011;108(3):428–32.
25. Gayed BA, Mally AD, Riley J, Ost MC. Resonance metallic stents do not effectively relieve extrinsic ureteral compression in pediatric patients. J Endourol. 2013;27(2):154–7.
26. Agrawal S, Brown CT, Bellamy EA, Kulkarni R. The thermo-expandable metallic ureteric stent: an 11-year follow-up. BJU Int. 2009;103(3):372–6.
27. Maan Z, Patel D, Moraitis K, El-Husseiny T, Papatsoris AG, Buchholz NP, Masood J. Comparison of stent-related symptoms between conventional Double-J stents and a new-generation thermoexpandable segmental metallic stent: a validated-questionnaire-based study. J Endourol. 2010;24(4):589–93.

28. Liu JS, Hrebinko RL. The use of 2 ipsilateral ureteral stents for relief of ureteral obstruction from extrinsic compression. J Urol. 1998;159(1):179–81.
29. Vogt B, Blanchet LH. 10-year experience with reinforced ureteral stents for malignant ureteral obstruction. Res Rep Urol. 2021;13:581–9.
30. Elsamra SE, Motato H, Moreira DM, Waingankar N, Friedlander JI, Weiss G, Smith AD, Okeke Z. Tandem ureteral stents for the decompression of malignant and benign obstructive uropathy. J Endourol. 2013;27(10):1297–302.

18

Comparison of vacuum-assisted sheaths and normal sheaths in minimally invasive percutaneous nephrolithotomy

Ling Zhu[1], Zhenghao Wang[2], Ye Zhou[2], Liping Gou[2], Yan Huang[1*] and Xiaofeng Zheng[2*]

Abstract

Background: A systematic review and meta-analysis was conducted to compare the safety and efficacy of vacuum-assisted sheaths and conventional sheaths in minimally invasive percutaneous nephrolithotomy (MPCNL) in the treatment of nephrolithiasis.

Methods: PubMed, Web of Science, Embase, EBSCO, and Cochrane Library databases (updated March 2021) were used to search for studies assessing the effect of vacuum-assisted sheaths in patients who underwent MPCNL. The search strategy and study selection processes were implemented in accordance with the PRISMA statement.

Result: Three randomized controlled trials and two case-controlled trials that satisfied the inclusion criteria were enrolled in this meta-analysis. Overall, the stone-free rate (SFR) in patients who underwent vacuum-assisted sheaths was significantly higher than that in patients who underwent conventional sheaths (RR 1.23, 95% CI 1.04, 1.46, $P=0.02$), with significant heterogeneity among the studies ($I^2=72\%$, $P=0.03$). In terms of the outcome of complications, vacuum-assisted sheath could bring a benefit to the postoperative infection rate (RR 0.48, 95% CI 0.33, 0.70, $P<0.00001$) with insignificant heterogeneity among the studies ($I^2=0\%$, $P=0.68$). There was no significant difference in the blood transfusion rate (RR 0.35, 95% CI 0.07, 1.73, $P=0.17$), with significant heterogeneity ($I^2=66\%$, $P=0.35$). Three studies contained operative time data, and the results indicated that the vacuum-assisted sheath led to a shorter operative time (MD = − 15.74; 95% CI − 1944, − 12.04, $P<0.00001$) with insignificant heterogeneity ($I^2=0\%$, $P=0.91$).

Conclusion: The application of a vacuum-assisted sheath in MPCNL improves the safety and efficiency compared to the conventional sheath. A vacuum-assisted sheath significantly increases the SFR while reducing operative time and postoperative infection.

Keywords: Nephrolithiasis, Minimally invasive percutaneous nephrolithotomy, Vacuum-assisted sheath, Conventional sheath, Meta-analysis

Background

Urolithiasis is the third most common disease of the urinary tract, and its prevalence has increased over the past decades [1]. The prevalence rate of kidney stones worldwide is approximately 1.7% to 8.8%, and kidney stones cost approximately $2.1 billion in 2020 alone [2]. Patients

*Correspondence: huangyanhy513@163.com; xiaofeng.zheng@wchscu.cn
[1] Health Management Center, West China Hospital, Sichuan University, Chengdu, China
[2] Department of Endocrinology and Metabolism, Center for Diabetes and Metabolism Research, West China Hospital, Sichuan University, Chengdu, China

with nephrolithiasis often suffer from short-term complications such as acute renal colic, nausea, vomiting, and hematuria and long-term complications such as chronic renal failure and hydronephrosis [3]. Therefore, treatment of calculi has always been the focus of surgeons. For renal stones > 2 cm in size, the American Urological Association recommends percutaneous nephrolithotomy (PCNL) as the primary treatment [4]. Previous studies have shown that standard PCNL is a highly effective approach [5]. However, it is often associated with major complications such as bleeding with the need for blood transfusion, postoperative fever, and pneumothorax [6].

In 2001, minimally invasive percutaneous nephrolithotomy (MPCNL), which involves the use of a small access sheath (i.e., 20F or less) was introduced in clinical practice [7, 8]. Despite the popularity of MPCL due to the lower risk of trauma and morbidities, it suffers from certain drawbacks. The efficiency of extraction of stone fragments and dust is lower than that of standard PCNL. Furthermore, the size of the sheath and the force of irrigation can lead to a higher incidence of infections due to the rise in renal intraluminal pressure and limitations in lithotripsy equipment [9]. With the development of new technologies, vacuum-assisted sheaths have emerged. Stone fragments and irrigation fluid can be sucked out continuously and contemporarily in the gap between the scope and sheath. Some studies on this issue have been conducted recently, but the outcomes of the effect and efficiency of MPCNL with a vacuum-assisted sheath are unsettled.

To date, there is still a lack of high-level evidence. The present write-up, therefore, aims to systematically review and perform a meta-analysis of the current studies to investigate the effectiveness and safety of vacuum-assisted sheaths for the treatment of nephrolithiasis.

Materials and methods

The systematic review and meta-analysis were carried out following the guidelines of the Preferred Reporting Items for Systematic Reviews and Meta-analysis (PRISMA) statement and the Cochrane Handbook for Systematic Reviews of Interventions [10]. Ethical approval and patient consent were not required, as all the analyses were performed in previously published studies.

Literature search and selection criteria

We systematically searched relevant published articles in several databases, including PubMed, Embase, Web of Science, EBSCO, and the Cochrane Library, from inception to March 2021 with the following keywords: "percutaneous nephrolithotomy," "minimally," "sheath," "evacuation," and "suction." The reference lists in the retrieved studies and relevant reviews were manually searched, and the above process was repeated to ensure that all eligible studies were identified.

The inclusion criteria were as follows: (1) the study design was a randomized controlled trial, (2) the patient had a history of kidney stones and underwent minimally invasive PCNL, (3) the intervention approach was a suctioning sheath versus a normal sheath, and (4) the entire text was available. Studies satisfying these inclusion criteria in all languages were included.

Data extraction and outcome measures

Baseline information extracted from the original studies included the first author, year of publication, number of patients, patient age and sex distributions, type of calcium stone, detailed methods for the two groups, and the evaluation of evidence level. Data were independently extracted by two investigators, and discrepancies were resolved by consensus.

The primary outcomes were stone-free rate (SFR) and perioperative complications (including postoperative infection rate, blood transfusion rate, and perforation rate). Secondary outcomes were operative time and hospitalization.

Quality assessment of individual studies

All assessments were performed independently by two researchers, with differences resolved by discussion. The methodological quality of each RCT was assessed according to the Jadad Score, which comprises the following three evaluation elements: randomization (0–2 points), blinding (0–2 points), and dropouts and withdrawals (0–1 points) [11]. One point was awarded for each element that was conducted and appropriately described in the original article. The total score varies from 0 to 5 points. An article with a Jadad score of ≤ 2 is considered to be of low quality, while a Jadad score of ≥ 3 indicates a high-quality study [12].

Statistical analysis

Risk ratios (RRs) with 95% confidence intervals (CIs) were calculated for dichotomous outcomes. Heterogeneity was evaluated using the I^2 statistic, with $I^2 > 50\%$ indicating significant heterogeneity [13]. Sensitivity analysis was performed to evaluate the influence of a single study on the overall estimate by omitting one study in turn or performing subgroup analysis. The random effects model was used for meta-analysis. Owing to the limited number of included studies (< 10), publication bias was not assessed. Statistical significance was accepted at $P < 0.05$. All statistical analyses were performed using Review Manager Software Version 5.3 (The Cochrane Collaboration, Software Update, Oxford, UK).

Result

Literature search, study characteristics, and quality assessment

A total of 126 articles were initially identified from the databases. After removing duplicates, 91 articles were retained. Then, 83 studies were excluded from the study due to unrelated abstracts and titles. One article with insufficient data, one article without full text, and three for not were also excluded from our analysis due to the study design. Finally, three randomized controlled trials (RCTs) with 857 patients who satisfied all inclusion criteria were subjected to the meta-analysis [14–16]. The article selection process was performed in accordance with the PRISMA statement (Fig. 1). The baseline characteristics of the three included studies are shown in Table 1. The studies included in this meta-analysis were published between 2016 and 2020. The JADAD score for three studies was 2, 3, and 4. One study was of low quality, as no blinding was used and the specific method of randomization was explained [14].

Primary outcomes

Stone-free rate

All studies included for the analysis reported the SFR, where stone-free was defined as stone fragments ≤ 4 mm (1 study using computed tomography (CT) scan and 2

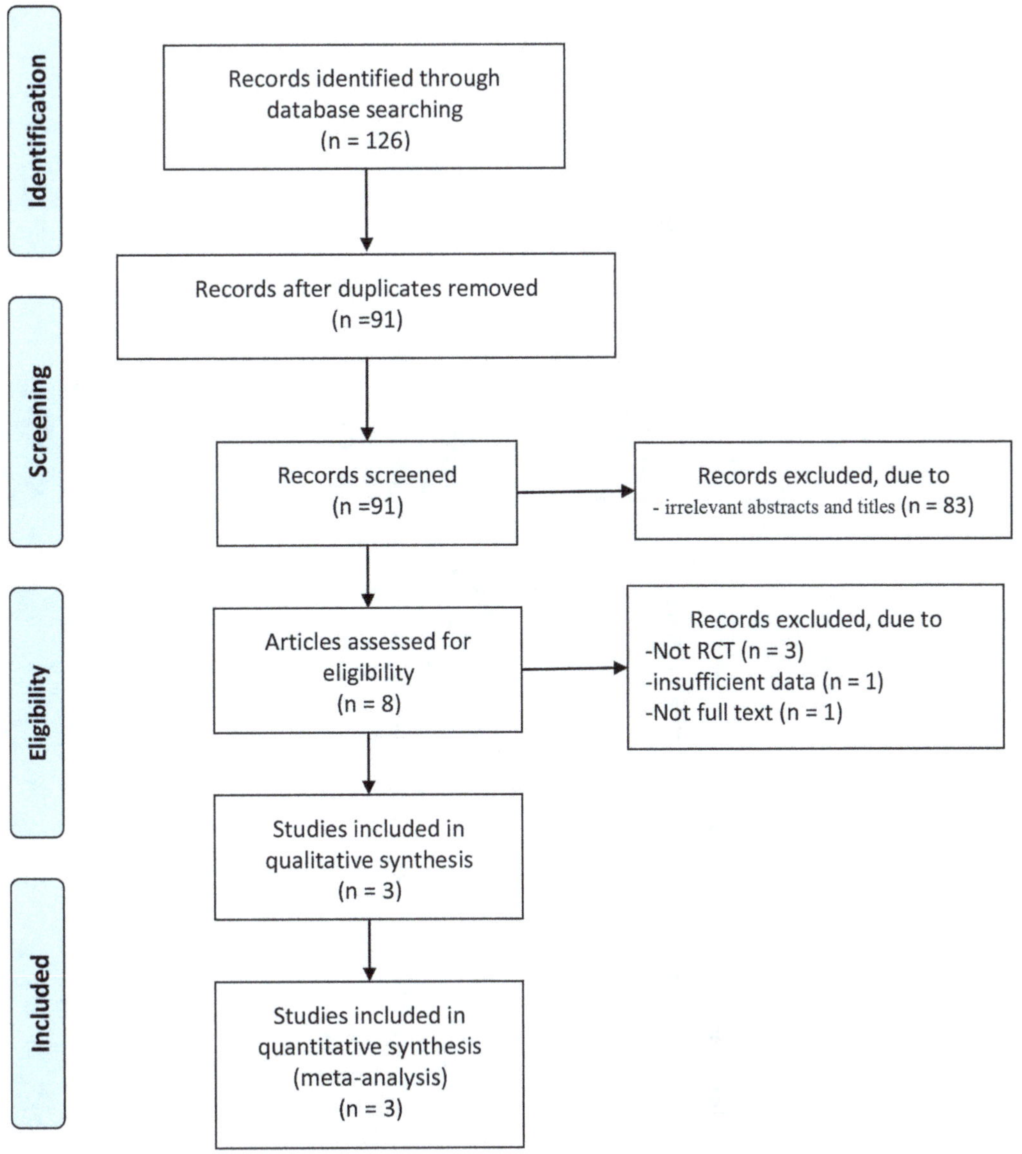

Fig. 1 Flow diagram of the study search and selection process

Table 1 Characteristics of included studies

No	Author	Year	Experimental group					Control group					Study design	Quality assessment
			Number (n)	Age (Mean ± SD)	Male (n)	Stone	Access sheath and lithotripsy energy	Number (n)	Age (Mean ± SD)	Male (n)	Stone size	Access sheath and lithotripsy energy		
1	Huang	2016	91	43.5 ± 2.9	53	Stone dimension 16.7 ± 5.8 mm	16F vacuum sheath/holmium laser	91	44.1 ± 3.2	51	15.1 ± 6.3 mm	16F peel-away sheath/holmium laser	RCT	3[a]
2	Du	2018	311	43.6 ± 17.4	187	Stone size 13.6 ± 5.2 cm^2	16-18F vacuum sheath/ultrasound	304	41.2 ± 16.9	181	13.9 ± 4.7 cm^2	16-18F peel-away sheath/ultrasound	RCT	2[a]
3	Xu	2020	30	52.1 ± 11.5	18	Stone diameter 4.2 ± 1.0 cm	20F vacuum sheath/pneumatic and holmium laser	30	51.8 ± 9.6	14	3.8 ± 1.4 cm	20F conventional sheath/pneumatic and holmium laser	RCT	4[a]

[a] Jadad score

studies using X-ray). Our results indicated that the SFR of the vacuum-assisted sheath group was significantly higher than that of the conventional sheath group (RR 1.23, 95% CI 1.04, 1.46, $P=0.02$), with significant heterogeneity among the studies ($I^2=72\%$, $P=0.03$) (Fig. 2).

Perioperative complications: postoperative infection rate, blood transfusion rate, and perforation rate

All the studies reported infection-related complications and blood transfusion rates. Three studies reported postoperative fever [14–16]. These results indicated that vacuum-assisted sheaths provided a benefit to the postoperative infection rate (RR 0.48, 95% CI 0.33, 0.70, $P<0.00001$), with insignificant heterogeneity among the studies ($I^2=0\%$, $P=0.68$) (Fig. 3). There was no significant difference in the blood transfusion rate (RR 0.35, 95% CI 0.07, 1.73, $P=0.17$), with significant heterogeneity ($I^2=66\%$, $P=0.35$) (Fig. 4) reported in the three studies [14–16]. Only one study reported perforation, and the vacuum-assisted sheath had a higher incidence of perforation (7/91 vs. 1/91; $P<0.001$).

Secondary outcomes

Operative time

Three studies containing operative time data [15, 16] were analyzed, and the results indicated that the operative time of the vacuum-assisted sheath group was significantly reduced compared to that of the conventional sheath group (MD = −15.74; 95% CI −1944, −12.04, $P<0.00001$), with insignificant heterogeneity ($I^2=0\%$, $P=0.91$) (Fig. 5).

Study or Subgroup	Experimental Events	Experimental Total	Control Events	Control Total	Weight	Risk Ratio M-H, Random, 95% CI
Xu 2020	24	30	16	30	14.2%	1.50 [1.03, 2.19]
Huang 2016	88	91	67	91	39.9%	1.31 [1.15, 1.49]
Du 2018	252	311	225	304	45.9%	1.09 [1.00, 1.19]
Total (95% CI)		**432**		**425**	**100.0%**	**1.23 [1.04, 1.46]**
Total events	364		308			

Heterogeneity: Tau² = 0.01; Chi² = 7.07, df = 2 (P = 0.03); I² = 72%
Test for overall effect: Z = 2.43 (P = 0.02)

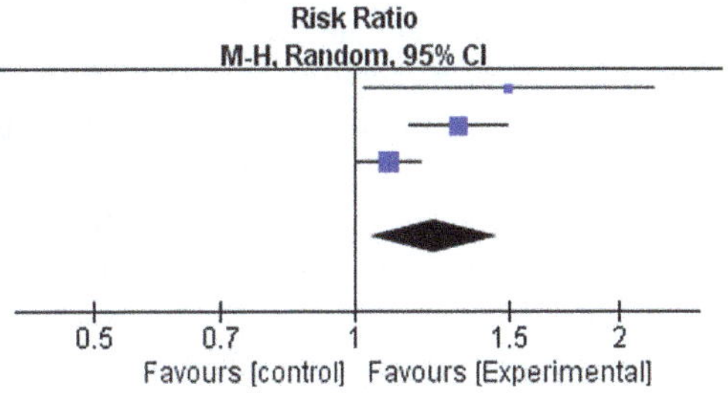

Fig. 2 Forest plot for the meta-analysis of stone free rate

Study or Subgroup	Experimental Events	Experimental Total	Control Events	Control Total	Weight	Risk Ratio M-H, Random, 95% CI
Du 2018	25	311	45	304	63.9%	0.54 [0.34, 0.86]
Huang 2016	10	91	25	91	30.2%	0.40 [0.20, 0.78]
Xu 2020	2	30	6	30	5.9%	0.33 [0.07, 1.52]
Total (95% CI)		**432**		**425**	**100.0%**	**0.48 [0.33, 0.70]**
Total events	37		76			

Heterogeneity: Tau² = 0.00; Chi² = 0.78, df = 2 (P = 0.68); I² = 0%
Test for overall effect: Z = 3.88 (P = 0.0001)

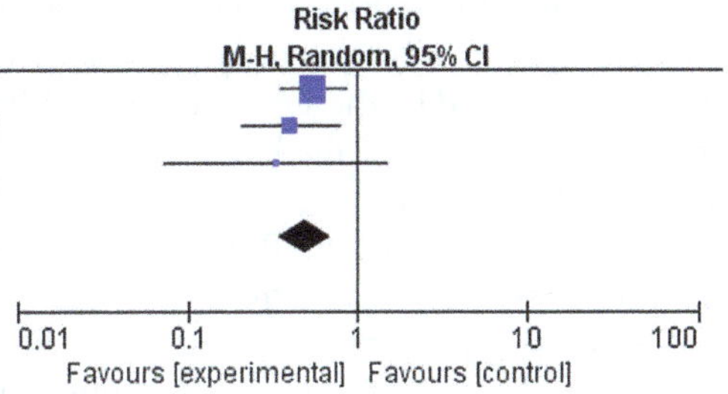

Fig. 3 Forest plot for the meta-analysis of postoperative infection

Study or Subgroup	Experimental Events	Experimental Total	Control Events	Control Total	Weight	Risk Ratio M-H, Random, 95% CI
Du 2018	11	311	14	304	46.4%	0.77 [0.35, 1.66]
Huang 2016	0	91	15	91	19.8%	0.03 [0.00, 0.53]
Xu 2020	2	30	4	30	33.8%	0.50 [0.10, 2.53]
Total (95% CI)		**432**		**425**	**100.0%**	**0.35 [0.07, 1.73]**
Total events	13		33			

Heterogeneity: Tau² = 1.25; Chi² = 5.95, df = 2 (P = 0.05); I² = 66%
Test for overall effect: Z = 1.28 (P = 0.20)

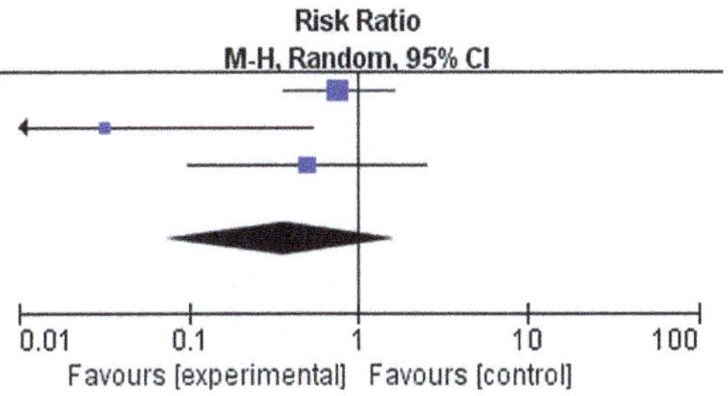

Fig. 4 Forest plot for the meta-analysis of transfusion

Hospitalization

Only studies reported hospitalization data, and the results showed that vacuum-assisted sheaths might prolong the hospitalization time compared to normal sheaths (10.6 ± 3.7 vs. 6.4 ± 2.3; $P < 0.001$).

Discussion

PCNL has been accepted as the gold standard for the treatment of large renal stones and is widely used in clinical practice [3, 17]. Although technological advances have ensured much progress in this field, many complications still exist [18]. To improve the safety and efficacy of this procedure, a small-size sheath was invented with the advent of mini-perc technology [19]. Due to the smaller size of the sheaths, MPCNL is associated with flaws such as longer operative time and infectious complications [20]. Recently, a sheath with irrigation and suctioning systems has been developed that can allow continuous infusion with saline intraoperatively [21]. Vacuum aspiration can be regulated manually or mechanically to keep the collecting system under negative pressure. Additionally, the nephroscope moves in and out conveniently through the movable sealing lid while preventing extremely high or low pressure [22]. To evaluate the effect and efficacy of the vacuum-assisted sheath, this meta-analysis was performed.

SFR is the main parameter for judging the efficacy of minimally invasive stone removal surgery [23]. Despite the difference in imaging modalities and follow-up time in the definition of SFR, our results show that vacuum-assisted sheaths have an improved stone clearance compared to normal sheaths. One possible explanation may be the low positive or low negative state of intrapelvic pressure controlled by the sheath while flushing and irrigation. In this situation, the kidney parenchyma shrank, tension in the renal pelvis decreased, and renal parenchymal compliance improved. Thus, the nephroscope can reach more renal calyces. Furthermore, when the calyceal neck is narrow or the angle is hard to reach, this sheath can perform lithotripsy and simultaneously suction out the fragments, making it a one-step procedure. Additionally, continuous negative pressure suction ensures a clear surgical field to avoid missing stone fragments, and therefore, a higher SFR is reached [14].

Xu et al. reported a higher incidence of postoperative fever [15]. Due to the small size of the sheath, high-pressure perfusion is very often performed. It is known that the limit of renal intrapelvic pressure is 30 mmHg [24]. Higher pressure can injure the integrity of the pelvic wall epithelium, leading to exposure of the lymphatic and venous systems [25]. In addition, tissue edema and congestion caused by urinary tract infection and stones are more likely to cause pelvic fluid absorption. When the bacteria along with the associated toxin reflux are absorbed, it may lead to infectious complications such as postoperative fever or sepsis [26]. By using the suction sheath, the renal pelvis is kept in a negative pressure state. Therefore, the infectious fluid flows smoothly, and the absorption of irrigation, bacteria, and toxin reflux is reduced. Du et al. found that MPCNL with a vacuum sheath has a low intrapelvic pressure compared to standard PCNL and MPCNL [14]. Xu et al. found that intrapelvic pressure ≥ 30 mmHg was achieved in the non-vacuum-sheath group [15].

Prolonged operative time is another independent risk factor for infectious complications [27]. The smaller size of access causing a limitation for more options for lithotripsy is a major inherent limitation of MPCNL. Another limitation is the small visual field in miniature endoscopes, which leads to a prolonged time to break the stones into smaller fragments [28]. Despite the different definitions of the operation time, present evidence indicates that vacuum-assisted sheaths can significantly shorten the operation time. The vacuum-assisted sheath could simultaneously suck out the small clots and fragments of stone in the gap. Furthermore, clearer vision was achieved during the procedure to shorten the surgery time [29]. Although a shorter operation time may decrease blood loss, this was not proven to be the case in our study, as it depends on many factors, such as puncture site, number, and size of the sheath [30].

Admittedly, there are a few limitations to this study. First, only three randomized controlled trials were included in our study, and the geographical region was single. Second, the impact of differences in puncture

Study or Subgroup	Experimental Mean	SD	Total	Control Mean	SD	Total	Weight	Mean Difference IV, Random, 95% CI
Huang 2016	54.4	14.5	91	70.2	11.7	91	93.5%	-15.80 [-19.63, -11.97]
Xu 2020	64.3	29.1	30	79.2	28.5	30	6.5%	-14.90 [-29.48, -0.32]
Total (95% CI)			**121**			**121**	**100.0%**	**-15.74 [-19.44, -12.04]**

Heterogeneity: Tau² = 0.00; Chi² = 0.01, df = 1 (P = 0.91); I² = 0%
Test for overall effect: Z = 8.33 (P < 0.00001)

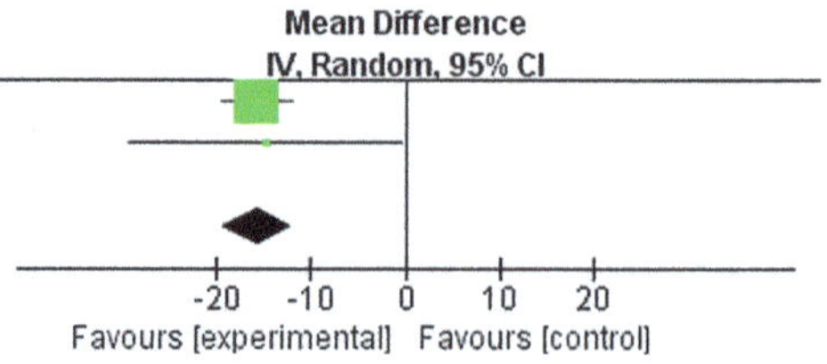

Fig. 5 Forest plot for the meta-analysis of operative time

kidney calices and depth in sheath placement was not assessed in the included studies. Finally, there are some unpublished data and missing negative data in the original reports, and because of this publication bias, our conclusion may be skewed.

The application of a vacuum-assisted sheath in MPCNL improves the safety and efficiency compared to the conventional sheath. A vacuum-assisted sheath significantly increases the SFR while reducing operative time and postoperative infection. Due to the inherent limitations of the included studies, large-scale, multiregion, multicenter, prospective RCTs should be performed in the future to validate our results.

Abbreviations

MPCNL: Minimally invasive percutaneous nephrolithotomy; SFR: Stone-free rate; PCNL: Percutaneous nephrolithotomy; PRISMA: Preferred Reporting Items for Systematic Reviews and Meta-analysis; MINORS: The Methodological Index for Nonrandomized Studies; CIs: Confidence intervals; RCTs: Randomized controlled trials; CCTs: Case-controlled trials; CT: Computed tomography.

Acknowledgements

Not applicable.

Authors' contributions

WZH, ZL, and ZXF participated in the design of this study. ZL drafted the manuscript. GLP and ZY collected and analyzed the data, and HY and ZXF critically revised the manuscript. All authors have read and approved the final manuscript.

Competing interests

The authors declare no competing interests.

References

1. Bouatia M, Benramdane L, Idrissi MOB, Draoui M. An epidemiological study on the composition of urinary stones in Morocco in relation to age and sex. Afr J Urol. 2015;21(3):194–7.
2. Antonelli JA, Maalouf NM, Pearle MS, Lotan Y. Use of the National Health and Nutrition Examination Survey to calculate the impact of obesity and diabetes on cost and prevalence of urolithiasis in 2030. Eur Urol. 2014;66(4):724–9. https://doi.org/10.1016/j.eururo.2014.06.036.
3. Torricelli FCM, Monga M. Staghorn renal stones: what the urologist needs to know. Int Braz J. 2020;46(6):927–33. https://doi.org/10.1590/s1677-5538.ibju.2020.99.07.
4. Pradère B, Doizi S, Proietti S, Brachlow J, Traxer O. Evaluation of guidelines for surgical management of urolithiasis. J Urol. 2018;199(5):1267–71. https://doi.org/10.1016/j.juro.2017.11.111.
5. Ghani KR, Andonian S, Bultitude M, Desai M, Giusti G, Okhunov Z, et al. Percutaneous nephrolithotomy: update, trends, and future directions. Eur Urol. 2016;70(2):382–96. https://doi.org/10.1016/j.eururo.2016.01.047.
6. Seitz C, Desai M, Häcker A, Hakenberg OW, Liatsikos E, Nagele U, et al. Incidence, prevention, and management of complications following percutaneous nephrolitholapaxy. Eur Urol. 2012;61(1):146–58. https://doi.org/10.1016/j.eururo.2011.09.016.
7. Ruhayel Y, Tepeler A, Dabestani S, MacLennan S, Petřík A, Sarica K, et al. Tract sizes in miniaturized percutaneous nephrolithotomy: a systematic review from the European Association of Urology Urolithiasis Guidelines Panel. Eur Urol. 2017;72(2):220–35. https://doi.org/10.1016/j.eururo.2017.01.046.
8. Feng MI, Tamaddon K, Mikhail A, Kaptein JS, Bellman GC. Prospective randomized study of various techniques of percutaneous nephrolithotomy. Urology. 2001;58(3):345–50. https://doi.org/10.1016/s0090-4295(01)01225-0.
9. Omar M, Noble M, Sivalingam S, El Mahdy A, Gamal A, Farag M, et al. Systemic inflammatory response syndrome after percutaneous nephrolithotomy: a randomized single-blind clinical trial evaluating the impact of irrigation pressure. J Urol. 2016;196(1):109–14. https://doi.org/10.1016/j.juro.2016.01.104.
10. Liberati A, Altman DG, Tetzlaff J, Mulrow C, Gøtzsche PC, Ioannidis JP, et al. The PRISMA statement for reporting systematic reviews and meta-analyses of studies that evaluate health care interventions: explanation and elaboration. PLoS Med. 2009;6(7): e1000100. https://doi.org/10.1371/journal.pmed.1000100.
11. Jadad AR, Moore RA, Carroll D, Jenkinson C, Reynolds DJ, Gavaghan DJ, et al. Assessing the quality of reports of randomized clinical trials: is blinding necessary? Control Clin Trials. 1996;17(1):1–12. https://doi.org/10.1016/0197-2456(95)00134-4.
12. Kjaergard LL, Villumsen J, Gluud C. Reported methodologic quality and discrepancies between large and small randomized trials in meta-analyse. Ann Intern Med. 2001;135(11):982–9.
13. Higgins JP, Thompson SG. Quantifying heterogeneity in a meta-analysis. Stat Med. 2002;21(11):1539–58. https://doi.org/10.1002/sim.1186.
14. Du C, Song L, Wu X, Fan D, Zhu L, Liu S, et al. Suctioning minimally invasive percutaneous nephrolithotomy with a patented system is effective to treat renal staghorn calculi: a prospective multicenter study. Urol Int. 2018;101(2):143–9. https://doi.org/10.1159/000488399.
15. Xu G, Liang J, He Y, Li X, Yang W, Lai D, et al. Comparison of two different minimally invasive percutaneous nephrostomy sheaths for the treatment of staghorn stones. BJU Int. 2020;125(6):898–904. https://doi.org/10.1111/bju.15031.
16. Huang J, Song L, Xie D, Li M, Deng X, Hu M, et al. A Randomized Study of Minimally Invasive Percutaneous Nephrolithotomy (MPCNL) with the aid of a patented suctioning sheath in the treatment of renal calculus complicated by pyonephrosis by one surgery. BMC Urol. 2016;16(1):71. https://doi.org/10.1186/s12894-016-0184-0.
17. Türk C, Petřík A, Sarica K, Seitz C, Skolarikos A, Straub M, et al. EAU guidelines on interventional treatment for urolithiasis. Eur Urol. 2016;69(3):475–82. https://doi.org/10.1016/j.eururo.2015.07.041.
18. Skolarikos A, Alivizatos G, de la Rosette JJ. Percutaneous nephrolithotomy and its legacy. Eur Urol. 2005;47(1):22–8. https://doi.org/10.1016/j.eururo.2004.08.009.
19. Sabnis RB, Ganesamoni R, Sarpal R. Miniperc: what is its current status? Curr Opin Urol. 2012;22(2):129–33. https://doi.org/10.1097/MOU.0b013e3283502fb4.
20. Wu C, Hua LX, Zhang JZ, Zhou XR, Zhong W, Ni HD. Comparison of renal pelvic pressure and postoperative fever incidence between standard- and mini-tract percutaneous nephrolithotomy. Kaohsiung J Med Sci. 2017;33(1):36–43. https://doi.org/10.1016/j.kjms.2016.10.012.
21. Chiancone F, Meccariello C, Fedelini M, Giannella R, Fedelini P. Four dilation techniques in percutaneous nephrolithotomy: a single-institute comparative analysis. Minerva urologica e nefrologica = The Italian journal of urology and nephrology. 2020. doi: https://doi.org/10.23736/s0393-2249.20.03836-9.
22. Lievore E, Boeri L, Zanetti SP, Fulgheri I, Fontana M, Turetti M, et al. Clinical comparison of minipercutaneous nephrolithotomy with vacuum cleaner effect or with a vacuum-assisted access sheath: a single center experience. J Endourol. 2020. https://doi.org/10.1089/end.2020.0555.
23. De S, Autorino R, Kim FJ, Zargar H, Laydner H, Balsamo R, et al. Percutaneous nephrolithotomy versus retrograde intrarenal surgery: a systematic review and meta-analysis. Eur Urol. 2015;67(1):125–37. https://doi.org/10.1016/j.eururo.2014.07.003.
24. Guohua Z, Wen Z, Xun L, Wenzhong C, Yongzhong H, Zhaohui H, et al. The influence of minimally invasive percutaneous nephrolithotomy on renal pelvic pressure in vivo. Surg Laparoscopy Endoscopy Percutaneous Tech. 2007;17(4):307–10. https://doi.org/10.1097/SLE.0b013e31806e61f4.
25. Goel P, Bajpai M, Kandasamy D. An enigmatic route to the contralateral pelvicalyceal system on antegrade pyelogram. J Indian Assoc Pediatr Surg. 2018;23(4):236–8. https://doi.org/10.4103/jiaps.JIAPS_139_18.
26. de la Rosette J, Denstedt J, Geavlete P, Keeley F, Matsuda T, Pearle M, et al. The clinical research office of the endourological society ureteroscopy global study: indications, complications, and outcomes in 11,885 patients. J Endourol. 2014;28(2):131–9. https://doi.org/10.1089/end.2013.0436.

27. Chen D, Jiang C, Liang X, Zhong F, Huang J, Lin Y, et al. Early and rapid prediction of postoperative infections following percutaneous nephrolithotomy in patients with complex kidney stones. BJU Int. 2019;123(6):1041–7. https://doi.org/10.1111/bju.14484.
28. Cheng F, Yu W, Zhang X, Yang S, Xia Y, Ruan Y. Minimally invasive tract in percutaneous nephrolithotomy for renal stones. J Endourol. 2010;24(10):1579–82. https://doi.org/10.1089/end.2009.0581.
29. Lai D, Chen M, Sheng M, Liu Y, Xu G, He Y, et al. Use of a novel vacuum-assisted access sheath in minimally invasive percutaneous nephrolithotomy: a feasibility study. J Endourol. 2020;34(3):339–44. https://doi.org/10.1089/end.2019.0652.
30. Sahan A, Cubuk A, Ozkaptan O, Ertaş K, Canakci C, Eryildirim B, et al. Safety of upper pole puncture in percutaneous nephrolithotomy with the guidance of ultrasonography versus fluoroscopy: a comparative study. Urol Int. 2020;104(9–10):769–74. https://doi.org/10.1159/000509448.

19

Augmentation uretero-enterocystoplasty for refractory urinary tract dysfunction: A long-term retrospective study

Xiaoqian Ying† and Limin Liao*†

Abstract

Objectives: To report the long-term efficacy and complications of the augmentation uretero-enterocystoplasty (AUEC), including augmentation cystoplasty with simultaneous ureteroplasty and ureteral anti-reflux implantation in a single center.

Methods: We retrospectively reviewed clinical records, video-urodynamic data, and magnetic resonance urography of 210 patients who underwent the procedure for refractory lower urinary tract dysfunction (LUTD) from 2003 to 2019. International vesicoureteral reflux (VUR) and upper urinary tract dilatation (UUTD) grading systems were applied to assess upper urinary tract function, and post-operative complications were assessed.

Results: Mean age was 28.1 years, with a mean follow-up time of 57.4 months. A total of 338 ureters were simultaneously re-implanted, and ureteroplasty was performed on all ureters. There was a significant postoperative improvement in the bladder capacity, intravesical pressure, and compliance ($P < 0.05$). VUR improvement rate was 97.7% and postoperative improvement of UUTD presented in 72.5% ureters. Mean serum creatinine (Scr) level was significantly improved compared to preoperative Scr values (226.0 ± 89.4 μmol/L vs. 217.5 ± 133.9 umol/L, $P < 0.05$). The 1.0% patients had unacceptably postoperative urinary incontinence and 85.4% preoperative megaureters were improved. Primary complications included metabolic acidosis (9.5%), vesicoureteral anastomosis stenosis (6.2%), persistent VUR (2.7%), urinary calculi (6.6%), and intestinal dysfunction requiring laparotomy (3.3%).

Conclusion: In the study, a large series of patients treated with a complex surgical procedure was reported. It is novel, as this case series represents patients with aggressive surgical correction of VUR, ureteral tortuosity and upper tract dilation at the time of AC. AUEC was shown to have a positive role in treating patients with refractory LUTD associated with hydronephrosis and ureteral dilatation, stenosis or obstruction, with or without high- or low-pressure VUR. It was effective in improving renal function and protecting the UUT function from further deterioration in most patients with renal insufficiency.

Keywords: Augmentation cystoplasty, Refractory bladder dysfunction, Ureteral re-implantation, Efficacy, Complications

Introduction

Augmentation cystoplasty (AC) was firstly performed in an experimental dog with ileum at the end of 19th century, then it was applied to the patients with neurogenic bladders and small tuberculous bladders [1]. Its aim is to increase bladder compliance and capacity, decrease

*Correspondence: lmliao@263.net
†Xiaoqian Ying and Limin Liao: co-first authors
Department of Urology, Beijing Boai Hospital, China Rehabilitation Research Centre; School of Rehabilitation of Capital Medical University, No 10. Jiaomen Beilu, Fengtai District, Beijing 100068, China

bladder pressure, preserve renal function, and sustain urinary continence after the failure of conservative urinary management [2]. Various indications and substitution, and surgical techniques have been described in patients and animals with lower urinary tract dysfunction (LUTD) in recent decades [3]. Laparoscopic and robot-assisted procedure in AC showed feasible and safe outcomes as well [4]. Nowadays the gold standard for AC is enterocystoplasty. However, there is no consensus regarding simultaneous ureteral re-implantation (URI) and its efficacy. High intravesical pressure may result in vesicoureteral reflux (VUR), which is an important factor for upper urinary tract dilatation (UUTD), pyelonephritis, renal scarring, and renal deterioration [5]. It was indicated that more than 50% patients with high-grade VUR (grades III–V) underwent AC without simultaneous URI had residual high-grade VUR [6]. VUR initiated at lower intravesical pressure was suggested to be corrected concomitantly during AC as well [7]. Nevertheless, other studies have shown that performing AC alone could resolved VUR in most patients, thus URI is unnecessary [8].

To improve LUTD and protect kidneys from damage, we performed a surgical procedure that combines AC with simultaneous ureteroplasty and ureteral anti-reflux implantation (UARI), which we called augmentation uretero-enterocystoplasty (AUEC). To describe and analyze the safety and efficacy of the procedure with simultaneous UARI, we carried out the retrospective study.

Materials and methods

Subjects and assessment

This is a retrospective case series, from the urological surgeons leading by Limin Liao at China Rehabilitation Research Center. After obtaining Institutional Review Board approval from our center, we retrospectively reviewed the medical records of total patients underwent AUEC from 2003 to 2019. Preoperative anti-muscarinic administration and clean intermittent catheterization (CIC) worked poorly in all these patients. Some cases also adopted other therapies. Eight patients (3.8%) failed to manage urinary tract symptoms via botulinum toxin A (BTX-A), five patients (2.4%) underwent sacral neuromodulation, nineteen patients (9.1%) in ureteral stenting, five patients (2.4%) suffered ureteral re-implantation without AC, and 2 patients (1%) underwent somatic-visceral nerve reconnection procedure. Five patients (2.4%) had suffered the unilateral kidney resection. Most patients had decreased bladder capacity, low compliance, high intravesical pressure, and normal or high urethral pressure. All video-urodynamics (VUD) studies, magnetic resonance urography (MRU), and serum creatinine (Scr) levels were analyzed. VUD studies were performed according to Good Urodynamics Practice [9] with a filling rate of 10 ml/min. Ureteral dilatation and hydronephrosis was evaluated according to MRU-UUTD system described by Liao [10, 11] and VUR was graded with the international grading system for vesicoureteral reflux [12]. The Scr level was derived from hematologic examination. Ureteral obstruction or stenosis were identified by radioactive renogram and MRU. Complications were recorded via medical records or telephone inquiries. MRU in 39 of 210 cases lost to follow-up, and no VUDS in 29 cases. All patients' Scr values and postop complications was obtained.

Surgical indications

To undergo AC, patients had to have at least one of the following conditions: (1) detrusor overactivity (DO) with high intravesical pressure (>40 cm H2O) during urinary storage phrase or lower bladder compliance (<10 ml/cm H_2O); (2) socially unacceptable urinary incontinence due to DO or severely decreased bladder capacity; (3) high-grade and/or low-pressure VUR with UUT deterioration; (4) high-grade UUTD with UUT deterioration; (5) infective or inflammatory disorders (e.g., tuberculous bladder contracture); or (6) a significant decrease in the Scr level (>1.5 mg/dL [132.6 umol/l]) after indwelling urethral catheterization in patients with chronic renal failure.

The indications for UARI during AC included at least one of the following conditions: (1) high-grade VUR (grade III–V) during urinary storage phrase [13]; (2) VUR at low intravesical pressures (<10 cm H_2O); and (3) high-graded UUTD (grade 3–4) according to MRU-UUTD system combined with ureteral tortuosity; (4) vesico-ureteral junction (UVJ) stenosis. The indication for ureteroplasty (ureterolysis and tailoring/shortening) during AUEC included megaureter, severely tortuous ureter, and stenosing ureteric stenosis.

Technique

AUEC with concomitant unilateral ureter treatment was performed with patients in the supine position (Fig. 1). We identified and detached the affected ureter from UVJ. About 25 cm sigmoid was isolated as a substitution.

The ends of the original intestine are anastomosed end-to-end. Anhydrous alcohol was used to deal with the isolated intestinal segment. The segment was detubularized along the border of the mesentery and it was sutured in a "U" (sigmoid) [14] shape to form a substitutable patch.

Urinary bladder was longitudinally incised and megaureters, severe tortuous ureters, or stenosing ureteric stenoses were performed simultaneous ureteroplasty, including ureterolysis and tailoring/shortening. Ureterolysis refers to mobilization and straightening of the ureter. Tailoring refers to shortening the length of

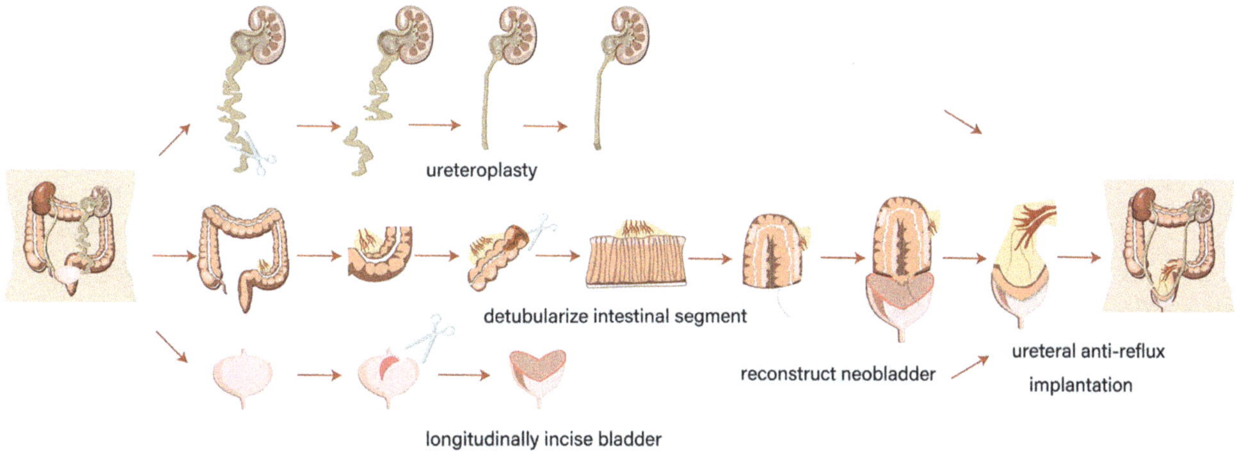

Fig. 1 Schematic diagram for AUEC involving the unilateral ureter (The copyright of Figure is attributed to Limin Liao. The manuscript has got permissions to use the image)

the ureter, and reducing the diameter of the megaureters, including ureterolysis and tailoring/shortening. Ureterolysis refers to mobilization and straightening of the ureter. Tailoring refers to shortening the length of the ureter, and reducing the diameter of the megaureters. We made a hemi-Kock nipple valve with original ureter, and the plastic ureter was re-implanted on the native bladder or bowel depend on the fibrotic tissue and the thickness of bladder wall, and bladder contracture. Double-J catheters were inserted for postoperative urinary drainage. A suprapubic catheter and two tubes were respectively placed for the postoperative neobladder, intra-abdominal and retropubic drainage. If the Mitrofanoff procedure was acceptable, it can be performed simultaneously.

Statistical analysis

Quantitative data are presented as the mean ± SD. The paired Student's t-test was used to compare preoperative with postoperative values. SPSS 21.0 was used, and a $P<0.05$ was considered statistically significant.

Results

Patient characteristics

Our study involved 153 males (72.9%) and 57 females (27.1%), and the mean age of these patients was 28.1 years (range: 4–67 years). The mean duration of their lower urinary tract symptoms was 13.5 years (range: 1–56 years). The mean follow-up was 57.4 months (range:1–151 months). Table 1 and Fig. 2 listed the etiologies of their clinical diagnoses.

Preoperative and postoperative VUD

Postoperative detrusor pressure decreased significantly ($P=0.001$), and a significant increase presented in postoperative bladder capacity and compliance compared to preoperative VUD parameters: mean detrusor pressure was decreased from 36.0 ± 28.0 cm H_2O to 17.2 ± 15.0 cm H_2O ($P=0.0001$); mean bladder capacity was increased from 220.8 ± 168.4 ml to 443.1 ± 161.2 ml ($P=0.001$); and compliance was increased from 8.9 ± 11.1 ml/cmH_2O to 42.7 ± 62.9 ml/cmH_2O ($P=0.001$). Mean intravesical pressure was decreased from 44.1 ± 26.3 cm H_2O to 24.5 ± 15.8 cm H_2O ($P=0.042$).

Table 1 Clinical diagnosis of 210 patients

Clinical diagnosis	No. Pts (%)
Neurogenic	176 (83.8)
Traumatic spinal cord injury	36 (17.1)
Neural tube defect*	102 (48.6)
Intraspinal tumor	21 (10.0)
Myelitis	1 (0.5)
Scoliosis	2 (1.0)
Pelvic and abdominal surgery	2 (1.0)
Pelvic fracture	2 (1.0)
Spinal vascular malformation	2 (1.0)
Complex etiology**	5 (2.4)
Lumbar disc herniation	3 (1.4)
Nonneurogenic	16 (7.6)
Congenital malformations of urinary system developmental defect	7 (3.3)
Infective or inflammatory disorders	9 (4.3)
Unclear etiology	18 (8.6)
Total	210

*Including myelomeningocele, spina bifida and tethered cord syndrome

**Complex etiology ≥ two clinical diagnoses

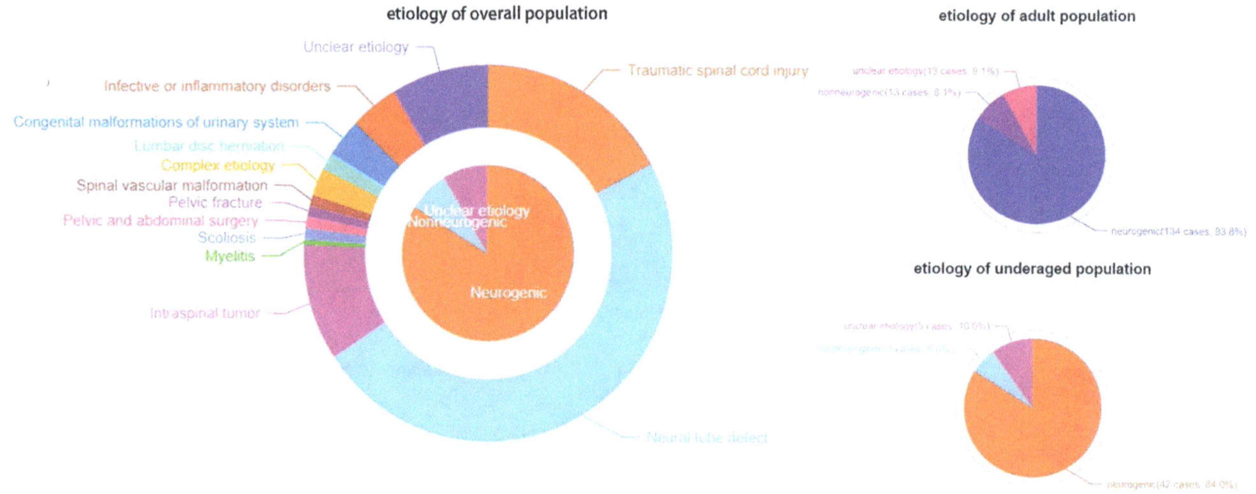

Fig. 2 Etiological characteristics of 210 patients

Hydronephrosis and ureteral dilatation improvement

We totally performed simultaneous UARI on 338 ureters during AC, and ureterolysis and/or cutting was performed on all ureters. According to MRU-UUTD system, significantly postoperative improvement of UUTD presented in 245 ureter units (72.5%), unchanged UUTD was observed in 66 ureter units (19.5%), and deterioration in 27 ureter units (8.0%).

Vesicoureteral reflux and improvement

Preoperative VUR was detected in 175 ureter units. According to postoperative VUD, residual VUR was observed in only 4 ureter units (2.3%), and the UARI improvement rate was as high as 97.7% (171 ureter units).

Renal function changes

Fifty-nine LUTD patients reported preoperative chronic renal insufficiency, and 74.6% of them had postoperative improvement according to the latest checkups. Mean Scr level was significantly improved compared to preoperative Scr values (226.0 ± 89.4 μmol/L vs. 217.5 ± 133.9 μmol/L, $P = 0.033$). Two (1.0%) patients with preoperative chronic renal insufficiency and required dialysis after 3 years, and a patient diagnosed with new onset uremia.

Urinary incontinence and megaureters

Before the operations, all these patients were diagnosed as varying degree of urinary incontinence and two patients (1.0%) had unacceptably postoperative urinary incontinence. They were treated with artificial urethral sphincter (AUS) implantation after AUEC. Totally 219 preoperative megaureters were observed and they were improved with a rate of 85.4% (187 ureters).

Complications

Metabolic acidosis

Twenty cases (9.5%) developed metabolic acidosis (CO_2 combining power < 22 mmol/L) accompanied by abnormally increased Scr values and serum chlorine (> 110 mmol/L). Only 8 (2.2%) cases reported new-onset postoperative metabolic acidosis among them. These patients recovered uneventfully after the oral bicarbonate or infusion administration.

Stenotic vesicoureteral anastomosis

Preoperative ureteral obstruction was detected in 179 ureters (53.0%). A postoperative vesicoureteral anastomotic stricture (VUAS) was observed in 14 ureters (4.1%) of 13 patients (6.2%). One of these cases had a large number of inflammatory polyps which obstructed the anastomosis of the bilateral ureteral orifices. Unilateral VUAS in the other 12 cases (3.6%). Among them, VUAS in 9 (2.7%) ureters was residual for incompletely solved obstruction and new onset VUAS in 5 (1.5%) ureters. The treatment included UARI again for 4 cases, the placement of D-J catheters or stents in 9 cases. Finally, VUAS in 12 ureters were improved apparently after above interventions. UUTD persisted for residual VUAS in 2 ureters of 2 cases and percutaneous nephrostomy was performed for.

Vesicoureteral reflux

There were 9 ureters (2.7%) with VUR within 1 year after the procedure, including residual VUR in 4 ureters (1.2%) and new-onset VUR in 5 ureters (1.5%). All these VUR was initiated at an intravesical pressure lower than 40 cm H_2O. After the treatment with anti-muscarinics and antibiotics or watchful waiting, VUR in 4 ureters solved and VUR in 5 ureters (1.5%) persisted at the final evaluation.

Urinary tract infection and stone formation

Preoperatively recurrent symptomatic urinary tract infection (UTI) was reported in 97 (46.2%) cases. Cases suffered postoperative symptomatic UTI is less than 20%, and 3 (1.4%) cases were diagnosed as epididymitis. Urinary calculi occurred to 14 (6.6%) cases, including bladder calculi in 6 cases (2.9%) and ureteral or renal calculi in 8 cases (3.8%). Ten cases were treated with endoscopic lithotripsy or removal and recovered uneventfully, and the other 4 cases were still under watchful waiting.

Bowel dysfunction and malignancy

Postoperative intestinal obstruction occurred in 7 (3.3%) cases. They were treated with laparotomy and recovered without any events. Changes in bowel habits were reported in 10 (4.7%) cases, including fecal incontinence in a case (0.5%), diarrhea in 6 (2.9%) cases and improved constipation in 3 (1.4%) cases. Malignancy in neobladder was not detected during follow up.

Discussion

Due to similar proportions of etiology (adults vs. underage: neurogenic 83.8% vs. 84.0%; nonneurogenic 8.1% vs. 6.0%; unclear 8.1% vs. 10.0%; Fig. 2), we analyzed data from adult and underage patients in combination. In the study, male patients were more than females and most patients suffered neurogenic bladder.

Patients with neurogenic bladder are at increased risk for the storage and emptying of bladder, hydronephrosis, and renal function deterioration [15]. According to the study of Adam and his colleagues, UUT alternations and renal damages was at low incidence within 8–11 years for multiple aggressive medical management [16]. As a surgical intervention, AC works to create a hypo-pressure storage reservoir, which facilitates increasing bladder capacity and compliance, protect against renal function damages, improving urinary continence and the quality of life. Various human tissues sources and synthetic materials in AC have been described, including bowel, stomach, ureters, peritoneum, omentum, polyvinyl sponge, gelatin sponge, collagen with polyglactin membrane and so on [17–19]. Due to the incidence of their complications, enterocystoplasty is the preferable choice and the commonly patches are from ileum and sigmoid. We preferred to use sigmoid segments for the large intestinal cavity, rich mesentery, thick intestinal wall, and available maneuverability [20]. The choice, however, comes with the disadvantages of numerous mucus secretion, high occurrence of urinary systems infections and stone formation. In the longer study, malignancy was reported as well. Ileum was adapted for being easily handled, abundant mesentery and blood supply. However, metabolic disturbances, significant anemia and bowel obstruction were common.

Simultaneously, URAI were performed with AC in these patients according to our indications. In addition to the significantly improvement in postoperative bladder capacity, compliance and intravesical pressure, 97.7% VUR and 72.5% UUTD improvement was observed. Postoperatively ameliorated renal function presented in 74.6% of patients with preoperative chronic renal insufficiency. AC alone plays a positive role in improving urodynamics, but the function of URI or URAI was controversial. VUR was considered as a crucial factor for complications of upper UTI and renal damages [21]. It was turned out that 0–47.3% of VUR was residual after AC alone [6, 7]. Simultaneous URAI could decrease the incidence to 4% [22]. In our study, only 2.3% residual VURs was observed. Some researchers suggested VUR was secondary to hypo-compliance and high intravesical pressure, thus VUR could be solved after AC alone. However, VUR at the low intravesical pressure made it less stringency, which was assumed relevant to ureterotrigonal insufficiency [7]. On the other hand, URAI was not encouraged to be performed in significant bladder contracture for increased technical difficulties and the risk of postoperative VUAS or obstruction from thickening or fibrosis of the bladder wall [23]. To avoid these risks, we commonly chose to perform URAI in the soft bowel patches fixed on the neobladder. Most urinary incontinence and megaureters was improved after AUEC. Merely unacceptable urinary incontinence was reported (1%), which was tightly relevant to low urethral closure pressure in the study. During AUEC, 5 cases (2.4%) had catheterisable channels created with appendix and ileum at the same time.

Commonly, complications were primarily associated with the sources of patches. Metabolic abnormalities were usually derived the usage of various patches. Reabsorption and secretion of bowel patches was the general underlying mechanism for electrolyte disturbances [24]. In other study, more than 15% patients were treated with oral bicarbonate for metabolic acidosis while it was less than 10% at our center. Baseline normal renal function of most patients may play a positive role for the outcomes. Postoperative VUAS was a structural complication, which often resulted from surgical techniques, the site URAI was performed and the perioperative local mucomembranous edema according to our experience. Timely individual interventions could solve it uneventfully. The postoperative VUR within 12 months was observed in other study as well [7]. It was hypothesized that augmented bowel need time to became expanded and more compliant in the early months after the procedure.

Symptomatic UTI in 22.7% of patients underwent AC with an ileal and 8% in patients suffered a gastrocystoplasty had been reported [25]. Symptomatic UTI included positive urine routine test and getting febrile in the article. More than 50% recurrent symptomatic UTI was solved after AUEC. About 6–52% patients underwent enterocystoplasty was detected with postoperative urinary calculi [26, 27]. Insufficient bladder emptying and urinary stasis increased the risks of urinary stone formation. Furthermore, bacteria, mucus secreted by bowel patches and metabolic abnormalities were very relevant to stone formation. To decrease the risks of UTI and stone formation, we administrated these patients with sufficient CIC and routine bladder irrigation.

The postoperative intestinal obstruction was 3.3%, which was similar with the reported data (3%-3.2%). As a fatal complication, spontaneous bladder perforation was not observed. Avoiding technical error and careful suture and fixation during the procedure was our experience. Although urinary bladder cancer has been reported, we didn't detect malignancy in these patients [28]. We presumed that 90% tumors were diagnosed after 10 years [29] and the follow-up time over 10 years of these patients was rare (3 cases, 1.4%). In the study, we were mainly aimed to recognize and report the effects of AUEC in all LUTD patients based our indications, no matter what causes were. Therefore, a small number of patients with nonneurogenic and unclear etiology were included in analysis. Generally, AUEC or AC for refractory LUTD resulting from various etiology (especially in tuberculous cystitis or urinary tract tuberculosis) was likely considered to produce different outcomes. However, the comparison between urinary tract tuberculosis causes and other etiology was rarely reported. A long term follow-up study (mean postoperative follow-up 11.1 ± 9.1 years) of de Figueiredo and colleagues suggested tuberculous cystitis patients obtained good bladder capacity, good compliance and normal sensation after AC with or without URI using detubularized sigmoid segments [30]. And preoperative renal function maintained in 80% cases. An Indian center also indicated AC with or without URI reconstruction could increases the bladder capacity and preserves UUTs [31]. In our study, nine cases underwent AUEC for indications resulting from inflammatory disorders. Of these cases, eight (88.9%) maintained preoperative renal function or got improvement. A case (11.1%) come into bad results for postoperative vesicoureteral anastomotic obstruction from bladder inflammatory polyps, although VUD parameters improvement had been observed. Mitrofanoff procedure was rarely performed in our center. Additionally, postoperative AUS implantation was tightly linked with originally low urethral pressure.

Whatever it goes, preoperative estimations for the capacity of CIC and long-term dynamic evaluations are still very important for patients treated with the procedure. In younger patients, CIC is performed by the nurses or their parents. The volume of CIC referred to the maximum bladder capacity from VUD.

Conclusions

We reported a large series of patients treated with a complex surgical procedure (AUEC). It is novel, as this case series represents patients with aggressive surgical correction of VUR, ureteral tortuosity and upper tract dilation at the time of AC. The results showed that AUEC procedure is safe and effective for most patients with refractory LUTD associated with hydronephrosis and ureteral dilatation, stenosis or obstruction, with or without high- or low-pressure VUR. It extends the indications for the AC. This technique played a positive role in stabilizing renal function and protecting the UUT function and residue renal function from further deterioration in most patients with renal insufficiency.

Abbreviations

AC: Augmentation cystoplasty; AUEC: Augmentation uretero-enterocystoplasty; AUS: Urethral sphincter; BTX-A: Botulinum toxin A; CIC: Clean intermittent catheterization; DO: Detrusor overactivity; LUTD: Lower urinary tract dysfunction; MRU: Magnetic resonance urography; Scr: Serum creatinine; URAI: Ureteral anti-reflux implantation; URI: Ureteral reimplantation; UTI: Urinary tract infection; UUTD: Upper urinary tract dilatation; UVJ: Vesico-ureteral junction; VUD: Video-urodynamics; VUAS: Vesicoureteral anastomotic stricture; VUR: Vesicoureteral reflux.

Acknowledgements

Thank Drs. G. Fu, G. Chen, J. Wu, Z. Xiong, F. Zhang, H. Cong, Y. Wang, L. Za, X. Li, D. Pang for the assistance during the procedure they performed for these patients.

Authors' contributions

L.L. Project development and data analysis. X.Y. Data management, analysis and manuscript writing. Both authors read and approved the final manuscript.

Competing interests

The authors declare that they have no competing interests.

References

1. Obermayr F, Szavay P, Schaefer J, Fuchs J. Outcome of augmentation cystoplasty and bladder substitution in a pediatric age group. Eur J Pediatr Surg. 2011;21(2):116–9.
2. Jednak R. The evolution of bladder augmentation: from creating a reservoir to reconstituting an organ. Front Pediatr. 2014; 2:10. Published 2014 Feb 10.
3. Biers SM, Venn SN, Greenwell TJ. The past, present and future of augmentation cystoplasty. BJU Int. 2012;109(9):1280–93.
4. Grilo N, Chartier - Kastler E, Grande P, et al. Robot-assisted supratrigonal cystectomy and augmentation cystoplasty with totally intracorporeal reconstruction in neurourological patients: technique description and preliminary results. Eur Urol. 2021;79: 858–65.
5. Cheng PJ, Myers JB. Augmentation cystoplasty in the patient with neurogenic bladder. World J Urol. 2020;38(12):3035–46.

6. Wang JB, Liu CS, Tsai SL, Wei CF, Chin TW. Augmentation cystoplasty and simultaneous ureteral reimplantation reduce high-grade vesicoureteral reflux in children with neurogenic bladder. J Chin Med Assoc. 2011;74(7):294–7.
7. Soygur T, Burgu B, Zümrütbas A, Süer E. The need for ureteric re-implantation during augmentation cystoplasty: video-urodynamic evaluation. BJU Int. 2010;105(4):530–2.
8. Soylet Y, Emir H, Ilce Z, Yesildag E, Buyukunal SN, Danismend N. Quo vadis? Ureteric reimplantation or ignoring reflux during augmentation cystoplasty. BJU Int. 2004;94(3):379–80.
9. Schäfer W, Abrams P, Liao L, et al. Good urodynamic practices: uroflowmetry, filling cystometry, and pressure-flow studies. Neurourol Urodyn. 2002;21(3):261–74.
10. Liao L, Zhang F, Chen G. New grading system for upper urinary tract dilation using magnetic resonance urography in patients with neurogenic bladder. BMC Urol. 2014;14:38. Published 2014 May 22.
11. Liao L. A new comprehensive classification system for both lower and upper urinary tract dysfunction in patients with neurogenic bladder. Urol Int. 2015;94(2):244–8.
12. Metcalfe CB, Macneily AE, Afshar K. Reliability assessment of international grading system for vesicoureteral reflux. J Urol. 2012;188(4 Suppl):1490–2.
13. Wang Z, Liao L. Effectiveness and complications of augmentation cystoplasty with or without nonrefluxing ureteral reimplantation in patients with bladder dysfunction: a single center 11-year experience. J Urol. 2018;199(1):200–5.
14. Hautmann RE, Volkmer B, Egghart G, et al. Functional outcome and complications following ileal neobladder reconstruction in male patients without tumor recurrence. More than 35 years of experience from a single center. J Urol. 2021;205(1):174–82.
15. Sripathi V, Mitra A. Management of neurogenic bladder. Indian J Pediatr. 2017;84(7):545–54.
16. Rensing AJ, Szymanski KM, Misseri R, et al. Radiographic abnormalities, bladder interventions, and bladder surgery in the first decade of life in children with spina bifida. Pediatr Nephrol. 2019;34(7):1277–82.
17. Budzyn J, Trinh H, Raffee S, Atiemo H. Bladder augmentation (Enterocystoplasty): the Current State of a Historic Operation. Curr Urol Rep. 2019;20(9):50. Published 2019 Jul 24.
18. Zhang F, Liao L. Tissue engineered cystoplasty augmentation for treatment of neurogenic bladder using small intestinal submucosa: an exploratory study. J Urol. 2014;192(2):544–50.
19. Mahan JD, Mentser MI, Koff SA. Complications of intestinal augmentation and substitution cystoplasty. Pediatr Nephrol. 1994;8(4):505–7.
20. Zhang F, Liao L. Sigmoidocolocystoplasty with ureteral reimplantation for treatment of neurogenic bladder. Urology. 2012;80(2):440–5.
21. Zaffanello M, Franchini M, Brugnara M, Fanos V. Evaluating kidney damage from vesico-ureteral reflux in children. Saudi J Kidney Dis Transpl. 2009;20(1):57–68.
22. Hayashi Y, Kato Y, Okazaki T, Lane GJ, Kobayashi H, Yamataka A. The effectiveness of ureteric reimplantation during bladder augmentation for high-grade vesicoureteric reflux in patients with neurogenic bladder: long-term outcome. J Pediatr Surg. 2007;42(12):1998-
23. Brereton RJ, Narayanan R, Ratnatunga C. Ureteric re-implantation in the neuropathic bladder. Br J Surg. 1987;74(12):1107–10.
24. Greenwell TJ, Venn SN, Mundy AR. Augmentation cystoplasty. BJU Int. 2001;88(6):511–25.
25. Metcalfe PD, Rink RC. Bladder augmentation: complications in the pediatric population. Curr Urol Rep. 2007;8(2):152–6.
26. Khoury AE, Salomon M, Doche R, et al. Stone formation after augmentation cystoplasty: the role of intestinal mucus. J Urol. 1997;158(3 Pt 2):1133–7.
27. DeFoor W, Minevich E, Reddy P, et al. Bladder calculi after augmentation cystoplasty: risk factors and prevention strategies. J Urol. 2004;172(5 Pt 1):1964–6.
28. Anderson JA, Matoso A, Murati Amador BI, et al. Invasive poorly differentiated adenocarcinoma of the bladder following augmentation cystoplasty: a multi-institutional clinicopathological study. Pathology. 2021;53:214–9.
29. Biardeau X, Chartier-Kastler E, Rouprêt M, Phé V. Risk of malignancy after augmentation cystoplasty: a systematic review. Neurourol Urodyn. 2016;35(6):675–82.
30. de Figueiredo, A. A., Lucon, A. M., Srougi. M. Bladder augmentation for the treatment of chronic tuberculous cystitis. Clinical and urodynamic evaluation of 25 patients after long term follow-up. Neurourol Urodyn.2006; 25: 433–440.
31. Singh V, Sinha RJ, Sankhwar SN, et al. Reconstructive surgery for tuberculous contracted bladder: experience of a center in northern India. Int Urol Nephrol. 2011;43:423–30.

20

Comparison of two different methods of establishment of canine urethroplasty model: An experimental trial

Jianpo Zhai[1†], Danhui Zhao[2†], Guanglin Huang[1], Libo Man[1], Guoqiang Yan[2] and Chengai Wu[2*]

Abstract

Background: Graft substitute urethroplasty is recommended for patients with long segment anterior urethral stricture. The therapeutic effects of the grafts need to be validated on the animal models. Therefore the aim of this study was to compared the operative time, blood loss, intra- and post- operative complications of two different methods of establishment of canine urethroplasty model.

Methods: Twelve Beagle dogs were randomly separated into control and experimental group using a random number table. Six animals in the control group received the conventional urethroplasty, while the other 6 in the experimental group received the modified procedures. Tube cystostomy and urethroplasty were performed in the control group. The cystostomy not the tube cystostomy were performed in the experimental group, and the testes were simultaneously removed with the scrotum. Per- and postoperative outcomes, complications were evaluated.

Results: The urethroplasty were successfully performed for all dogs and all of these procedures were done by the same surgeon. The median operative time in the control and experimental groups was 186.8 min and 188.7 min respectively. The blood loss in the control and experimental groups was 40.8 ml and 45.8 ml respectively. No intraoperative complications occurred. 3 animals in the control group developed acute urinary retention after the accidental removal of suprapubic bladder tube and the cystostomy was done again. There was no occurrence of urinary retention in the experimental group. 4 animals in the control group developed the perineal hematoma, in which one animal had the urine leakage and incision infection. Perineal hematoma occurred in only one animal in the experimental group.

Conclusion: The occurrence of urinary retention and perineal hematoma decreased in the modified group, in which the cystostomy not the tube cystostomy were performed and the testes with the scrotum were simultaneously removed.

Keywords: Urethroplasty, Animal model, Canine model, Urethral construction

Background

The treatment of severe urethral stricture has always been a challenge even for skilled urologists [1, 2]. Substitution urethroplasty is recommended for patients with long anterior segmental urethral stricture [3]. Several autologous grafts or flaps from genital and extragenital skin or mucosa have been recommended for patients with anterior urethral stricture [4–7]. Till now, the buccal mucosa is still the most commonly used substitute material. However, the autologous tissues are limited in quantity [8]. Furthermore, significant donor site morbidity

*Correspondence: drogon982007@163.com
†Jianpo Zhai and Danhui Zhao have contributed equally to this article.
[2] Beijing Research Institute of Traumatology and Orthopaedics, No. 31 Xinjiekou East Street, Xicheng District, Beijing 100035, China

has also been reported after its harvesting (16–32% for buccal mucosa grafts), therefore alternative therapeutic options are needed to improve the long-term outcomes [9, 10]. Tissue engineered urethra may overcome some of the aforementioned disadvantages by providing a temporary template to guide the urethral regeneration [11].

The therapeutic effects of the tissue engineered urethra need to be validated on the animal models. Large-animal models, such as the canine model, were preferred because large-animal urethral reconstruction closely mimics the scale and structure of human urethra [12]. In the substitute urethroplasty, the cystostomy has to be done simultaneously to prevent the postoperative urinary retention. The tube cystostomy is the most commonly performed in the conventional surgical procedures [13, 14]. However, the incidence of accidental removal of the cystostomy tube is high in animal studies. Moreover, several other defects of the techniques were still remained, including postoperative urinary retention, urinary leakage, perineal hematoma and incision infection. We currently modified the conventional techniques and compared the safety and effectiveness of two different methods of establishment of canine urethroplasty model.

Methods

The study was conducted with the approval of the Ethics Committee of Beijing Jishuitan Hospital. 12 Beagle dogs (at an average age of 1.2 y, 10.5 kg in weight), purchased from Beijing Marshall Biotechnology Co. Ltd, were used in the study. The dogs were randomly separated into control and experimental group using a random number table. Six animals in the control group received the conventional urethroplasty, while the other 6 in the experimental group received the modified procedures. The scaffold used in the experimental trial is the decellularized artery.

Dogs were fasted for 12 h and were walked prior to each anesthetic episode and procedure. The animals were sedated with acepromazine (0.05 mg/kg intramuscularly) and anesthesia was induced using a combination of ketamine (5 mg/kg intravenous) and diazepam (0.25 mg/kg intravenous). The animals were intubated and maintained under isoflurane (1–2%) anesthesia. The ventral abdomen from the xiphoid process to the scrotum was clipped, and the prepuce was flushed. A standard preparation scrub was performed on the ventral abdomen with iodophor. The surgical site was isolated using sterile drapes.

Preparation of scaffold

Carotid arteries were harvested from sacrificed beagle dogs, which were also purchased from Beijing Marshall Biotechnology Co. Ltd, and cut into 4.5-cm-long segments. Decellularized artery was then processed as below. First the carotid arteries were placed in the 0.625% glutaraldehyde solution for fixation for 4 h. Then the glutaraldehyde solution was replaced by a fresh solution of 1.0 M NaOH and 0.5% SDS to remove cells and virus-inactivated was carried out. Thirdly, Decellularized arteries were washed thoroughly by 0.1 M PBS at 4 °C for 48 h to remove residual substances. Finally the processed arteries were aseptically packed after histological examination to determine that it contained no cellular components, and stored at 0–4 °C.

Cystostomy

Conventional tube cystostomy: A midline incision was made in the skin of the lower abdomen (Fig. 1A). The skin, subcutaneous tissue and muscle were incised layer by layer, and the peritoneum was dissected to expose the bladder. A purse string suture was placed in the dome of the bladder, an incision was made within the purse string loop to allow the placement of a 16F tube and then the suture was tightened (Fig. 1B). After confirming that there was no leak around the tube, the bladder was secured to the ventral abdominal wall with four interrupted 3–0 sutures, placed left, right, cranial and caudal to the entrance of the tube into the bladder. The peritoneum and skin was closed with a 3–0 polypropylene suture. The tube was cut off with only 2–3 cm length left outside the body and secured to the skin with a finger-trap suture (Fig. 1C).

Modified cystostomy procedures: the bladder was also exposed through the midline abdominal incision (Fig. 1D). The intended entrance site of bladder was pulled out through the incision with an Allis forceps. The adjacent part of the entrance site was attached to the abdominal wall by interrupted sutures (Fig. 1E). Then the entrance site of the bladder wall was incised and 8 interrupted stitches were placed around the incision. In each stitch, the 3–0 suture passed through the entire thickness of bladder wall, the peritoneum and abdominal wall successively, then the sutures were tightened and tied (Fig. 1F). At last, a F16 tube was inserted into the bladder through the cystostomy and secured with the finger-trap suture.

Urethroplasty

Conventional urethroplasty procedures: A 6Fr urethral catheter was inserted into the urethra and a longitudinal incision was made over the penoscrotal junction segment of urethra (Fig. 2A). The corpora cavernosa was separated in the midline. In the tubular substitute urethroplasty, a segment of urethra with pre-set length (3 cm) was exposed and dissected (Fig. 2B, C), and the tubularized scaffold was anastomosed with the native ends of the urethral tissues using 5–0 vicryl sutures (Fig. 2D). In the

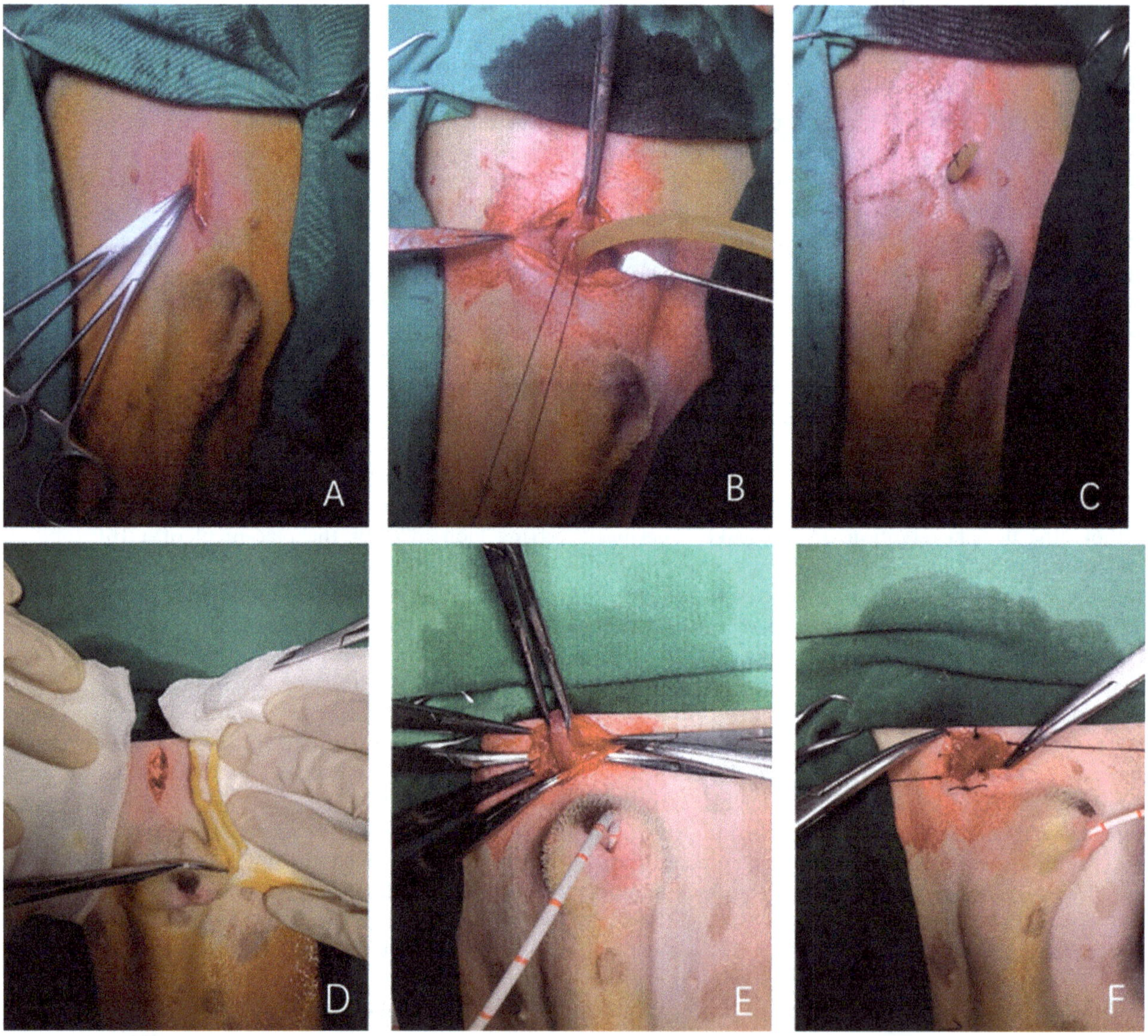

Fig. 1 Conventional and modified cystostomy **A** midline incision of lower abdomen. **B** Purse-string suture in the dome of the bladder with a F16 tube inserted into the bladder. **C** Subcutaneous and skin layers closed routinely with the tube secured with a finger-trap suture. **D** Midline incision of lower abdomen. **E** The intended entrance site of bladder pulled out through the incision. **F** The entrance site of the bladder wall incised and 8 interrupted stitches placed around the incision

patch substitute urethroplasty, the ventral surface of the urethra was exposed and a segment with pre-set length (3 cm) including half of the urethral circumference was excised. A part of the same length and width of the graft was sutured to the edges of the remaining normal urethra using 5–0 vicryl sutures. Identification nonabsorbable sutures were introduced at the distal and proximal ends of the anastomosis. The wound was closed in layers in a routine fashion (Fig. 2E, F). The 6F urethral catheter was fixed to the external urethral meatus by 3–0 silk suture and the mean duration of the catheter inside the urethra was 14 days.

Modified urethroplasty procedures: the longitudinal incision was also made over the penoscrotal junction segment of urethra after a 6Fr urethral catheter was inserted into the urethra (Fig. 3A). The corpora cavernosa was separated in the midline. Tunica vaginalis on the both sides were incised, and the testes were isolated and removed after the bilateral ligation of the vas deferens (Fig. 3B). Then the substitute urethroplasty was carried out (Fig. 3C, D). After that, the skin of the scrotum

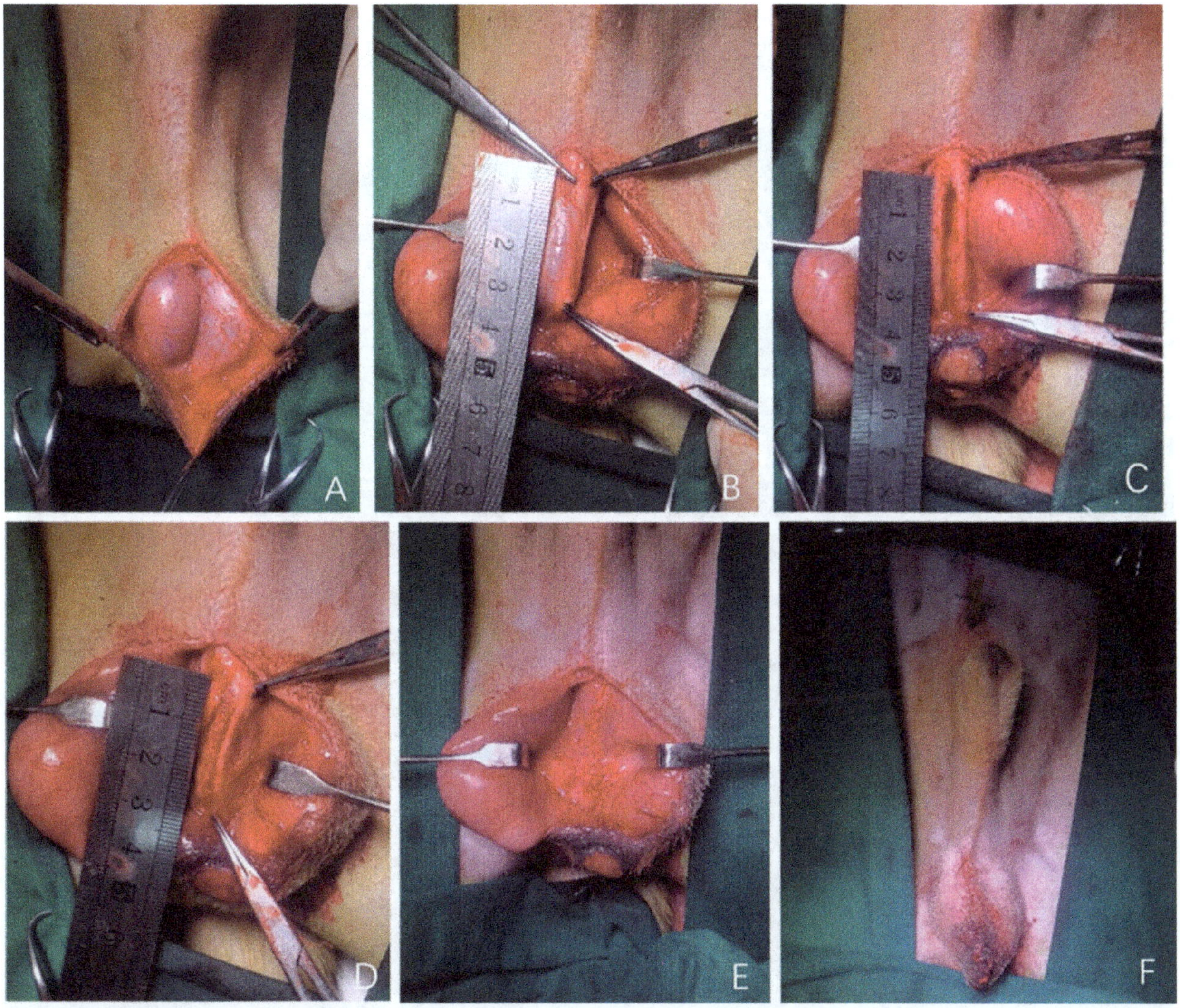

Fig. 2 Conventional urethroplasty **A** longitudinal incision over the penoscrotal junction segment of urethra. **B** The corpora cavernosa separated in the midline. **C** A segment of urethra with pre-set length was exposed and dissected. **D** Tubularized scaffold anastomosed to the native ends of the urethra and identification nonabsorbable sutures taken at the distal and proximal ends of the anastomosis. **E** The wound closed in layers. **F** The tube fixed to the external urethral meatus

and tunica vaginalis were removed (Fig. 3E) and then the incision was closed in layers with interrupted sutures (Fig. 3F).

Postoperative care

The dogs were housed individually in stainless steel cages. Free access to water and food (Beijing Keaoxieli Feed Co. Ltd.) was provided. The Elizabethan collar was used to prevent the dog from removing the cystostomy tube or urethral catheter. All dogs were given subcutaneous antibiotics (enrofloxacin, 0.1 mg/kg) and analgesic (lornoxicam, 0.27 mg/kg) daily for 3 days. Urethrogram was done 1 month postoperatively and then the experimental animals were humanely killed with intravenous injection of 3–4 ml ketamine. The urethra and bladder were removed from the body and analyzed grossly and histologically.

Statistical analysis

The Statistical Package for Social Sciences 21.0 software (SPSS 21.0, Chicago, IL, USA) was used for statistical analysis. The characteristics of the two groups were compared with the Mann–Whitney *U* test for continuous variables. The Fisher's exact or Pearson Chi-square

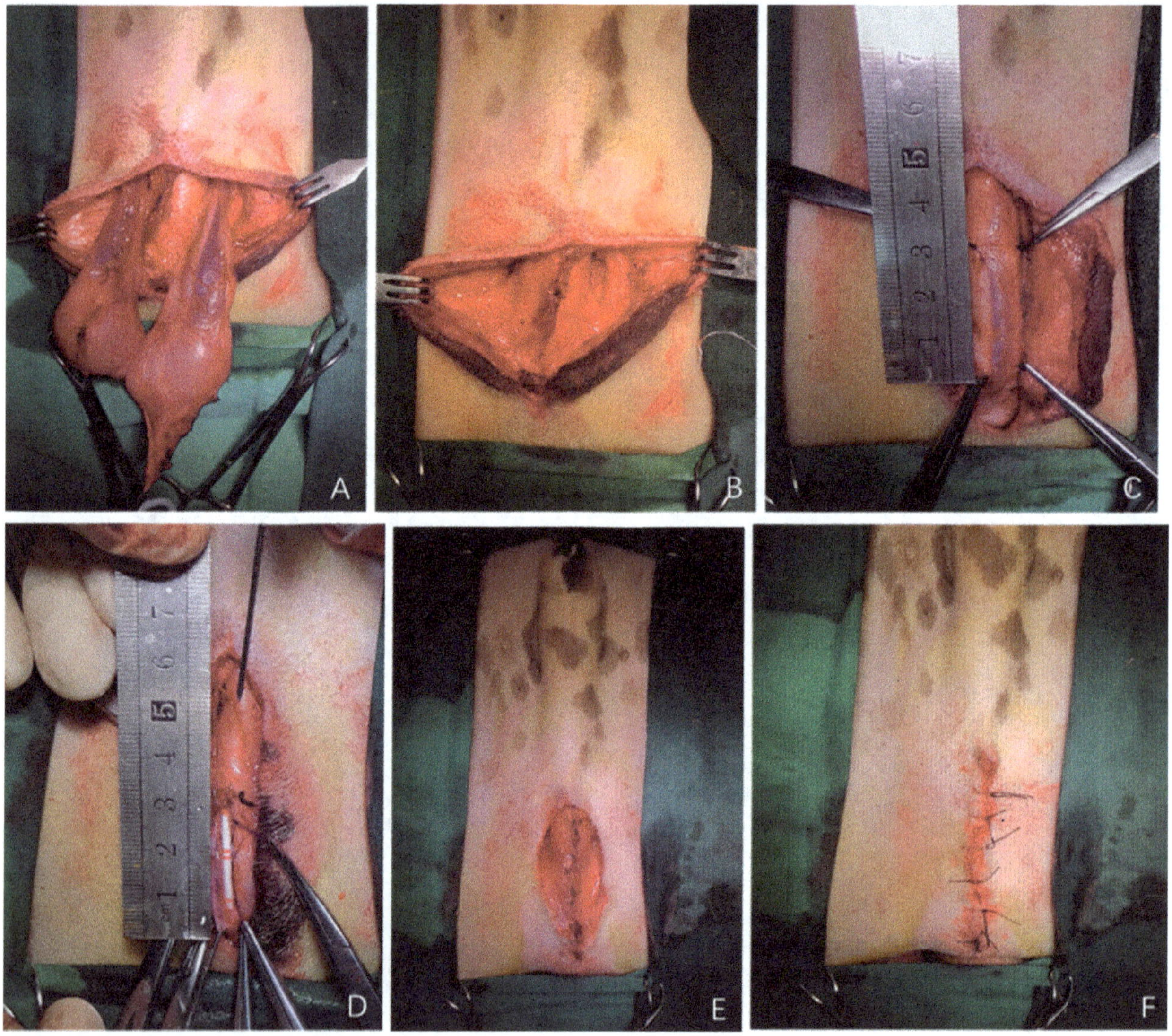

Fig. 3 Modified urethroplasty **A** longitudinal incision over the penoscrotal junction segment of urethra. **B** The testes isolated and removed. **C** A segment of urethra with pre-set length was exposed and dissected. **D** Scaffold sutured to the native edges of the urethra. **E** The scrotum and tunica vaginalis removed. **F** The incision closed in layers with interrupted sutures

tests were used for categorical variables. $P < 0.05$ considered as statistically significant.

Results

Operative time and blood loss

The urethroplasty were successfully performed for all dogs and all of these procedures were done by the same surgeon. The median operative time in the control and experimental groups was 186.8 min and 188.7 min respectively ($P = 0.706$). The blood loss in the control and experimental groups was 40.8 ml and 45.8 ml respectively ($P = 0.455$) (Table 1).

Table 1 Animals' characteristics and perioperative complications

Variations	Conventional (*N*:6)	Modified (*N*:6)	*P* value
Weight (kg)	8.5 ± 0.3	8.6 ± 0.3	0.807
Operative time (min)	186.8 ± 7.3	188.7 ± 8.9	0.706
Blood loss (ml)	40.8 ± 12.4	45.8 ± 9.7	0.455
Intestinal damage	0	0	
Urinary retention	3	0	0.182
Incision infection	1	0	1.000
Perineal or scrotal hematoma	4	1	0.242
Die	0	0	

Perioperative complications

All experimental dogs survived to the date of harvest. No intraoperative complications occurred. Three animals in the control group developed acute urinary retention after the accidental removal of suprapubic bladder tube and the cystostomy was done again. There was no occurrence of urinary retention in the experimental group. 4 animals in the control group developed the perineal hematoma, in which one animal had the urine leakage and incision infection. Perineal hematoma occurred in only one animal in the experimental group (Table 1).

Discussion

Tissue engineering and regenerative medicine studies have led to the development of various bioscaffolds that can be used for urethral repair, such as synthetic materials, collagen, and acellular matrix [15–17]. Results from the study of Orabi and De Filippo demonstrated that collagen scaffolds seeded with cells can be used for longer urethral replacement [12, 18]. Therefore, the scaffolds and seeded-cells are the two critical components of tissue engineering urethra [19–21]. A good blood supply and sterile environment, which can only be provided in good animal models, are essential for the survival both of the scaffolds and the seeded-cells after its transplantation.

It is essential to keep the catheter and tube in place after the urethroplasty. Cystostomy tube can drain the urine out of the body timely, preventing the inflammation caused by the urine leakage [22]. Urethral catheter can provide the support for the substitute grafts, favoring the urethral regeneration [23, 24]. Dogs tend to interfere with the foreign material after surgery, such as all kinds of tubes, dressings, sterile gauzes and so on. Post-operative accidental removal of tubes and catheters can cause the urinary retention and influence the results of the surgery. The occurrence of urinary retention decreased in the modified group. 3 animals in the control group developed the urinary retention, while no animal in the modified group developed. However, the difference was not statistically significant, possibly because of the small sample size. In the tube cystostomy group, it is difficult to insert the cystostomy tube back into the bladder after its accidentally removal, because of the closure of the cystostomy site, therefore cystostomy had to be performed again. While in the modified group, the entrance site of bladder will not closed after the accidental removal of the cystostomy tube and therefore the tube can be easily reinserted into the bladder.

The accidental removal of cystostomy tube or urethral catheter in this study were caused by the bite of the experimental animals. The dogs slipped their neck collars and removed the tubes. In order to avoid the accidental removal of tubes, the neck collars should be firmly worn. Secondly, the tubes or catheters should be secured firmly with the finger-trap suture. Moreover, the exposed portion of the tube should be as short as possible to reduce the interference with the experimental animals.

The occurrence of perineal hematoma decreased in the modified group. 4 animals in the control group and 1 animal in the modified group developed the perineal hematoma. However, these results failed to achieve statistical significance due to the small sample size of the study. In the conventional group, the exudates and bleeding are accumulated in the loose connective tissue due to the elasticity of the scrotum skin, and contributed to the development of the hematoma. While in the modified group, hemostasis can be effectively achieved by local compression that can be easily implemented after the resection of testes and scrotum.

This study provides a good canine model of urethroplasty, in which the occurrence of urinary retention and perineal hematoma were decreased. However, one limitation to this study is the small number of experimental animals. Another limitation is that further investigation is required to clarify the effect of bilateral orchiectomy on the urethral reconstruction.

Conclusion

The occurrence of urinary retention and perineal hematoma decreased in the modified group, in which the cystostomy not the tube cystostomy were performed and the testes with the scrotum were simultaneously removed.

Acknowledgements

Not applicable.

Authors' contributions

JZ, GH: Protocol/project development, conduction of experiments, data collection and management, data analysis, manuscript and figure writing. DZ, GY: conduct of experiments, data collection and management. LM, CW: Protocol/project development, manuscript and figure writing/editing, supervision. All authors read and approved the final version of the manuscript.

Competing interests

The authors declare that they have no competing interest.

Author details

[1]Department of Urology, Beijing Jishuitan Hospital, No. 68, Huinanbei Road, Changping District, Beijing 100096, China. [2]Beijing Research Institute of Traumatology and Orthopaedics, No. 31 Xinjiekou East Street, Xicheng District, Beijing 100035, China.

References

1. Fossati N, Barbagli G, Larcher A, Dell'Oglio P, Sansalone S, Lughezzani G, Guazzoni G, Montorsi F, Lazzeri M. The surgical learning curve for one-stage anterior urethroplasty: a prospective single-surgeon study. Eur Urol. 2016;69(4):686–90.
2. Kuo TL, Venugopal S, Inman RD, Chapple CR. Surgical tips and tricks during urethroplasty for bulbar urethral strictures focusing on accurate localisation of the stricture: results from a tertiary centre. Eur Urol. 2015;67(4):764–70.
3. Zumrutbas AE, Ozlulerden Y, Celen S, Kucuker K, Aybek Z. The outcomes of Kulkarni's one-stage oral mucosa graft urethroplasty in patients with panurethral stricture: a single centre experience. World J Urol. 2020;38(1):175–81.
4. Pagura EJ, Cavallo JA, Zinman LN, Vanni AJ. Rectal mucosa graft take in staged urethroplasty. Urology. 2019;127:e1–2.
5. Madden-Fuentes RJ, Belsante MJ, Granieri MA, Peterson AC. Contemporary analysis of management of isolated pendulous urethral strictures using pedicled skin flap urethroplasty repair. World J Urol. 2019;37(12):2769–74.
6. Kojovic V, Djordjevic ML, Vuksanovic A. Single-stage repair of obliterated anterior urethral strictures using buccal mucosa graft and dorsal penile skin flap. Int J Urol. 2019;26(1):90–5.
7. Granieri MA, Zhao LC, Breyer BN, Voelzke BB, Baradaran N, Grucela AL, Marcello P, Vanni AJ. Multi-institutional outcomes of minimally invasive harvest of rectal mucosa graft for anterior urethral reconstruction. J Urol. 2019;201(6):1164–70.
8. Lumen N, Vierstraete-Verlinde S, Oosterlinck W, Hoebeke P, Palminteri E, Goes C, Maes H, Spinoit AF. Buccal versus lingual mucosa graft in anterior urethroplasty: a prospective comparison of surgical outcome and donor site morbidity. J Urol. 2016;195(1):112–7.
9. Lacy JM, Madden-Fuentes RJ, Dugan A, Peterson AC, Gupta S. Short-term complication rates following anterior urethroplasty: an analysis of national surgical quality improvement program data. Urology. 2018;111:197–202.
10. Chapple CR. Oral pain and morbidity with buccal mucosa grafts for substitution urethroplasty: closure or not. Eur Urol. 2018;73(6):923–4.
11. Versteegden LRM, de Jonge P, IntHout J, van Kuppevelt TH, Oosterwijk E, Feitz WFJ, de Vries RBM, Daamen WF. Tissue engineering of the urethra: a systematic review and meta-analysis of preclinical and clinical studies. Eur Urol. 2017;72(4):594–606.
12. Orabi H, AbouShwareb T, Zhang Y, Yoo JJ, Atala A. Cell-seeded tubularized scaffolds for reconstruction of long urethral defects: a preclinical study. Eur Urol. 2013;63(3):531–8.
13. Xie M, Xu Y, Song L, Wang J, Lv X, Zhang Y. Tissue-engineered buccal mucosa using silk fibroin matrices for urethral reconstruction in a canine model. J Surg Res. 2014;188(1):1–7.
14. Hu X, Xu Y, Song L, Zhang H. Combined buccal and lingual mucosa grafts for urethroplasty: an experimental study in dogs. J Surg Res. 2011;169(1):162–7.
15. Pederzoli F, Joice G, Salonia A, Bivalacqua TJ, Sopko NA. Regenerative and engineered options for urethroplasty. Nat Rev Urol. 2019;16(8):453–64.
16. Mangir N, Wilson KJ, Osman NI, Chapple CR. Current state of urethral tissue engineering. Curr Opin Urol. 2019;29(4):385–93.
17. Chapple C. Tissue engineering of the urethra: where are we in 2019? World J Urol. 2019;38:2101.
18. De Filippo RE, Yoo JJ, Atala A. Urethral replacement using cell seeded tubularized collagen matrices. J Urol. 2002;168(4 Pt 2):1789–92 (**discussion 1792-1783**).
19. Culenova M, Ziaran S, Danisovic L. Cells involved in urethral tissue engineering: systematic review. Cell Transplant. 2019;28(9–10):1106–15.
20. De Filippo RE, Kornitzer BS, Yoo JJ, Atala A. Penile urethra replacement with autologous cell-seeded tubularized collagen matrices. J Tissue Eng Regen Med. 2015;9(3):257–64.
21. Djordjevic ML. Graft surgery in extensive urethral stricture disease. Curr Urol Rep. 2014;15(8):424.
22. Moncrief T, Gor R, Goldfarb RA, Jarosek S, Elliott SP. Trauma, urologic reconstruction network of S: urethral rest with suprapubic cystostomy for obliterative or nearly obliterative urethral strictures: urethrographic changes and implications for management. J Urol. 2018;199(5):1289–95.
23. Poelaert F, Oosterlinck W, Spinoit AF, Lumen N. Duration of urethral catheterization after urethroplasty: how long is enough? Minerva Urol Nefrol. 2017;69(4):372–6.
24. Sussman RD, Hill FC, Koch GE, Patel V, Venkatesan K. Novel pericatheter retrograde urethrogram technique is a viable method for postoperative urethroplasty imaging. Int Urol Nephrol. 2017;49(12):2157–65.

21

Risk factors and prediction model of urosepsis in patients with diabetes after percutaneous nephrolithotomy

Jun Liu[1,2†], Qingya Yang[3†], Jiayi Lan[1,2], Yang Hong[1,2], Xiaobo Huang[1,2] and Bo Yang[1,2*]

Abstract

Objective: To analyze the risk factors of patients with diabetes mellitus (DM) and urosepsis after percutaneous nephrolithotomy (PCNL) for upper urinary tract stones and to develop a nomogram to predict postoperative urosepsis according to the risk factors.

Methods: The data of patients with type 2 diabetes who underwent one-stage PCNL due to upper urinary tract stones were retrospectively analyzed. The risk factors of patients with postoperative urosepsis were evaluated by univariate and multivariate logistic regression analysis, and the nomogram prediction model was developed according to the regression coefficient.

Results: One-stage PCNL was successfully completed in 241 patients with DM, and urosepsis occurred in 41 (17.0%) patients after PCNL. Based on multivariate logistic regression analysis, the independent risk factors associated with postoperative urosepsis included preoperative leukocyte elevation (OR = 3.973, P = 0.005), positive urine nitrite (OR = 3.697, P = 0.010), and positive urine culture (OR = 3.562, P = 0.002). According to the results of the logistic regression analysis model, staghorn stones (OR = 2.049, P < 0.1) and complete intraoperative stone clearance (OR = 0.431, P < 0.1), were used to develop the nomogram. Internal validation of the nomogram showed that the concordance index (C-index) was 0.725. Additionally, the Hosmer–Lemeshow test was performed, P = 0.938 > 0.05.

Conclusion: Preoperative leukocyte elevation, positive urine nitrite, and positive urine culture are independent risk factors for urosepsis after one-stage PCNL for patients with DM with upper urinary tract stones. The nomogram, which is based on independent risk factors that combine stone morphology and intraoperative stone clearance, can help predict the risk of postoperative urosepsis.

Keywords: PCNL, Diabetes, Urosepsis, Risk factors, Nomogram

Introduction

After decades of development, percutaneous nephrolithotomy (PCNL) has become one of the main surgical methods for upper urinary tract stones, especially those with kidney stones or upper ureteral stones larger than 2 cm [1]. However, it is important to consider the potential postoperative complications caused by PCNL [2, 3].

Urosepsis is a serious postoperative complication of PCNL. If it is not properly treated in a timely manner, it can cause septic shock and can be lethal [4]. Clinical studies have shown that diabetes mellitus was independently associated with increased risk of infectious complications after PCNL(OR = 14.6, P = 0.001) [5]. Therefore, when implementing PCNL in patients with

*Correspondence: boyoung1971@163.com
†Jun Liu and Qingya Yang have contributed equally to this work
[1] Urology and Lithotripsy Center, Peking University People's Hospital, 133 Fuchengmen Inner Street, Xicheng District, Beijing 100034, People's Republic of China

DM, early detection of patients with potential urosepsis risk is extremely important. This study retrospectively analyzed clinical data of patients with DM submitted for primary PCNL treatment for upper urinary tract stones at the Urology and Lithotripsy Center of Peking University People's Hospital, as well as the independent risk factors for urosepsis after PCNL. Subsequently, a prediction model for postoperative urosepsis was developed for early detection of urosepsis in patients with DM when performing PCNL, as well as prevention and early intervention.

Materials and methods

Patients

We retrospectively analyzed the data of patients who underwent one-stage PCNL for upper urinary tract stones and were preoperatively diagnosed with type 2 diabetes mellitus(T2DM) at the Urology and Lithotripsy Center of Peking University People's Hospital between June 2012 and December 2019. Diagnosis of T2DM was defined by 2-h PG(two-hour 75-g postload plasma glucose level) $\geq$ 11.1 mmol/L on OGTT(oral glucose tolerance test) or FPG(fasting plasma glucose) $\geq$ 7.0 mmol/L according to ADA(American Diabetes Association) criteria, or a previous diagnosis of T2DM. Exclusion criteria included (1) patients who underwent bilateral endoscopic lithotripsy for one-stage surgery; (2) patients with severe systemic diseases, namely, American Society of Anesthesiologists (ASA) class IV-VI status; (3) solitary kidney and patients undergoing nephrectomy; and (4) patients with missing data. Clinical data of 241 consecutive patients were collected.

Clinical data

Preoperative preparation included blood cell count, serum biochemical parameters, renal ultrasound, abdominal X-ray examination, and urinary CT examination if necessary. After perineal cleaning, midstream urine was collected for routine urine test and urine culture. Positive urine white blood cells (WBC) were defined as WBC 10 per high power field ($\times$ 400). For patients with positive WBC or nitrite in urine, antibiotics were given immediately for 3–7 days and adjusted according to the results of the urine culture and drug sensitivity test during treatment. Regardless of whether the preoperative urine culture was positive or negative, all patients received a single dose of antibiotic prophylaxis 30 min before PCNL and continued to use it 48 h after surgery if the urine culture was positive. Body temperature, blood pressure, respiration, heart rate, white blood cells, and serum creatinine were closely monitored after PCNL.

Upper urinary tract stones occurring in the renal pelvis and extending to at least two calyces are classified as staghorn stones. All patients were followed up with systemic inflammatory response syndrome (SIRS) criteria after surgery (white blood cell count $< 4000 \times 10^9$/L or $> 12{,}000 \times 10^9$/L; fever > 38 °C or < 36 °C; heart rate > 90 beats/min; respiratory rate > 20 breaths/min), and blood culture was tested if necessary [6]. SIRS was diagnosed in patients who met two or more criteria. Urosepsis diagnostic criteria included both urinary tract infections and SIRS, while other site infections were excluded [4, 7].

Surgical methods

All patients received spinal anesthesia. A retrograde 5-Fr ureteral catheter (BARD, USA) was inserted into the affected side, with a 22-Fr cystoscope in the lithotomy position and a 16-Fr ureteral catheter was inserted for bladder drainage. After ureteral catheter insertion, the patient was placed in a prone position and underwent renal puncture under the guidance of 3.5 MHz ultrasound at the 11th intercostal space, or the 12th subcostal space, using a 18-gauge puncture needle. After observing urine flow through the needle, a J-shaped guide wire was placed into the collection system through a puncture needle, and the nephrostomy tract was dilated with a nested metal dilator until a 24 Fr Amplatz sheath was inserted. A 20.8Fr rigid nephroscope (Richard Wolf, Knittlingen, Germany) combined with ultrasonic and pneumatic lithotripsy (Swiss lithotripter, EMS, Nyon, Switzerland) was used for stone fragmentation in all cases. Intraoperative ultrasonography, or X-ray fluoroscopy, was used to check whether the kidney stones were completely cleared, and stone clearance was defined in cases in which fragments of stones were less than 4 mm. A 6-Fr double J catheter and a 14-Fr nephrostomy tube (BD Medical System, Franklin Lake, New Jersey, USA) were placed at the end of each surgery. Additionally, vital signs were monitored 24 h after PCNL and fasting peripheral blood routines were performed the next morning to help diagnose SIRS. The duration of the surgery was obtained from the patient's surgical anesthesia record sheet, in which the start of the procedure consisted of the ultrasound-guided renal puncture and the end of the surgery consisted of the placement of the indwelling nephrostomy tube.

Statistical methods

The data were statistically analyzed using SPSS20.0 software. Continuous variables were tested for normality, and those conforming to normal distribution were expressed by mean $\pm$ standard deviation and analyzed by independent sample *t*-test; those not conforming to normal distribution were expressed by median (minimum, maximum), together with ordered categorical variables, and the comparison between groups was expressed by

Mann–Whitney U-test analysis. The chi-square test analysis was used for comparison between groups of disordered categorical variables; univariate and multivariate logistic regression analysis was used for risk factor analysis. A $P < 0.05$ was considered statistically significant.

Based on the results of the logistic regression analysis model, and combined with clinically significant variables, the nomogram prediction model was constructed using the RMS software package of R software (R 3.6.2 Institute of Statistics and Mathematics, Vienna, Austria). The bootstrap method was used to sample 1000 times repeatedly, and the nomogram model was verified internally. Model accuracy was evaluated by calculating the consistency index (C-index), drawing the calibration curve, and by the Hosmer–Lemeshow goodness-of-fit test [8].

Results

Clinical data and surgical outcome

One-stage PCNL was successfully completed in 241 patients with DM, including 135 males and 106 females, with ages ranging from 28 to 81 years, with mean age of 57 years, mean stone size of 2.96 ± 2.18 cm, and a median operative time of 70 (20–175) min. Urosepsis occurred in 41 (17.0%) patients after PCNL. All cases of urosepsis occurred within 24 h postoperatively, and all cases improved after anti-infection treatment. The patients were classified in one of two groups: the urosepsis group and the non-urosepsis group, based on postoperative occurrence of urosepsis. The comparison of clinical parameters between the two groups is shown in Table 1. Compared with the non-urosepsis group, patients in the urosepsis group had a higher preoperative white blood cell count ($\times 10^9$/L) (8.8 ± 2.9 vs. 7.1 ± 2.3, $P < 0.001$) and longer hospital stay (13.7 ± 5.5 vs. 11.2 ± 5.2, $P = 0.006$). Also, we observed an increased incidence of urosepsis in female patients versus male patients ($P < 0.05$), and an increased incidence of urosepsis in patients with staghorn stones and residual stones ($P < 0.05$). Notably, there were no significant differences between the two groups regarding age, BMI index, blood glucose level, duration of surgery, and number of channels.

Logistic regression analysis of clinical features and urosepsis

In univariate analysis, we analyzed potential predictors based on three aspects, including patient, stone and surgery (Table 2). The results showed that the factors significantly correlated with postoperative urosepsis in univariate analysis included female ($OR = 2.032$, $P = 0.042$), preoperative WBC elevation ($OR = 2.750$, $P = 0.019$), preoperative positive urine culture ($OR = 3.667$, $P < 0.001$), positive urinary nitrite ($OR = 3.697$, $P < 0.001$), staghorn stones ($OR = 2.269$, $P = 0.024$), and intraoperative stone clearance ($OR = 0.337$, $P = 0.009$). These factors were included in the multivariate logistic regression analysis. The results showed that there were three variables that could be used as independent risk factors of postoperative urosepsis: preoperative WBC elevation ($OR = 3.973$, $P = 0.005$), positive urinary nitrite ($OR = 3.697$, $P = 0.010$), and positive urine culture ($OR = 3.562$, $P = 0.002$).

Nomogram for predicting the probability of postoperative urosepsis following PCNL

Based on multivariate logistic analysis, we included two parameters related to calculi, staghorn calculi ($OR = 2.049$, $P < 0.1$) and complete intraoperative stone clearance ($OR = 0.431$, $P < 0.1$), in the development of the nomogram (Fig. 1). Additionally, we performed the bootstrap method repeated sampling 1000 times and determined the internal validation of the nomogram model, with consistency index (C-index) of 0.725, and by drawing the Calibration curve. Calibration of the nomogram was close to the standard curve (Fig. 2), and the Hosmer–Lemeshow goodness-of-fit test was performed ($P = 0.938 > 0.05$), which indicated that the nomogram model could accurately predict the risk of urosepsis in patients with DM after PCNL surgery, and had good consistency with the actual risk.

NOMOGRAM USE INSTRUCTION: Use the corresponding points on each index axis on the nomogram to make a vertical line on the scoring scale to get the score of the index. After calculating the sum of the scores of each index, correspond downward to determine the risk of urosepsis in this patient after PCNL.

Culture: Preoperative urine culture; WBC positive: Preoperative blood WBC $\geq 10X10^9$/L; NIT: Preoperative urine nitrite; Staghorn: staghorn stone; Clearance: stone clearance.

Discussion

The main objective of this retrospective study was to construct, and internally validate, a nomogram to predict the incidence of urosepsis after PCNL in patients with DM. To our knowledge, this is the first clinical retrospective study of a population of patients with DM undergoing PCNL, in which the associated risk factors can be obtained in the first postoperative period, leading to an earlier assessment of the risk of postoperative urosepsis for early intervention and treatment.

In recent years, with the development of minimally invasive technology, the safety and effectiveness of PCNL has improved; however, postoperative infection is still one of the major complications. Studies have shown that the incidence of infectious complications after PCNL surgery is 2.8–32.1% [9]. If postoperative infection is

Table 1 Comparison of clinical data between patients with and without postoperative urosepsis

Items	Non-urosepsis	Urosepsis	P value
Gender, n(%)			
Male	118	17	0.039
Female	82	24	
Age/years	57.3±9.7	55.4±10.9	0.272
BMI (kg/m^2)	26.2±4.0	26.1±4.2	0.814
Hypertension			
Yes	133	30	0.407
No	67	11	
Staghorn stone			
Yes	44	16	0.022
No	156	25	
Preoperative urine WBC			
Positive	173	40	0.045
Negative	27	1	
Preoperative urine nitrite			
Positive	27	15	0.0004
Negative	173	26	
Preoperative urine culture			
Positive	74	28	0.0002
Negative	126	13	
Preoperative blood WBC (109/L)	7.1±2.3	8.8±2.9	0.0001
Preoperative hemoglobin (g/L)	134.4±18.5	132.7±20.1	0.608
Preoperative serum creatine (μmol/L)	84.5±39.6	92.4±55.8	0.285
Preoperative blood glucose (mmol/L)	6.9±2.1	7.2±2.1	0.352
ASA			
I–II	187	35	0.079
III	13	6	
Operative time/min	60 (20–145)	75 (20–175)	0.349
Tract			
Single	174	31	0.063
Multiple	26	10	
Stone clearance			
Yes	178	30	0.007
No	22	11	
Hospital stay (days)	11.2±5.2	13.7±5.5	0.006

BMI body mass index, *WBC* white blood cell, *ASA* American Society of Anesthesiologists

not detected in time and there is no active anti-infective treatment, septic shock can result. Indeed, in different regions and countries, mortality rates for severe sepsis and septic shock vary among medical centers, with reported results ranging from 22 to 76% based on available epidemiological data [10]. Urosepsis refers to sepsis due to urinary tract and/or infections of the male reproductive system [4, 7]. In recent years, research on risk factors of urosepsis caused by urinary calculi has increased significantly. However, most studies have focused on risk factors for urosepsis after endoscopic lithotripsy, such as procalcitonin levels, stone culture, and postoperative WBC levels [11, 12]. Kumar et al. demonstrated the importance of time as a prognostic factor: initiating empirical antibiotic therapy within an hour of diagnosis of sepsis was associated with 80% survival. For each hour of delayed antibiotic use, the survival rate decreased by an average of 7.6% (79.9% for 1–2 h, 42.0% for 5–6 h, and 25.4% for 9–12 h) [13]. Therefore, early identification and treatment of urosepsis have important clinical significance, which is also the aim of this study.

Table 2 Univariate and multivariate logistic regression analysis of clinical data and urosepsis

Variables	Univariate analysis			Multivariate analysis		
	OR	95% CI	P value	OR	95% CI	P value
Gender						
Male	Ref			Ref		
Female	2.032	1.027 to 4.019	0.042	0.681	0.271 to 1.710	0.413
Age						
>60	Ref					
≤60	0.981	0.948 to 1.015	0.271			
BMI						
>26	Ref					
≤26	0.990	0.909 to 1.077	0.813			
Preoperative blood glucose (mmol/L)						
<7.0	Ref					
≥7.0	1.076	0.923 to 1.254	0.352			
Preoperative urine WBC						
Negative	Ref					
Positive	6.243	0.824 to 47.3134	0.076			
Preoperative urine nitrite						
Negative	Ref			Ref		
Positive	3.697	1.739 to 7.856	0.0007	3.697	1.360 to 10.050	0.010
Preoperative urine culture	Ref			Ref		
Negative						
Positive	3.667	1.789 to 7.517	0.0004	3.562	1.584 to 8.011	0.002
Preoperative WBC (≥ 10X109/L)						
No	Ref			Ref		
Yes	2.750	1.182 to 6.395	0.019	3.973	1.519 to 10.394	0.005
Staghorn stone						
No	Ref			Ref		
Yes	2.269	1.114 to 4.621	0.024	2.049	0.891 to 4.712	0.092
Stone clearance						
No	Ref			Ref		
Yes	0.337	0.148 to 0.766	0.009	0.431	0.162 to 1.142	0.091

In our study, all patients were diabetic, with an overall incidence of urosepsis of 17.0%. Compared with 7.6–14.3% reported in the general population [4, 14], the incidence is relatively high, and it is currently believed that the reason for the increased incidence of postoperative infection caused by diabetes may be related to the following mechanisms. First, diabetes-related microvascular disease reduces oxygen and nutrient delivery to peripheral tissues [15]. Also, hyperglycemic status impairs the function of leukocytes and monocytes [16]. Additionally, peripheral neuropathy alters neuropeptide-mediated inflammatory response [17]. Therefore, for patients with DM receiving PCNL, it is important to identify the preoperative and intraoperative risk factors independently related to urosepsis after surgery in order to identify and implement the appropriate treatment as early as possible. Unfortunately, we did not find a statistical difference in preoperative blood glucose levels between the two groups. This result may be due to the fact that all patients with DM had their preoperative blood glucose level adjusted over a prolonged period of time before surgery, with surgery only being performed when the blood glucose level reached an acceptable range.

In this study, positive preoperative urine culture results were an independent risk factor for predicting urosepsis after PCNL in patients with DM (OR = 3.562, P = 0.002). However, current studies have confirmed that the sensitivity of preoperative midstream urine culture results for predicting postoperative SIRS is only 50% compared with pelvic urine culture and stone culture, and that it cannot predict the occurrence of postoperative SIRS [18]. However, both pelvic urine and stone culture require specimens to be obtained during surgery, and there is an

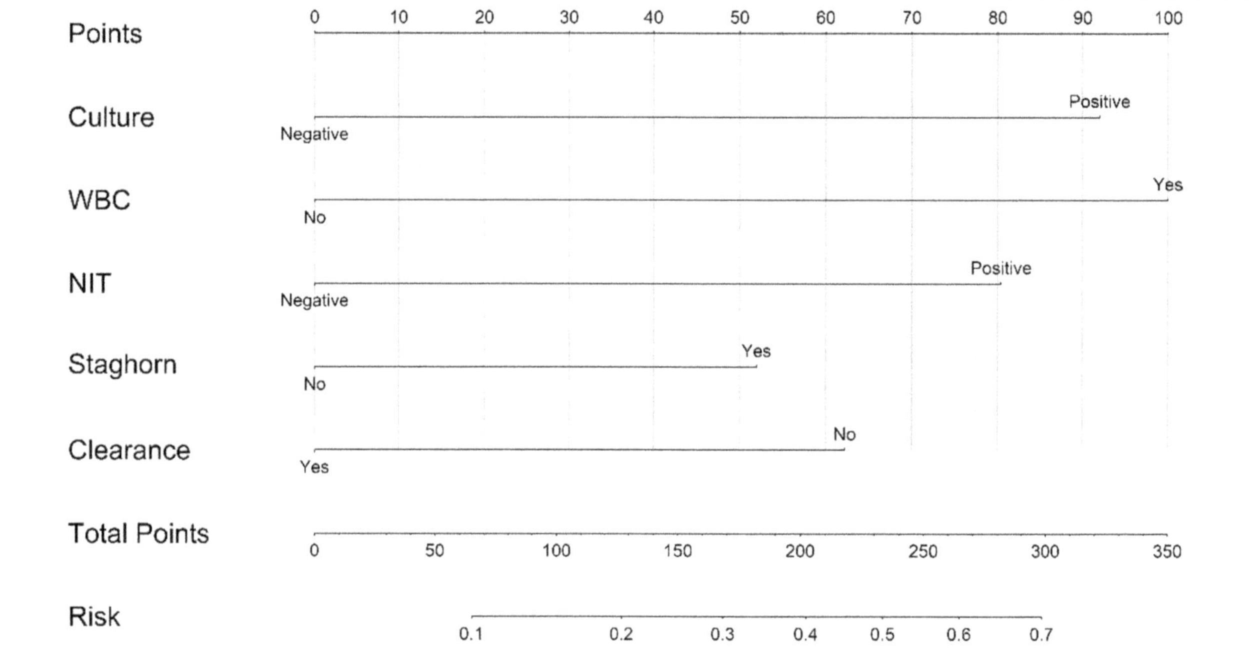

Fig. 1 Nomogram for predicting the probability of postoperative urosepsis following PCNL in patients with DM

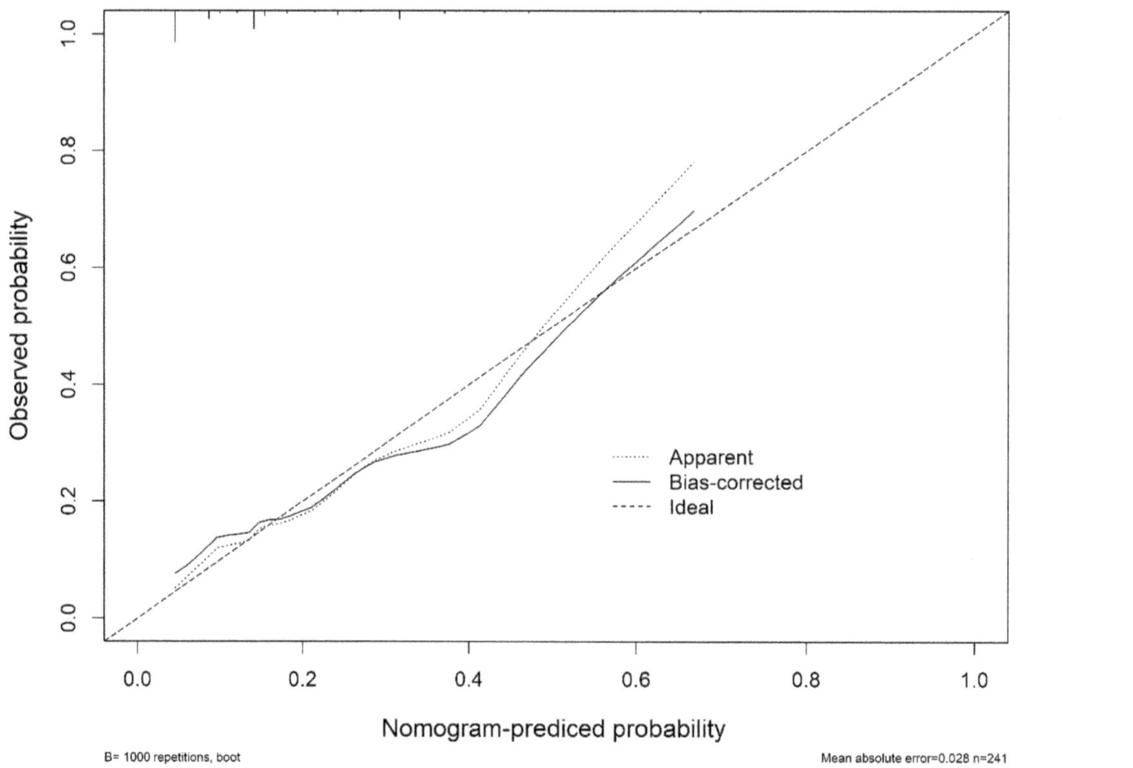

Fig. 2 Calibration curve of the prediction model for postoperative urosepsis following PCNL in patients with DM

increased wait time for results after surgery; therefore, effective intervention in cases of postoperative infection cannot be made in a timely manner, which limits the clinical application value of pelvic urine and stone cultures. Additional studies have shown that the significance of preoperative midstream urine culture cannot be ignored. Indeed, Gutierrez studied 865 patients undergoing PCNL and found that positive preoperative midstream urine culture ($OR = 2.12$, $P < 0.05$) was an independent risk factor for fever after PCNL [19]. Similarly, a multivariate analysis of 496 patients receiving ureteroscopic laser lithotripsy by Uchida et al. showed that obstructive pyelonephritis, positive preoperative bladder urine culture results, and female gender were associated with postoperative SIRS [20]. Our results are in line with results of previous studies that have demonstrated that positive preoperative midstream urine culture results are significantly associated with increased risk of urosepsis after surgery. Additionally, this result can be obtained preoperatively, which is extremely important for predicting the risk and for prevention of infection after PCNL.

In this study, multivariate analysis found that patients with preoperative $WBC \geq 10 \times 10^9/L$ had a 3.973-fold higher risk of urosepsis than patients with normal preoperative WBC ($P = 0.005$). Liang et al. conducted a retrospective analysis of 287 patients who underwent stone surgery and found that preoperative WBC ($WBC > 10 * 10^{9/L}$) ($P = 0.027$), type of surgery ($P = 0.009$), intraoperative hypotension ($P < 0.001$), and emergency surgery ($P < 0.001$) were associated with intraoperative and postoperative urosepsis in calculous pyonephrosis patients.[4] In addition, the same study also found that urine nitrite (NIT) positive patients had a 3.697-fold higher postoperative risk of urosepsis than NIT (–) patients ($P = 0.010$); therefore, urine nitrite status may help predict urinary tract infection and the need for subsequent treatment. Fan et al. conducted a multivariate logistic analysis of 156 patients undergoing minimal PCNL surgery and showed that preoperative positive NIT status ($OR = 10.570$, $P = 0.025$), stone size ($OR = 11.512$, $P = 0.009$), and postoperative leukopenia ($OR = 0.009$, $P < 0.001$) were independently associated with uroseptic shock [21]. These results are consistent with the results of this study, which provide a good reference for our early detection of urosepsis after PCNL.

In our study, staghorn stones and stone clearance were not independent risk factors for urosepsis after PCNL in multivariate regression analysis. Nevertheless, staghorn stones have always been difficult to treat in PCNL surgery. Also, the morphology of staghorn stones is complex, involving multiple calyces. It may take longer stone removal by lithotripsy during surgery, and it also increases the possibility of multiple tracts. Rivera analyzed several infectious factors after PCNL surgery and found that in multivariate analysis, the presence of staghorn stones alone was independently associated with an increased risk of postoperative infectious complications ($OR = 3.14$; $P = 0.02$) [22]. Similar studies in people with DM undergoing PCNL also reached the same conclusion. For example, Wei et al. showed by logistic regression analysis that diabetic complications and complete comorbidity of staghorn stones were independent risk factors for postoperative infectious complications [23]. Residual stones may contain bacteria and endotoxins and increase the risk of infectious complications after PCNL surgery [24]. The occurrence of intraoperative residual stones may be caused by various reasons, such as staghorn stones, renal structural abnormalities, calyceal neck stenosis, intraoperative bleeding, etc. The pursuit of full clearance may also increase the operation time and irrigating pressure, resulting in increased complications of infection. Therefore, while controlling the operation time and irrigating pressure, the stones should be completely removed as far as possible. To judge whether the stone is completely removed, we can use intraoperative ultrasonography and X-ray fluoroscopy to determine the need for interventions of anti-urosepsis after PCNL.

Based on the results of the above multivariate analysis, we included five risk factors associated with the occurrence of urosepsis after PCNL, including preoperative urine culture ($P = 0.002$), preoperative WBC elevation ($P = 0.005$), preoperative NIT ($P = 0.010$), staghorn stones ($P = 0.092$), and stone clearance ($P = 0.091$).These five factors may be interconnected; therefore, we constructed a nomogram according to the relative risk of each factor, which is convenient for rapid clinical reference and application. After internal verification, the C-index of this nomogram is 0.725, which has good conformity. The aforementioned five risk factors can be obtained in the first postoperative period; therefore, the risk of urosepsis in high-risk patients needs to be fully considered when making surgical plans. The application of this tool not only contributes to clinical decision-making and timely intervention for patients with potentially severe infections but also provides a referable digital basis for surgical prognosis and facilitates preoperative communication with patients regarding surgical options and possible risks, which is extremely important for perioperative management of the diabetic population. This study is also the first study to investigate the occurrence of urosepsis after PCNL in patients with DM.

This study has some limitations. First, this is a retrospective study and selection bias cannot be avoided. However, we carefully selected the inclusion criteria and collected sufficient clinical samples to enable patients in both the experimental and control groups to acquire an accurate representation of disease occurrence. Second, the data from the prediction model was obtained from a single center. Although we used patient samples from different periods, evidence from other centers is needed to validate the model. Therefore, we intend to carry out a multicenter study and provide sufficient clinical data to further evaluate and externally validate our prediction model. Despite these limitations, to our knowledge, this study presents the most critical assessment to date of urosepsis secondary to PCNL surgery in patients with DM and, for the first time, provides a nomogram that can be used in the first postoperative period.

Conclusion

Preoperative WBC elevation, positive urine culture, and urine NIT(+) were independent risk factors for urosepsis in patients with DM after one-stage PCNL. We constructed a nomogram to predict urosepsis postoperatively, which can provide help predict the risk of urosepsis after PCNL in patients with DM and help individualized treatment of upper urinary tract stones.

Abbreviations

DM: Diabetes mellitus; PCNL: Percutaneous nephrolithotomy; T2DM: Type 2 diabetes mellitus; 2-h PG: Two-hour 75-g postload plasma glucose level; OGTT : Oral glucose tolerance test; FPG: Fasting plasma glucose; ADA: American Diabetes Association; CT: Computed tomography; WBC: White blood cells; SIRS: Systemic inflammatory response syndrome; NIT: Urine nitrite.

Acknowledgement

We are very grateful to Dr. Haifeng Song of Tsinghua University, for statistical help.

Authors' contributions

Conception and design: JL, QY, administrative support: XH, provision of study materials or patients: XH, BY, collection and assembly of data: JL, YH, data analysis and interpretation: JL, QY, manuscript writing. All authors final approval of manuscript.

Competing interests

The authors have no conflicts of interest to declare.

Author details

[1]Urology and Lithotripsy Center, Peking University People's Hospital, 133 Fuchengmen Inner Street, Xicheng District, Beijing 100034, People's Republic of China. [2]Peking University Applied Lithotripsy Institute, Peking University, Beijing 100034, People's Republic of China. [3]Department of Urology, Qilu Hospital (Qingdao), Cheeloo College of Medicine, Shandong University, Qingdao 266035, People's Republic of China.

References

1. Pradère B, Doizi S, Proietti S, Brachlow J, Traxer O. Evaluation of guidelines for surgical management of urolithiasis. J Urol. 2018;199(5):1267–71.
2. Kyriazis I, Panagopoulos V, Kallidonis P, Özsoy M, Vasilas M, Liatsikos E. Complications in percutaneous nephrolithotomy. World J Urol. 2015;33(8):1069–77.
3. Kallidonis P, Panagopoulos V, Kyriazis I, Liatsikos E. Complications of percutaneous nephrolithotomy: classification, management, and prevention. Curr Opin Urol. 2016;26(1):88–94.
4. Liang X, Huang J, Xing M, et al. Risk factors and outcomes of urosepsis in patients with calculous pyonephrosis receiving surgical intervention: a single-center retrospective study. BMC Anesthesiol. 2019;19(1):61.
5. Lorenzo Soriano L, Ordaz Jurado DG, Pérez Ardavín J, et al. Predictive factors of infectious complications in the postoperative of percutaneous nephrolithotomy. Actas Urol Esp. 2019;43(3):131–6.
6. Levy MM, Fink MP, Marshall JC, Abraham E, Angus D, Cook D, et al. 2001 SCCM/ESICM/ACCP/ATS/SIS international sepsis definitions conference. Crit Care Med. 2003;31:1250–6.
7. Wagenlehner FM, Pilatz A, Naber KG, Weidner W. Therapeutic challenges of urosepsis. Eur J Clin Investig. 2008;38(Suppl 2):45–9.
8. Harrell FE Jr, Lee KL, Mark DB. Multivariable prognostic models: issues in developing models, evaluating assumptions and adequacy, and measuring and reducing errors. Stat Med. 1996;15(4):361–87.
9. Seitz C, Desai M, Hacker A, et al. Incidence, prevention, and management of complications following percutaneous nephrolitholapaxy. Eur Urol. 2012;61:146–58.
10. Levy MM, Artigas A, Phillips GS, et al. Outcomes of the Surviving Sepsis Campaign in intensive care units in the USA and Europe: a prospective cohort study. Lancet Infect Dis. 2012;12(12):919–24.
11. Zheng J, Li Q, Fu W, et al. Procalcitonin as an early diagnostic and monitoring tool in urosepsis following percutaneous nephrolithotomy. Urolithiasis. 2015;43(1):41–7.
12. Gao X, Lu C, Xie F, et al. Risk factors for sepsis in patients with struvite stones following percutaneous nephrolithotomy. World J Urol. 2020;38(1):219–29.
13. Kumar A, Roberts D, Wood KE, et al. Duration of hypotension before initiation of effective antimicrobial therapy is the critical determinant of survival in human septic shock. Crit Care Med. 2006;34(6):1589–96.
14. Koras O, Bozkurt IH, Yonguc T, et al. Risk factors for postoperative infectious complications following percutaneous nephrolithotomy: a prospective clinical study. Urolithiasis. 2015;43(1):55–60.
15. Klein R. Hyperglycemia and microvascular and macrovascular disease in diabetes. Diabetes Care. 1995;18:258–68.
16. Turina M, Fry DE, Polk HC Jr. Acute hyperglycemia and the innate immune system: clinical, cellular, and molecular aspects. Crit Care Med. 2005;33:1624–33.
17. Gibran NS, Jang YC, Isik FF, et al. Diminished neuropeptide levels contribute to the impaired cutaneous healing response associated with diabetes mellitus. J Surg Res. 2002;108:122–8.
18. Mariappan P, Smith G, Bariol SV, Moussa SA, Tolley DA. Stone and pelvic urine culture and sensitivity are better than bladder urine as predictors of urosepsis following percutaneous nephrolithotomy: a prospective clinical study. J Urol. 2005;173(5):1610–4.
19. Gutierrez J, Smith A, Geavlete P, et al. Urinary tract infections and post-operative fever in percutaneous nephrolithotomy. World J Urol. 2013;31(5):1135–40.
20. Uchida Y, Takazawa R, Kitayama S, Tsujii T. Predictive risk factors for systemic inflammatory response syndrome following ureteroscopic laser lithotripsy. Urolithiasis. 2018;46(4):375–81.
21. Fan J, Wan S, Liu L, et al. Predictors for uroseptic shock in patients who undergo minimally invasive percutaneous nephrolithotomy. Urolithiasis. 2017;45(6):573–8.
22. Rivera M, Viers B, Cockerill P, Agarwal D, Mehta R, Krambeck A. Pre- and postoperative predictors of infection-related complications in patients undergoing percutaneous nephrolithotomy. J Endourol. 2016;30(9):982–6.
23. Wei W, Leng J, Shao H, Wang W. Diabetes, a risk factor for both infectious and major complications after percutaneous nephrolithotomy. Int J Clin Exp Med. 2015;8(9):16620–6.
24. Degirmenci T, Bozkurt IH, Celik S, Yarimoglu S, Basmaci I, Sefik E. Does leaving residual fragments after percutaneous nephrolithotomy in patients with positive stone culture and/or renal pelvic urine culture increase the risk of infectious complications? Urolithiasis. 2019;47(4):371–5.

22

Denonvilliers' fascia acts as the fulcrum and hammock for continence after radical prostatectomy

Xuwei Lu[1,2], Chang He[1], Sihong Zhang[2], Fan Yang[1], Zhuifeng Guo[1], Jiaqi Huang[1], Minke He[1], Jiawen Wu[1], Xia Sheng[3], Wenyao Lin[4], Jie Cheng[4], Jianming Guo[2*] and Hang Wang[2*]

Abstract

Background: Radical prostatectomy (RP) is the primary treatment of localized prostate cancer. Immediate urinary incontinence post-RP was still common and depressing without specific reason.

Methods: A multicenter cohort of 154 consecutive patients from 2018 to 2020, who was diagnosed with localized prostate cancer underwent either modified mini-incision retropubic radical prostatectomy (Mmi-RRP) or laparoscopic radical prostatectomy (LRP) or robotic-assisted radical prostatectomy (RARP). Seventy-two patients with Denonvilliers' fascia (DF) spared were included in DFS (Denonvilliers' fascia sparing) group. Whereas eighty-two patients with DF completely or partially dissected were set as Group Control. The primary outcome was immediate continence (ImC). Continuous data and categorical data were analyzed with *t*-test and *Chi*-square test, respectively. Odds ratios (*ORs*) were calculated with logistic regression.

Results: Urinary continence of Group DFS was significantly better than that of Group Control at each time point within one year after operation. Incidence rate of continence in Group DFS and Group Control were 83.3% vs 13.4% ($P < 0.01$) for ImC, 90.3% vs 30.5% ($P < 0.01$) at 3 months, 91.7% vs 64.6% ($P < 0.01$) at 6 months, and 93.1% vs 80.5% ($P = 0.02$) at 1 year after operation, respectively. Positive surgical margin (PSM) showed no significant difference (20.8% vs 20.7%, $P = 1.0$). In multivariate analysis, DFS showed importance for ImC post RP ($OR = 26.4$, $P < 0.01$).

Conclusions: Denonvilliers' fascia acted as the fulcrum and hammock for continence post RP. Preservation of DF contributed to better continence after RP without increase of PSM.

Trail registration Our research was conducted retrospectively and approved by the ethical committees of Minhang Hospital, but not registered.

Keywords: Prostate cancer, Prostatectomy, Denonvilliers' fascia, Urinary continence, Positive surgical margin

Introduction

Prostate cancer (PCa) is the top-ranking malignant tumor for men worldwide [1]. Radical prostatectomy (RP) is the primary therapeutic choice for localized PCa. Dramatic improvement of surgery technique and more application of newer devices have reduced the incidence of severe complications for RP. Unfortunately, incontinence after RP, which haunted patients extremely hard, is still a huge challenge. The morbidity of incontinence one-year after

*Correspondence: guo.jianming@zs-hospital.sh.cn; wang.hang@zs-hospital.sh.cn
[2] Department of Urology, Zhongshan Hospital, Fudan University, Fenglin Rd 130, Shanghai 200032, China

RP remains up to 21%, regardless whether open radical prostatectomy (ORP) or laparoscopic radical prostatectomy (LRP) or robotic-assisted radical prostatectomy (RARP) has been taken [2]. Although many researchers have proposed many factors that might matter such as sphincter, length of membrane urethra, bladder neck preservation, neurovascular bundle (NVB) sparing, and Denonvilliers' fascia (DF) as well, that is still uncertainty about the mechanism of post RP continence [3].

Furthermore, most literatures reported continent rate of short-term, mid-term and long-term post RP. As to immediate continence (ImC), few reports could be found. We have applied a new technique as DF-sparing (DFS) since 2018 in RP with excellent urinary continence, especially the ImC. Because of the encouraging outcome of urinary control, there must be something worth thinking about. So, we analyzed the data to explore the mechanism of continence post RP and the role of DF in it, as well as the feasibility and safety of DFS.

Methods

From January 2018 to October 2020, 154 consecutive patients with localized prostate cancer underwent RP in Zhongshan Hospital, Minhang Hospital and Xuhui Hospital, FUDAN University. All the patients were given bone scan or PET-CT and excluded with metastasis before operation. The majority of patients completed MRI before operation except for those with contraindications including metal implantation and claustrophobia. Any suspicious sign showing that prostate capsule was invaded whether in radiology or in surgery, especially at the lateral-posterior direction, DF sparing was not recommended. If tumor was localized and prostate capsule wasn't invaded, DFS technique was available. Seventy-two cases that underwent either modified mini-incision retropubic radical prostatectomy (Mmi-RRP) or LRP or RARP with DFS were included in Group DFS. Group Control included 82 cases received Mmi-RRP/LRP/RARP with DF completely or partially dissected.

All the procedures were completed by three experienced surgeons. Due to puncture approach, local invasion or neoadjuvant therapies, DFS was applied to appropriate patients. Urinary catheter was removed 5–7 days after operation. All the patients were followed up for 2–26 (14.5 ± 6.9) months.

The primary outcome was ImC. All the continence status were assessed by outpatient follow-up. Continent status reported by patients was collected at 1-week, 3-month, 6-month, and 1-year after urethral catheter was discarded. We defined continence as usage of ≤ 1 pad per 24 h. Considering that urine leakage caused by multiple factors was prevalent shortly after catheter removal, most of which was transient and could recover soon without treatment, we defined ImC as regaining continence within 1-week after urinary catheter removal [4].

Surgery and post-surgery protocol

All the procedures were operated out of peritoneal under general anesthesia. The surgical approaches were decided by financial conditions and personal preferences of patients with full knowledge of benefits and risks. Mmi-RRP was operated with an approximate 7 cm longitudinal suprapubic incision, whereas LRP or RARP was with 3–4 poles. DF was thought to be composed of multiple layers and ensheathed both seminal vesicles and vas deferens into the anterior layer. After isolation of seminal vesicles, anterior layer of DF was isolated at the level of seminal vesicle triangle, and the dissection was located between prostate capsule (PC) and DF towards prostate apex in order to keep DF intact (Figure 1, Figure 2f–h). For the sake of cavernous nerves protection, blunt dissection was preferred. In consideration of potential nerve fiber damage, energy devices were seldom used during dissection near prostate.

Unfortunately, it was difficult to keep DF intact sometimes. In locally advanced PCa cases, the tight junction between DF and prostate added extra difficulty to LRP procedures. In these situations, DF would be resected partially or completely together with prostate (Fig. 2a–d). As to NVB sparing, careful dissection along PC in post-lateral direction should be enforced in some suitable cases.

No bladder neck and anterior and/or posterior reconstruction were conducted in our procedures. It was necessary to dissect close to prostate and keep bladder neck intact. But some situations, for example, locally advanced PCa, big prostate volume, and irregularly shaped prostate could make it hard to keep bladder neck intact. Under these circumstances, reconstruction of bladder neck was made to restore anastomosis, always by suturing bladder neck at 6 o'clock position.

Statistical analysis

The pathology images were processed with K-viewer version 1.5.3.1 (KFBIO, Zhejiang, CHINA). The continuous data and categorical data were analyzed with *t*-test and *Chi*-square test, respectively. Kaplan–Meier method was used to compute urinary continence curve. Binary logistic regression analysis was applied to screen predictors for ImC. All data analyses were performed using SPSS 22.0 statistical software (IBM SPSS, Chicago, IL, USA). In all analysis, $P < 0.05$ was considered statistically significant.

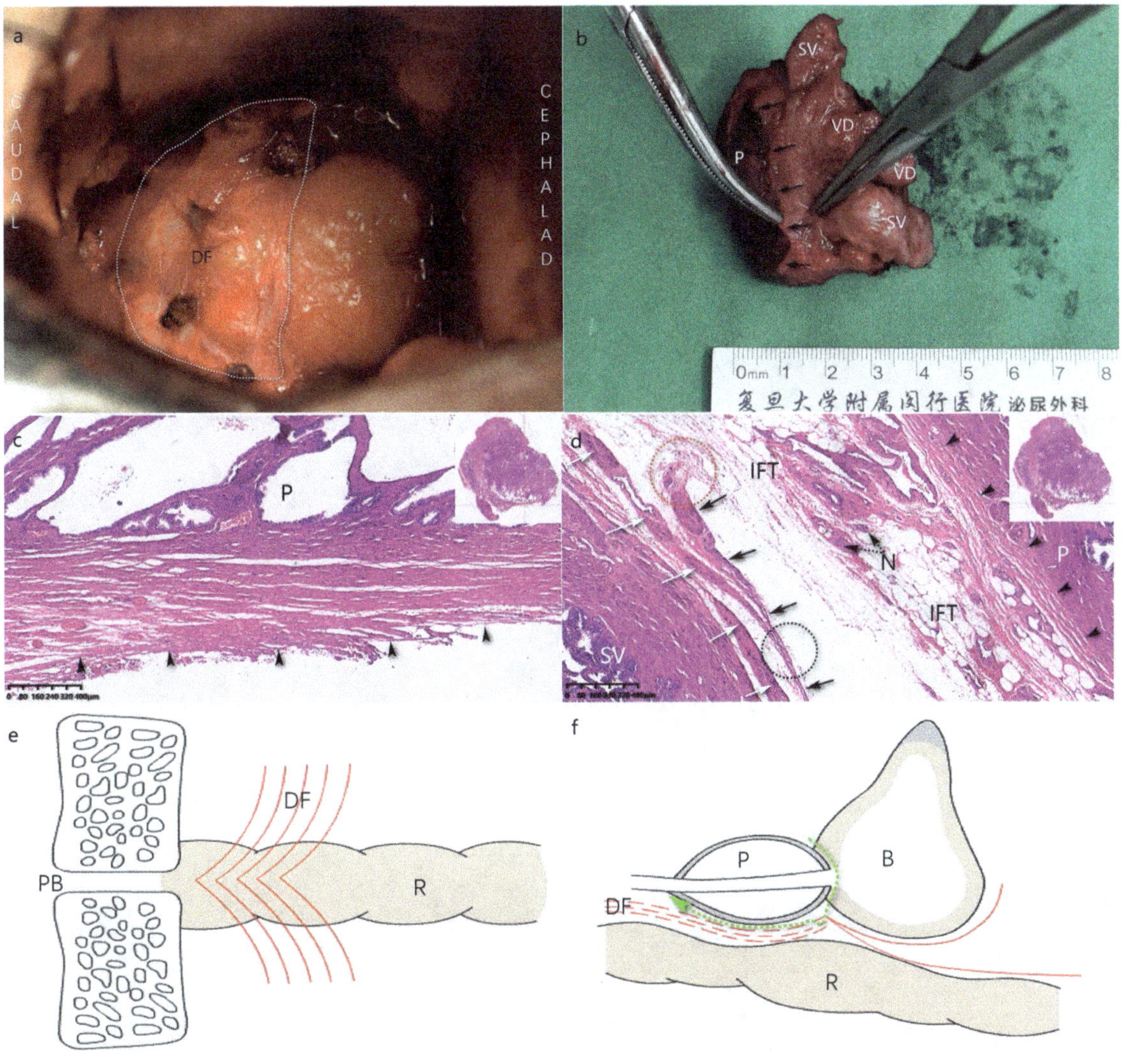

Fig. 1 Scenes of Mmi-RRP procedure with DFS technique and pathological section through paramedian of prostate, stained by HE. **a** DF (white dot line area) kept intact after prostate removal, also shown on schematic drawing (**e**). **b** Anterior layer of DF cut open at seminal vesicles triangle level. Dissection was kept between DF and PC towards apex of prostate. Black arrows exhibited the cut-line of DF's anterior layer. **c** No DF structure in the backward direction of prostate. **d** The cut-line of DF on the pathological section (red dot line circle), fused with seminal vesicle fascia propria (black dot line circle). **e, f** Schematic drawing OF dissecting bladder and prostate junction (green dot line). B: bladder; HE: hematoxylin and eosin; IFT: inter fascial tissue; N: nerve; P: prostate; PB: pubic bone; PC: prostate capsule; R: rectum; SV: seminal vesicles; VD: vas deferens. Black arrow: DF; Black arrow head: PC; White arrow: seminal vesicle fascia propria

Results

All the 154 consecutive patients completed RRP successfully and were followed-up for (14.5 ± 6.9) months, ranging from 2 to 26 months. The demographic and tumor characteristics of patients were shown in Table 1, while the details of procedures and pathology in Table 2. There was shorter duration of surgery ($P < 0.01$), more NVB sparing ($P < 0.01$), and less seminal vesicle invasion ($P = 0.04$) in Group DFS vs Group Control. Especially, the post-surgery continence condition was better in Group DFS than in Group Control at each time point from ImC to 3 months, 6 months ($P < 0.01$) and 12 months ($P = 0.02$), showed in Fig. 3.

In univariate analysis, surgery type ($OR = 1.2$–13.0, $P < 0.01$), surgery duration ($OR = 1.0$, $P < 0.01$), IIEF-5 Q2 pre-surgery ($OR = 1.4$, $P = 0.03$), Gleason score ($OR = 0.7$, $P = 0.02$), SV invasion ($OR = 0.2$, $P < 0.01$), NVB sparing (OR = 2.1–4.8, $P = 0.01$) and DF sparing ($OR = 32.3$, $P < 0.01$) were significantly related with ImC. While in multivariate analysis, only DF sparing was proved to be statistically significant for ImC, $OR = 26.4$, $P < 0.01$ (Table 3).

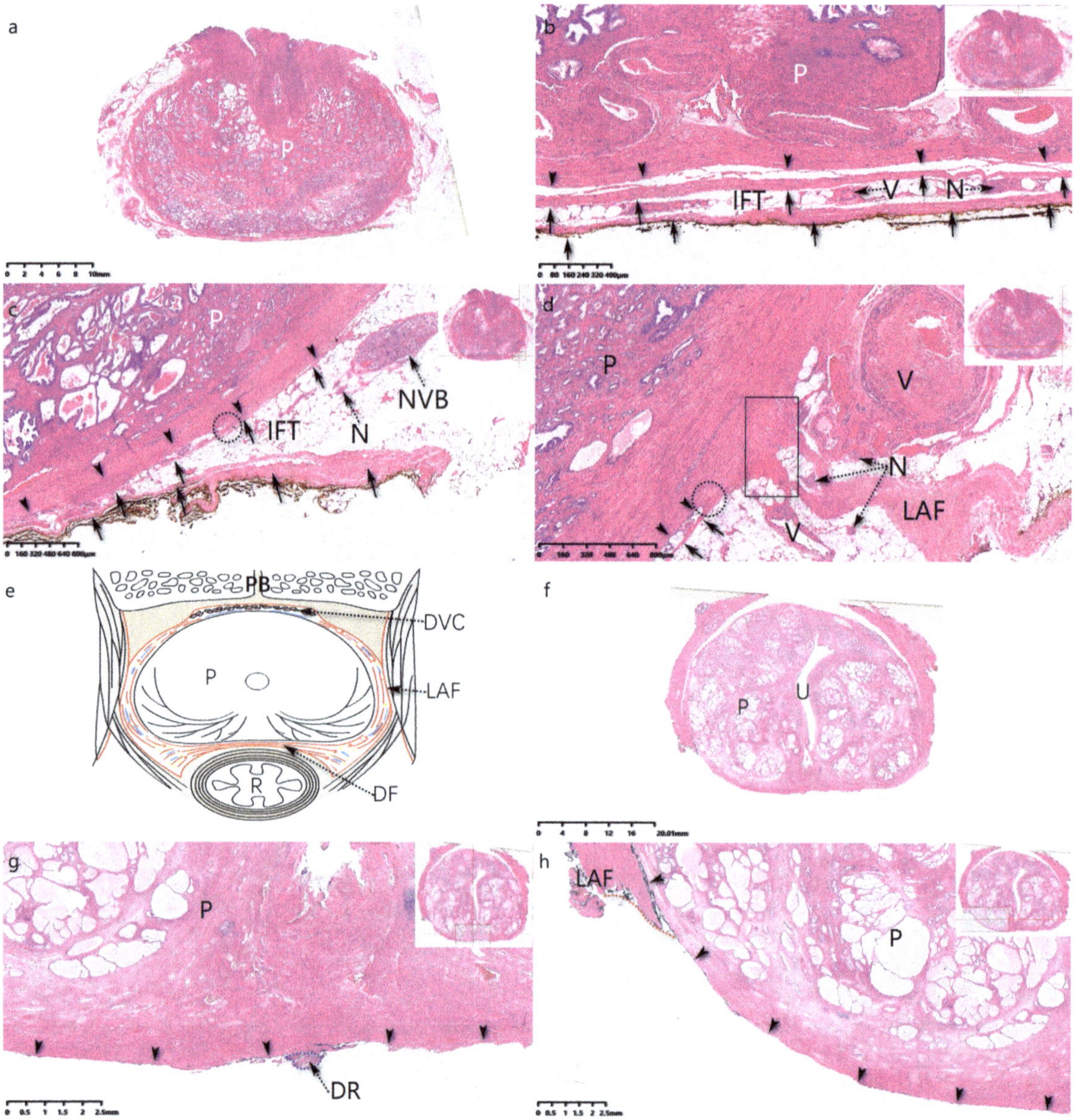

Fig. 2 Transverse sections at mid-prostate in Group Control (**a**–**d**) and Group DFS (**f**–**h**), both stained by HE. **a** Overall vision of pathological section from Group Control. **b** In 6-o'clock direction of prostate, two layers of DF were dissected with prostate. **c** In 4-o'clock direction, anterior layer of DF extended anterolaterally alongside with prostate capsule, sometime fused together (show in black dot line circle). Middle layer of DF and NVB were removed with prostate. **d** Anterior layer of DF extended anterolaterally and connected with levator ani fascia (LAF) at 3-o'clock direction. **e** Schematic drawing simulated peri-prostate fascia structure including DF and LAF. **f** Overall vision of pathological section from Group DFS. **g** In 6-o'clock direction of prostate, few DR fragments without DF layers. **h** In 8-o'clock direction, DF was spared successfully with no DF structure visible in the specimen. DR: dorsal raphe; DVC: dorsal vascular complex; IFT: inter fascial tissue; LAF: levator ani fascia; N: nerve; P: prostate; PB: pubic bone; R: rectum; V: vessel. Black arrow: DF; Black arrow head: PC; Black rectangle: anterior layer of DF adhered with LAF; Red dot line: cut line of LAF

As to definition of sexual dysfunction, we used cutoff value between response 2 and 3 for question NO.2 in IIEF-5 [2]. There were more potent patients in Group DFS than in Group Control at 12 months post-surgery, (34.7% *vs* 17.1%, $P=0.01$). No statistical difference of PSM was found between two groups (20.8% *vs* 20.7%, $P=1.0$, Table 2).

Discussion

Tumor control, urinary continence and sexual potency make up the Trifecta of RP. Post-surgery incontinence is one of the most functionally devastating complications, which could make patients too depressed to maintain social relationship and can even lead to suicide. Albkri A et al. [5] figured out that 28.1% patients regretted for

Table 1 Demographics and tumor characteristics of patients

	Group DFS (n = 72)	Group Control (n = 82)	*P*
Mean ± Std (Range)			
Age, years	67.8 ± 5.0 (58–79)	69.3 ± 6.5 (54–80)	0.1
BMI	24.5 ± 2.6 (17.4–30.9)	24.5 ± 2.7 (16.8–30.3)	0.9
Diagnosis PSA, ng/ml	16.0 ± 12.5 (0.4–61.0)	38.9 ± 114.7 (4.1–946.6)	0.1
Prostate volume, ml	49.2 ± 15.8 (13.5–100.7)	51.5 ± 18.5 (16.7–122.5)	0.4
Clinical stage, n (%)			0.8
T1	30 (41.7)	33 (40.2)	
T2	38 (52.8)	46 (56.1)	
T3	4 (5.6)	3 (3.7)	
Diagnosis Gleason, n (%)			0.2
≤6	31 (43.1)	26 (31.7)	
7	31 (43.1)	37 (45.1)	
≥8	10 (13.9)	19 (23.2)	
Diagnosis method, n (%)			0.5
Biopsy	66 (91.7)	78 (95.1)	
TURP	6 (8.3)	4 (4.9)	
IIEF-5 $Q_2 \geq 3$ pre-surgery, n (%)	49 (68.1)	47 (57.3)	0.2
Comorbid condition, n (%)			
CAD	9 (12.5)	10 (12.2)	1.0
DM	12 (16.7)	17 (20.7)	0.5
HBP	38 (52.8)	39 (47.6)	0.5
COPD	8 (11.1)	4 (4.9)	0.2
CVD	4 (5.6)	6 (7.3)	0.8

BMI body mass index, *CAD* coronary artery disease, *COPD* chronic obstruction pulmonary diseases, *CVD* cerebrovascular diseases, *DM* diabetes mellitus, *HBP* high blood pressure, *TURP* transurethral resection of prostate

IIEF-5 Q2: International Index of Erectile Function-5, question NO.2. "When you had erections with sexual stimulation, how often was your erection hard enough for penetration during the last 3 months?" The following responses were available: "No sexual activity" (0); "Almost never or never" (1); "A few times (much less than half the time)" (2); "Sometimes (about half the time)" (3); "Most times (much more than half the time)" (4); and "Almost always or always" (5)

RP decision because of complications. Unfortunately, there is so far no universal definition of continence up to now, which makes the morbidity of continence post-RP vary [6]. As literatures reported, ImC varied from 18 [7] to 63.5% [8], while continence at 3 months from 45 [9] to 82% [10], and continence at 12 months from 79.8 [2] to 91% [11]. In consideration of urinary consequences on record, morbidity of incontinence after RP in real world could probably be higher than reported [12]. Grivas N et al. [13] pointed out that continence at 12 months post-surgery was only 49.2% with strict definition.

The debate between cancer free and continence still lacks conclusion. Routinely, the more tissue near the tumor incised, the better tumor control. But it also means more potential functional structures to be cut, and incontinence is more likely to happen. Therefore, the discovery of landmark structure for urinary continence is needed. There are many hypotheses, such as membrane urethra length, urethral sphincter complex, detrusor apron of bladder neck, pelvic floor musculature, DVC, and NVB [3], etc. Asimakopoulos AD et al. [14] preferred complete periprostatic anatomy preservation to protect maximal functional structure and got 100% continence (≤1 pad per day) just at the time of catheter removal. However, this procedure may not be suitable for patients with higher tumor stage. Here we suppose DF to be the answer, particularly for the early-term and mid-term urinary control after RP.

DF has been demonstrated to be a multiple-layer structure both in cadaveric studies [15, 16] and histologic studies [17, 18] on specimen of RP. At the central-post direction of prostate and proximal of urethra, DF's fascicles tend to fuse and adhere with PC to form a dorsal raphe (DR) [16, 18]. The tendinous DR, which extends distally to prostate apex and ends at perineal tendon, may act as a fulcrum to support prostate and proximal urethra [19]. At the lateral-post direction of prostate, DF disperses to connect with LAF (Fig. 2). Dalpiaz et al. [19] described DF as part of musculofascial suspension system, stabilizing prostate apex and proximal urethra. Interestingly, there was similar view on stress urinary incontinence (SUI) of females. DeLancey [20]

Table 2 Outcomes of surgery

Group	DFS, n (%)	Control, n (%)	*P*
Mean ± Std (Range)			
Surgery duration, min	153.2 ± 66.4 (100–400)	188.3 ± 65.1 (90–480)	< 0.01
Blood loss, ml	143.1 ± 107.2 (20–800)	132.4 ± 136.9 (20–1000)	0.6
NVB sparing			< 0.01
Bilateral	27 (37.5)	24 (29.3)	
Unilateral	13 (18.1)	2 (2.4)	
None	32 (44.4)	56 (68.3)	
LND	63 (87.5)	74 (90.2)	0.6
pT			0.5
T0	1 (1.4)	0 (0)	
T2	53 (73.6)	57 (69.5)	
T3	18 (25.0)	25 (30.5)	
Gleason scores			0.1
0	1 (1.4)	0 (0)	
≤6	17 (23.6)	9 (11)	
7	38 (52.8)	50 (61)	
≥8	16 (22.2)	23 (28)	
Positive LN	0 (0)	3 (3.7)	0.2
SV invasion	7 (9.7)	18 (22)	0.04
PSM	15 (20.8)	17 (20.7)	1.0
Sites of PSM			0.3
One-site (*location; %*)	13 (*5 basal, 7 apical, 1 post-lateral; 18%*)	11 (*2 basal, 8 apical, 1 post-lateral; 13.4%*)	
Multiple-sites (*locations; %*)	2 (*2 apical and post-lateral; 2.8%*)	6 (*5 apical and basal, 1 apical, basal and post-lateral; 7.3%*)	
Post-lateral PSM	3 (4.2%)	2 (2.4%)	0.7
IIEF-5 $Q_2 \geq 3$ post-surgery	25 (34.7)	14 (17.1)	0.01
Continence			< 0.01
Immediate	60 (83.3)	11 (13.4)	< 0.01
3 months-	65 (90.3)	25 (30.5)	< 0.01
6 months-	66 (91.7)	53 (64.6)	< 0.01
12 months-	67 (93.1)	66 (80.5)	0.02

LND lymph node dissection, *NVB* nerve vascular bundle, *PSM* positive surgical margin, *SV* seminal vesicles

delineated endopelvic fascia and anterior vaginal wall as the hammock-like supportive layer of urethra, which could stabilize and help to close urethra during cough. Sling, placing a supportive material behind urethra, had been a staple procedure for SUI and withstood the test of time [21]. Back to continence after RP, we hypothesized "hammock theory" still work on and preferred DF to be the critical structure (Figs. 1, 2 and 4), which could uplift vesicourethral anastomosis. Meanwhile, DR just acted as the fulcrum beneath urethra and contributed to closure of it when abdomen pressure increased. Hence, together with DR (also part of DF), DF was supposed to be the critical landmark for continence post RP. Our research also proved that DFS could significantly improve ImC ($OR = 26.4$, $P < 0.01$). However, because of individual difference, DF or DR could not be kept intact in every operation. So, we proposed a grading system for DFS procedure and our study showed that different grades can indicate different continence prognosis after RP (Fig. 4).

Considering that the scattering neurovascular plexus, which innervates corpora cavernosa and sphincter complex, is embedded in the multiple-layers of DF [3, 22], there was a minority of nerve fibers located in front of DF which would be dissected inevitably [23], while most of them are located in post-lateral and post regions of prostate [3] (Fig. 1). Tewari et al. [24] proposed a nerve-sparing (NS) grading system based on "landmark vein (LV)" lateral to prostate. An intra-fascial dissection was defined as grade-1, while an extra-fascial dissection was defined as grade-4. Srivastava et al. [25] demonstrated that grade-1 achieved more early continence than grade-4 (71.8% *vs* 43.5%), which may account for incomplete continence situation with intact DF.

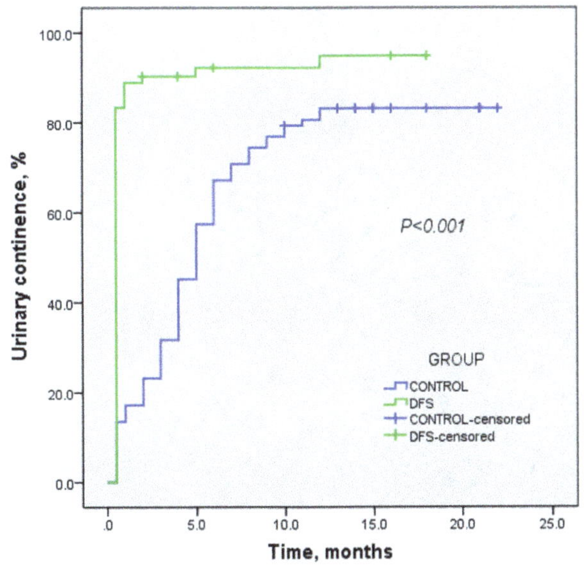

Fig. 3 Kaplan–Meier analysis for time to urinary continence post-surgery

Table 3 Logistic regression analysis for predictors of immediate continence

ImC	Univariate		Multi-variate	
	OR (95%CI)	*P*	*OR* (95%CI)	*P*
Surgery type		<0.01		0.6
Mmi-RRP *vs* LRP	13.0 (5.7–29.7)	<0.01	1.9 (0.4–8.7)	0.4
RARP *vs* LRP	1.2 (0.4–4.0)	0.7	0.8 (0.2–3.6)	0.7
LND, Yes *vs* No	0.7 (0.3–2.0)	0.6		
Gleason score	0.7 (0.5–0.9)	0.02	0.9 (0.5–1.6)	0.8
SV invasion, Yes *vs* No	0.2 (0.1–0.7)	<0.01	0.3 (0.1–1.3)	0.1
PSM, Yes *vs* No	0.9 (0.4–1.9)	0.8		
TURP before, Yes *vs* No	1.2 (0.3–4.3)	0.8		
Diagnosis PSA	1.0 (0.992–1.003)	0.4		
IIEF-5 Q_2 pre-surgery	1.4 (1.0–1.9)	0.03	1.6 (0.9–2.7)	0.1
Prostate volume	1.0 (0.98–1.01)	0.6		
Age	1.0 (0.91–1.02)	0.2	1.0 (0.9–1.1)	0.6
BMI	0.9 (0.8–1.1)	0.3		
Surgery duration	1.0 (0.98–0.99)	<0.01	1.0 (0.981–1.002)	0.1
Blood loss	1.0 (0.996–1.001)	0.3		
NVB sparing		0.01		0.9
Unilateral vs No	4.8 (1.4–16.4)	0.01	0.8 (0.1–4.3)	0.8
Bilateral vs No	2.1 (1.1–4.3)	0.04	1.1 (0.3–3.8)	0.9
DF sparing, Yes *vs* No	32.3 (13.3–78.4)	<0.01	26.4 (8.4–83. 3)	<0.01

BMI body mass index, *CI* confidence interval, *ImC* immediate continence, *LND* lymph node dissection, *NVB* nerve vascular bundle, *OR* odds ratio, *PSM* positive surgical margin, *SV* seminal vesicles

DF-sparing technique doesn't equal to complete periprostatic anatomy preservation or intra-fascial dissection. DFS procedure emphasizes dissecting before anterior layer of DF to protect the whole DF fascicles and the majority of neurovascular fibers, which is a procedure with a specific target to be spared, making the incision area selective but thorough. Whereas complete peri-prostate sparing technique aims to preserve functional structure as much as possible [14]. However, good functional recovery may sacrifice safety of tumor control. DF-targeted sparing procedure provides a compromised solution to the dilemma of urinary- or tumor-control.

With the same aim at preserving continence, Retzius-sparing (RS) technique puts more emphasis on preserving the structure in front of prostate [26]. RS was supposed to suspend and stabilize the bladder and anastomosis which might contribute to fast recovery of continence [26]. Compared with standard RP, lots of researches reported Retzius-sparing RP (RSRP) with better continence in short term, especially ImC [27, 28]. Given that more neurovascular plexus located post-lateral direction [3, 23], DFS might result in better continence from another perspective theoretically, but more prospective randomized controlled studies were needed to clarify that.

In our research, Group DFS achieved 83.3% ImC, 90.3% continence in 3 months, 91.7% in 6 months, 93.1% in 12 months (Fig. 3), better than Group Control at every time point with no difference in PSM (20.8% *vs* 20.7%, $P=1.0$), especially no difference of PSM in post-lateral direction of prostate (4.2% *vs* 2.4%, $P=0.7$).

Another key point to protect neurovascular plexus is the limited usage of energy devices, such as ultrasonic or electronic scalpels, bipolar coagulator, especially during prostate apex anatomy [29], in which nerve fibers penetrate DF or periprostatic tissue to innervate urethral sphincter. The electrical and thermal conduction may cause extra damage to neurovascular fibers nearby. Thereby, "blunt", or "cold" dissection for prostate apex with finger, forceps, or scissors is preferred. The NS grading system proposed by Patel et al. [30] proved the idea. In Patel's system, grade 5 NS was performed between "landmark artery (LA)" lateral to prostate and PC with neither sharp dissection nor energy devices, which resulted in complete nerve sparing (>95%). Grade 4 NS (75%) was also performed between LA and PC with sharp dissection but without energy devices.

Last but not least, we preferred to pay more attention to ImC post RP. Temml et al. [31] testified that QoL wasn't related to duration of incontinence but frequency and degree of incontinence, need for pads, etc. Coyne et al. [32] pointed out remarkable prevalence of 19.1% anxiety and 6.6% depression in patients with urinary

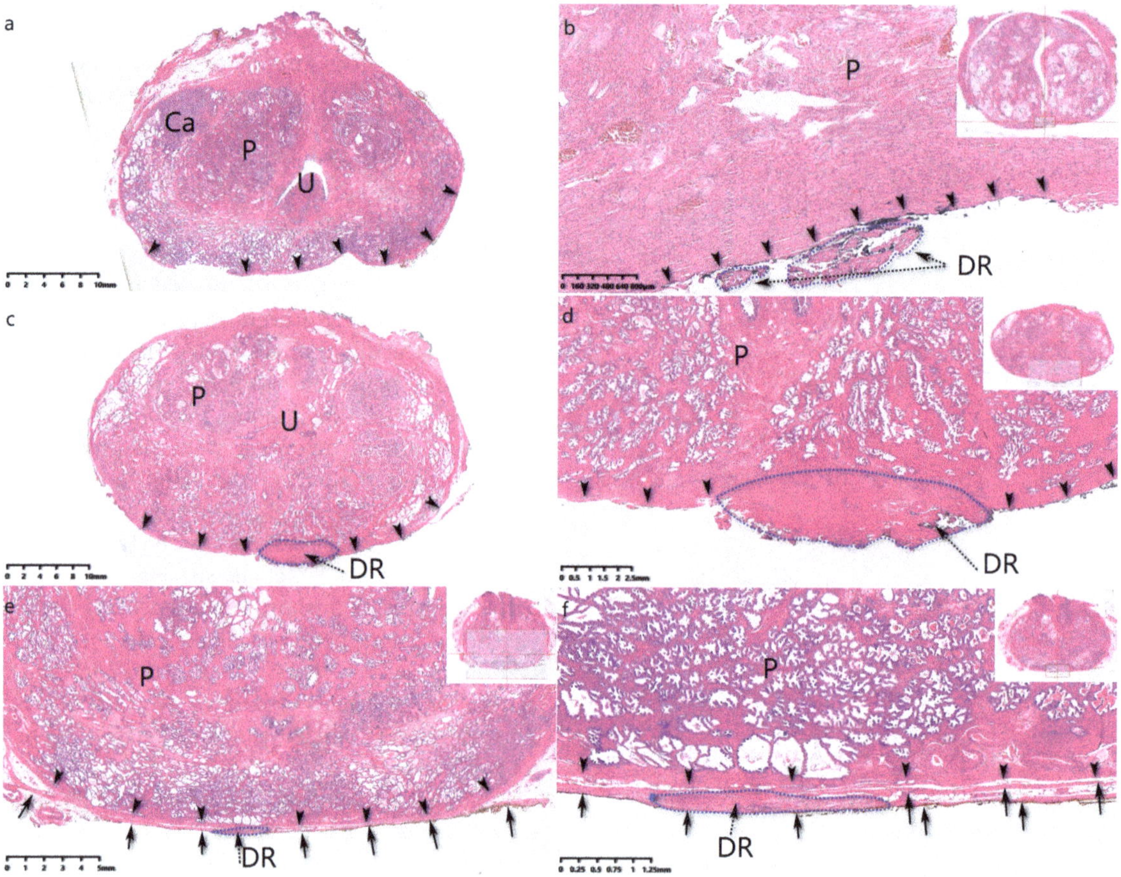

Fig. 4 Different grades of DFS in RP, stained by hematoxylin and eosin. **a** In Grade-1 DF sparing procedure, neither DF nor DR was cut with prostate. **b** In Grade-2 DFS procedure, DF was preserved while DR fragments removed with prostate. **c, d** In Grade-2 DFS procedure, DF spared successfully while DR was totally cut away. **e–f** Grade-3 DFS was defined as neither DF nor DR spared. Black arrow head: prostate capsule; Ca: prostate cancer; DR: dorsal raphe (show in blue dot line circle); P: prostate; U: urethra. Black arrow: DF; Black arrow head: PC

incontinence (UI). Anxiety may trigger and aggravate UI in return. So better ImC may guarantee not only "extra" better continence in the future but also positive mental health.

Indeed, there are limitations in present research including small sample size, retrospective, and lack of randomization. Therefore, a prospective randomized controlled study with larger sample size should be organized for further verification.

Conclusion

Denonvilliers' fascia was supposed to act as the fulcrum and hammock for urinary control after RP. We recommend to preserve DF, minimize utility of energy devices during dissecting, which could probably contribute to best continence after RP without increase of PSM.

mellitus; DF: Denonvillier's fascia; DFS: DF-sparing; DR: Dorsal raphe; DVC: Dorsal vascular complex; HBP: High blood pressure; HE: Hematoxylin and eosin; IFT: Inter fascial tissue; IIEF-5: International Index of Erectile Function-5; ImC: Immediate continence; LAF: Levator ani fascia; LND: Lymph node dissection; LRP: Laparoscopic radical prostatectomy; Mmi-RRP: Mini-incision retropubic radical prostatectomy; NVB: Neurovascular bundle; ORP: Open radical prostatectomy; PC: Prostate capsule; PSM: Positive surgical margin; RARP: Robotic-assisted radical prostatectomy; RP: Radical prostatectomy; RS: Retzius sparing; RSRP: Retzius sparing radical prostatectomy; TURP: Transurethral resection of prostate; SUI: Stress urinary incontinence; SV: Seminal vesicles; VD: Vas deferens.

Acknowledgements

We sincerely thank Ms. Miao Gong for production of pathological sections, and Dr. Yuan Ji for support in pathological image scanning and enlightening advices.

Authors' contributions

Project developed by HW, JMG. Manuscript written by XWL, edited by HW, CH and SHZ. Data collected by FY, ZFG, WYL and JC, analyzed by JQH, MKH and JWW. Pathological section managed and analyzed by XS.

Abbreviations

BMI: Body mass index; CAD: Coronary artery disease; COPD: Chronic obstruction pulmonary diseases; CVD: Cerebrovascular diseases; DM: Diabetes

Competing interests

The authors declare that they have no competing interests.

Author details

[1]Department of Urology, Minhang Hospital, Fudan University, Shanghai 201199, China. [2]Department of Urology, Zhongshan Hospital, Fudan University, Fenglin Rd 130, Shanghai 200032, China. [3]Department of Pathology, Minhang Hospital, Fudan University, Shanghai 201199, China. [4]Department of Urology, Xuhui Hospital, Fudan University, Shanghai 200031, China.

References

1. Siegel RL, Miller KD, Jemal A. Cancer statistics, 2019. CA Cancer J Clin. 2019;69(1):7–34. https://doi.org/10.3322/caac.21551.
2. Haglind E, Carlsson S, Stranne J, Wallerstedt A, Wilderäng U, Thorstein sdottir T, et al. Urinary incontinence and erectile dysfunction after robotic versus open radical prostatectomy: a prospective, controlled, nanrandomised trial. Eur Urol. 2015;68(2):216–25. https://doi.org/10.1016/j.eururo.2015.02.029.
3. Walz J, Epstein JI, Ganzer R, Graefen M, Guazzoni G, Kaouk J, et al. A critical analysis of the current knowledge of surgical anatomy of the prostate related to optimisation of cancer control and preservation of continence and erection in candidates for radical prostatectomy: an update. Eur Urol. 2016;70(2):301–11. https://doi.org/10.1016/j.eururo.2016.01.026.
4. Grasso AA, Mistretta FA, Sandri M, Cozzi G, De Lorenzis E, Rosso M, et al. Posterior musculofascial reconstruction after radical prostatectomy: an updated systematic review and a meta-analysis. BJU Int. 2016;118(1):20–34. https://doi.org/10.1111/bju.13480.
5. Albkri A, Girier D, Mestre A, Costa P, Droupy S, Chevrot A. Urinary incontinence, patient satisfaction, and decisional regret after prostate cancer treatment: a French national study. Urol Int. 2018;100(1):50–6. https://doi.org/10.1159/000484616.
6. Liss MA, Osann K, Canvasser N, Chu W, Chang A, Gan J, et al. Continence definition after radical prostatectomy using urinary quality of life: evaluation of patient reported validated questionnaires. J Urol. 2010;183(4):1464–8. https://doi.org/10.1016/j.juro.2009.12.009.
7. John H, Hauri D. Seminal vesicle-sparing radical prostatectomy: a novel concept to restore early urinary continence. Urology. 2000;55(6):820–4. https://doi.org/10.1016/s0090-4295(00)00547-1.
8. Moinzadeh A, Shunaigat AN, Libertino JA. Urinary incontinence after radical retropubic prostatectomy: the outcome of a surgical technique. BJU Int. 2003;92(4):355–9. https://doi.org/10.1046/j.1464-410x.2003.04348.x
9. Hollabaugh RS, Dmochowski RR, Kneib TG, Steiner MS. Preservation of putative continence nerves during radical retropubic prostatectomy leads to more rapid return of urinary continence. Urology. 1998;51(6):960–7. https://doi.org/10.1016/s0090-4295(98)00128-9.
10. Walsh PC, Marschke PL. Intussusception of the reconstructed bladder neck leads to earlier continence after radical prostatectomy. Urology. 2002;59(6):934–8. https://doi.org/10.1016/s0090-4295(02)01596-0.
11. Coughlin GD, Yaxley JW, Chambers SK, Occhipinti S, Samaratunga H, Zajdlewicz L, et al. Robot-assisted laparoscopic prostatectomy versus open radical retropubic prostatectomy: 24-month outcomes from a randomised controlled study. Lancet Oncol. 2018;19(8):1051–60. https://doi.org/10.1016/S1470-2045(18)30357-7.
12. Nelson JB. The ongoing challenge of urinary incontinence after radical prostatectomy. J Urol. 2017;198(6):1223–5. https://doi.org/10.1016/j.juro.2017.09.053.
13. Grivas N, van der Roest R, Schouten D, Cavicchioli F, Tillier C, Bex A, et al. Quantitative assessment of fascia preservation improves the prediction of membranous urethral length and inner levator distance on continence outcome after robot-assisted radical prostatectomy. Neurourol Urodyn. 2018;37(1):417–25. https://doi.org/10.1002/nau.23318.
14. Asimakopoulos AD, Annino F, D'Orazio A, Pereira CF, Mugnier C, Hoepffner JL, et al. Complete periprostatic anatomy preservation during robot-assisted laparoscopic radical prostatectomy (RALP): the new pubovesical complex-sparing technique. Eur Urol. 2010;58(3):407–17. https://doi.org/10.1016/j.eururo.2010.04.032.
15. Ghareeb WM, Wang X, Chi P, Wang W. The "multilayer" theory of Denonvilliers' fascia: anatomical dissection of cadavers with the aim to improve neurovascular bundle preservation during rectal mobilization. Colorectal Dis. 2020;22(2):195–202. https://doi.org/10.1111/codi.14850.
16. Xu Z, Chapuis PH, Bokey L, Zhang M. Denonvilliers' fascia in men: a sheet plastination and confocal microscopy study of the prerectal space and the presence of an optimal anterior plane when mobilizing the rectum for cancer. Colorectal Dis. 2017. https://doi.org/10.1111/codi.13906.
17. Secin FP, Karanikolas N, Gopalan A, Bianco FJ, Shayegan B, Touijer K, et al. The anterior layer of Denonvilliers' fascia: a common misconception in the laparoscopic prostatectomy literature. J Urol. 2007;177(2):521–5. https://doi.org/10.1016/j.juro.2006.09.028.
18. Kiyoshima K, Yokomizo A, Yoshida T, Tomita K, Yonemasu H, Nakamura M, et al. Anatomical features of periprostatic tissue and its surroundings: a histological analysis of 79 radical retropubic prostatectomy specimens. Jpn J Clin Oncol. 2004;34(8):463–8. https://doi.org/10.1093/jjco/hyh078.
19. Dalpiaz O, Anderhuber F. The fascial suspension of the prostate: a cadaveric study. Neurourol Urodyn. 2017;36(4):1131–5. https://doi.org/10.1002/nau.23073.
20. DeLancey JO. Structural support of the urethra as it relates to stress urinary incontinence: the hammock hypothesis. Am J Obstet Gynecol. 1994;170(6):1713–20. https://doi.org/10.1016/s0002-9378(94)70346-9.
21. Schreiner G, Beltran R, Lockwood G, Takacs EB. A timeline of female stress urinary incontinence: how technology defined theory and advanced treatment. Neurourol Urodyn. 2020;39(6):1862–7. https://doi.org/10.1002/nau.24407.
22. Muraoka K, Hinata N, Morizane S, Honda M, Sejima T, Murakami G, et al. Site-dependent and interindividual variations in Denonvilliers' fascia: a histological study using donated elderly male cadavers. BMC Urol. 2015;15:42. https://doi.org/10.1186/s12894-015-0034-5.
23. Kinugasa Y, Murakami G, Uchimoto K, Takenaka A, Yajima T, Sugihara K. Operating behind Denonvilliers' fascia for reliable preservation of urogenital autonomic nerves in total mesorectal excision: a histologic study using cadaveric specimens, including a surgical experiment using fresh cadaveric models. Dis Colon Rectum. 2006;49(7):1024–32. https://doi.org/10.1007/s10350-006-0557-7.
24. Tewari AK, Srivastava A, Huang MW, Robinson BD, Shevchuk MM, Durand M, et al. Anatomical grades of nerve sparing: a risk-stratified approach to neural-hammock sparing during robot-assisted radical prostatectomy (RARP). BJU Int. 2011;108(6 Pt 2):984–92. https://doi.org/10.1111/j.1464-410X.2011.10565.x.
25. Srivastava A, Chopra S, Pham A, Sooriakumaran P, Durand M, Chughtai B, et al. Effect of a risk-stratified grade of nerve-sparing technique on early return of continence after robot-assisted laparoscopic radical prostatectomy. Eur Urol. 2013;63(3):438–44. https://doi.org/10.1016/j.eururo.2012.07.009.
26. Galfano A, Ascione A, Grimaldi S, Petralia G, Strada E, Bocciardi AM. A new anatomic approach for robot-assisted laparoscopic prostatectomy: a feasibility study for completely intrafascial surgery. Eur Urol. 2010;58(3):457–61. https://doi.org/10.1016/j.eururo.2010.06.008.
27. Rosenberg JE, Jung JH, Edgerton Z, Lee H, Lee S, Bakker CJ, et al. Retzius-sparing versus standard robot-assisted laparoscopic prostatectomy for the treatment of clinically localized prostate cancer. BJU Int. 2021;128(1):12–20. https://doi.org/10.1111/bju.15385.
28. Umari P, Eden C, Cahill D, Rizzo M, Eden D, Sooriakumaran P. Retzius-sparing versus standard robot-assisted radical prostatectomy: a comparative prospective study of nearly 500 patients. J Urol. 2021;205(3):780–90. https://doi.org/10.1097/JU.0000000000001435.
29. Tewari A, Takenaka A, Mtui E, Horninger W, Peschel R, Bartsch G, et al. The proximal neurovascular plate and the tri-zonal neural architecture around the prostate gland: importance in the athermal robotic technique of nerve-sparing prostatectomy. BJU Int. 2006;98(2):314–23. https://doi.org/10.1111/j.1464-410X.2006.06266.x.

30. Schatloff O, Chauhan S, Sivaraman A, Kameh D, Palmer KJ, Patel VR. Anatomic grading of nerve sparing during robot-assisted radical prostatectomy. Eur Urol. 2012;61(4):796–802. https://doi.org/10.1016/j.eururo.2011.12.048.
31. Temml C, Haidinger G, Schmidbauer J, Schatzl G, Madersbacher S. Urinary incontinence in both sexes: prevalence rates and impact on quality of life and sexual life. Neurourol Urodyn. 2000;19(3):259–71.
32. Coyne KS, Kvasz M, Ireland AM, Milsom I, Kopp ZS, Chapple CR. Urinary incontinence and its relationship to mental health and health-related quality of life in men and women in Sweden, the United Kingdom, and the United States. Eur Urol. 2012;61(1):88–95. https://doi.org/10.1016/j.eururo.2011.07.049.

23

Predicting Gleason sum upgrading from biopsy to radical prostatectomy pathology: A new nomogram and its internal validation

Xiaochuan Wang†, Yu Zhang†, Fengbo Zhang, Zhengguo Ji, Peiqian Yang and Ye Tian*

Abstract

Background: To explore the rate of Gleason sum upgrading (GSU) from biopsy to radical prostatectomy pathology and to develop a nomogram for predicting the probability of GSU in a Chinese cohort.

Methods: We retrospectively reviewed our prospectively maintained prostate cancer (PCa) database from October 2012 to April 2020. 198 patients who met the criteria were enrolled. Multivariable logistic regression analysis was performed to determine the predictors. Nomogram was constructed based on independent predictors. The receiver operating curve was undertaken to estimate the discrimination. Calibration curve was used to assess the concordance between predictive probabilities and true risks.

Results: The rate of GSU was 41.4%, whilst GS concordance rate was 44.4%. The independent predictors are prostate specific antigen (PSA), greatest percentage of cancer (GPC), clinical T-stage and Prostate Imaging Reporting and Data System (PI-RADS) score. Our model showed good discrimination (AUC of 0.735). Our model was validated internally with good calibration with bias-corrected C-index of 0.726.

Conclusions: Utilization of basic clinical variables (PSA and T-stage) combined with imaging variable (PI-RADS) and pathological variable (GPC) could improve performance in predicting actual probabilities of GSU in the 24-core biopsy scheme. Our nomogram could help to assess the true risk and make optimal treatment decisions for PCa patients.

Keywords: Prostatic neoplasms, Neoplasm grading, Biopsy, needle, Prostatectomy, Nomograms

Background

Gleason score is a critical factor for both risk stratification and disease management in prostate cancer (PCa). However, it was reported that the concordance of Gleason score between initial biopsy and final radical prostatectomy (RP) pathology was barely satisfactory [1]. Gleason sum upgrading (GSU) may affect assessment of the true PCa risk and treatment options for PCa patients. For instance, active surveillance is recommended for patients with Gleason 6 or 3+4 but not appropriate for patients with Gleason 4+3 or above [2]. Patients with organ-confined tumors of Gleason 8 or above should underwent RP followed by lymph node dissection and other ancillary therapies in case of PSA failure [3]. Similarly, external beam radiation therapy is recommended to be combined with androgen deprivation therapy in patients with Gleason 4+3 or above [4]. It has been demonstrated in large-scale studies that patients with GSU were significantly associated with biochemical recurrence, distant metastasis and death from PCa [5, 6].

To address this matter, our study aimed to examine the rate of GSU between biopsy and final pathology and determine independent predictors for GSU. Moreover, our study developed a nomogram including clinical,

*Correspondence: tianye166@126.com
†Xiaochuan Wang and Yu Zhang have contributed to the study consistently
Department of Urology, Capital Medical University Affiliated Beijing Friendship Hospital, No. 95, Yongan Road, Xicheng District, Beijing, People's Republic of China

imaging and pathologic variables based on Chinese population. We therefore expect to help reassess the risk after biopsy and select optimal treatment modalities for PCa patients after a comprehensive evaluation.

Methods

Data acquisition and patient selection

From our prospectively maintained institutional review board-approved prostate biopsy database, we identified 2039 consecutive men who underwent biopsy at our institution (1st October 2012 to 30th April 2020). 212 patients who underwent RP at our institution met the inclusion criteria. The exclusion criteria were as follows: (1) patients treated with neoadjuvant therapy before RP; (2) patients with missing data. Finally, 198 eligible patients entered into our study cohort. Two researchers independently browsed the database, extracted the data and cross-checked. This study did not contain any human participants or animals and it received ethics approval from Capital Medical University affiliated Beijing Friendship Hospital Ethics Committee for database access (2019-P2-081-01).

Clinical evaluation

Prostate volume (PV) was calculated using anterior–posterior diameter, superior-inferior diameter and left–right diameter which were obtained from multiparametric magnetic resonance imaging (mpMRI). Prostate specific antigen (PSA) was measured before digital rectal examination (DRE) and biopsy. Clinical T-stage was assigned according to the 2017 TNM system which relied on findings of biopsy, DRE and mpMRI.

As recommended [7], the prostate mpMRI was performed before biopsy at a 3-T (T) system. MpMRI protocol consisted of T2-weighted imaging (T2WI), diffusion-weighted imaging (DWI) with apparent diffusion coefficient map (ADC), and dynamic contrast-enhanced (DCE) sequences and calculated b value of 1000 or above. Urological radiologists who were experienced with PI-RADS score and were blinded to pathology as well as clinical data evaluated all the images and performed scoring.

Biopsy and pathological evaluation

Patients received 18-gauge transperineal needle biopsy under general anesthesia in a dorsal lithotomy position. The biopsy was performed under the guidance of transrectal ultrasonography (TRUS) utilizing an 24-core extended scheme. There were twenty needles in the peripheral zone (PZ) from apex and mid to posterior base and four needles in the transitional zone (TZ). Each core was submitted in a separate container. 24-core systematic biopsy was a standard practice across our center performed by experienced urologists. Gleason sum was assigned core by core by a specialized team of urogenital pathologists using global Gleason score. All RP specimens were examined for prostatectomy Gleason sum by the same team. Hence, non-uniform interpretation of reports between pathologists and clinicians could be avoided [8]. Tertiary patterns were included in biopsy, but not included in prostatectomy specimens. GSU was defined as any Gleason sum upgrading from biopsy to RP. GPC (greatest percentage of cancer in a single core) and fraction of positive cores (FPC) were applied to measure tissue tumor extent (TTE) in biopsy cores [9].

Statistical analysis

The patients were divided into two groups as those with GSU and those without GSU. Age, metabolic status, body mass index (BMI), interval from biopsy to RP, PV, PSA, PSA density (PSAD), clinical T-stage, PI-RADS score and biopsy specimen features were analyzed in all patients. Normality of distribution of the variables was checked using the Shapiro–Wilk tests and P–P plots. Normally distributed numerical variables were analyzed by the student *t* tests. Mann–Whitney U tests were applied to determine the significance of nonnormally distributed numerical variables. Chi-square tests were used for categorical variables. Univariable regression analysis was performed followed by the multivariable analysis. Variables that were found statistically significant in univariable analysis entered the multivariable analysis in a forward stepwise selection (probability of 0.05). The nomogram was constructed with validated independent predictors. The performance of the prediction model was evaluated from the aspect of discrimination and calibration. Discrimination was measured using the receiver operating curve (ROC) with the area under the curve (AUC) value. Calibration was assessed by visually inspecting the plots of predicted probability and actual probability. Bias-corrected C-index was also calculated to be compared with original C-index (AUC value). Internal validation was performed by bootstrap resampling ($n = 1000$) to evaluate the accuracy estimates and to reduce overfit bias. Tests were 2 sided and $P < 0.05$ was the threshold for statistical significance. Statistical tests were performed using computer software of SPSS version 24.0 and R version 4.0.2.

Results

A statistical significance was met when it came to variables: cT-stage, PI-RADS score, PSA and GPC (all $P < 0.05$). Patients in GSU subgroup had a higher ratio for $T_{2b\text{-}2c}$ cancers (66.3%) and PI-RADS score of 4–5 (89.9%), higher PSA level (15.7 ng/ml) and higher GPC (90.0%). Other demographic details were shown in Table 1.

Table 1 Demographics of patients underwent biopsy followed by prostatectomy in total and subgroups

Variables	Total (n = 198)	GSU (n = 89)	Non-GSU (n = 109)	*P* value
Age at biopsy (year), M(IQR)	67.0(63.0–71.0)	67.0 (62.0–71.0)	67.0 (63.0–71.0)	0.496[a]
MS (n, %)	–	–	–	0.150
Absence	156(78.8)	66 (74.2)	90 (82.6)	–
Presence	42(21.2)	23 (25.8)	19 (17.4)	–
BMI, M(IQR) (kg/m^2)	24.7(22.9–26.9)	25.0(23.1–27.2)	24.6(22.3–26.7)	0.345[a]
Interval from biopsy to RP, M(IQR) (d)	21.0(14.0–34.3)	21.0(14.0–31.5)	21.0(14.0–35.0)	0.771[b]
PV, M(IQR) (ml)	39.0(28.1–53.0)	38.8(28.7–52.8)	39.2(23.9–53.4)	0.801[b]
Pre-biopsy PSA level, M(IQR) (ng/ml)	14.2(8.6–28.7)	15.7(9.1–35.9)	13.1(7.8–23.6)	0.032[b]
Pre-biopsy PSAD, M(IQR) (ng/ml^2)	0.37(0.21–0.79)	0.46(0.23–1.01)	0.34(0.20–0.74)	0.061[b]
Clinical T-stage (n, %)	–	–	–	0.002
T_{1c-2a}	63(31.8)	18 (20.2)	45 (41.3)	0.001[c]
T_{2b-2c}	105(53.0)	59 (66.3)	46 (42.2)	0.117[d]
T_{3a-3b}	30(15.2)	12(13.5)	18 (16.5)	0.270[e]
PI-RADS score (n, %)	–	–	–	< 0.001
2–3	51(25.8)	9 (10.1)	42 (38.5)	–
4–5	147(74.2)	80 (89.9)	67 (61.5)	–
Cores obtained (n, %)	–	–	–	0.480
12–23	16(8.1)	9(10.1)	7(6.4)	–
24	165(83.3)	74(83.1)	91(83.5)	–
25–30	17(8.6)	6(6.7)	11(10.1)	–
FPC, M(IQR) (%)	25.0(13.0–42.0)	25.0(12.5–48.0)	25.0(13.0–42.0)	0.906[b]
GPC, M(IQR) (%)	70.0(30.0–90.0)	90.0(50.0–90.0)	50.0(30.0–90.0)	0.001[b]
Experience in biopsy (n, %)	–	–	–	0.886
Senior	79(39.9)	36(40.4)	43 (39.4)	–
Junior	119(60.1)	53 (59.6)	66 (60.6)	–

GSU Gleason sum upgrade, *M* median, *IQR* interquartile range, *MS* metabolic syndrome, *RP* radical prostatectomy, *BMI* body mass index, *PV* prostate volume, *PSA* prostate specific antigen, *PSAD* PSA density, *PI-RADS* prostate Imaging Reporting and Data System, *FPC* fraction of positive cores, *GPC* the greatest percentage of cancer

[a] Analyzed by the student *t* test

[b] Analyzed by the Mann–Whitney U test

[c] Comparison between T_{1c-2a} and T_{2b-2c}

[d] Comparison between T_{2b-2c} and T_{3a-3b}

[e] Comparison between T_{1c-2a} and T_{3a-3b}

Table 2 Distribution in Gleason scores between the biopsy cores and RP specimens

Biopsy Gleason sum	RP Gleason sum						
	6	3+4	4+3	8	9	10	Total
6	28	28	4	6	3		69
3+4	3	24	9	13	4		53
4+3	1	7	13	10	1		32
8		2	9	7	9		27
9		1	2		9	1	13
10				1	2	1	4
Total	32	62	37	37	28	2	198

We found that concordance rate between initial biopsy pathology and final RP specimens was 41.4% (82/198), whilst GSU was 44.4% (88/198). Downgrading was found in 14.1% (28/198) of patients (Table 2). Our study further divided the entire cohort into three groups according to the biopsy Gleason sum (6, 7, ≥ 8). The percentage of GSU was highest in patients with Gleason sum 6, while the concordance rate was highest in patients with Gleason sum 7. The percentage of downgrading was highest in patients with Gleason sum 8–10 (Fig. 1).

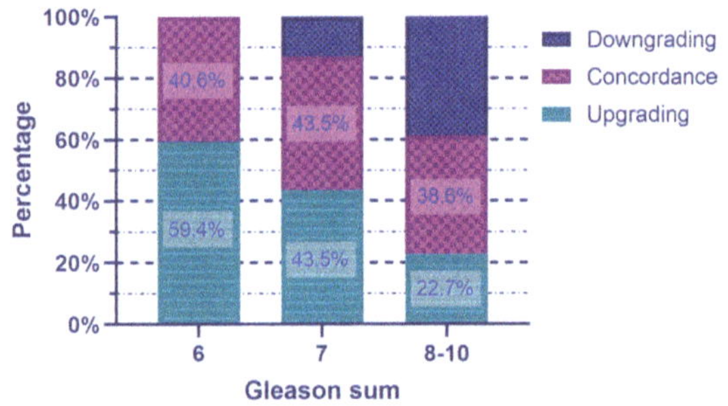

Fig. 1 Stacked bar chart of the distribution and magnitude of Gleason sum change from biopsy to prostatectomy pathology in three cohorts of men with different Gleason sum

Univariate analysis revealed that PSA, PSAD, GPC, cT-stage and PI-RADS score were the predictors of GSU (all $P < 0.05$). Multivariate analysis confirmed that PSA, GPC, cT-stage and PI-RADS score were independent predictors of GSU (all $P < 0.05$) (Table 3). Additionally, we managed to find whether there were predictors for downgrading and consequently no significant factor was found in regression analysis. The nomogram was constructed based on four predictors of multivariable analysis. The AUC of GPC, PSA, PI-RADS score and cT-stage were 0.636, 0.589, 0.642 and 0.579 respectively. The AUC of GSU model was 0.735, which showed good performance of discrimination (Figs. 2, 3).

Our internally validated calibration plot demonstrated virtually ideal predictions that the rate of predicted probabilities closely paralleled the observed rate (nearly corresponded to the 45° line) with bias-corrected C-index of 0.726 (Fig. 4). Our model predicting GSU might underestimate the risk at the probability range of 53–64% and below 41%. The overestimate risk was at the range of 42–52% and above 64%.

Discussion

A systematic review including 14,839 patients reported that concordance rate was 63%, while overall upgrading was found in 30% [1]. Based on British Association

Table 3 Predictors of Gleason sum upgrading from biopsy to RP

Variables	Univariable analysis		Multivariable analysis	
	OR (95% CI)	*P* value	OR (95% CI)	*P* value
Age at biopsy	0.98(0.94–1.03)	0.494	–	–
MS, presence vs absence	1.65 (0.83–3.28)	0.152	–	–
BMI	1.05 (0.95–1.15)	0.343	–	–
Interval from biopsy to RP	1.00(0.99–1.00)	0.253	–	–
PV	1.00(0.99–1.01)	0.713	–	–
Pre-biopsy PSA level	1.01(1.00–1.02)	0.009	1.02(1.00–1.03)	0.007
Pre-biopsy PSAD	1.42(1.01–2.01)	0.044	0.41(0.14–1.12)	0.522
Clinical T-stage	–	–	–	–
T1c-2a	1.00(Reference)	-	1.00(Reference)	–
T2b-2c	3.21(1.64–6.26)	0.001	4.13(1.82–7.24)	0.042
T3a-3b	1.67(0.67–4.15)	0.272	2.39(0.86–4.85)	0.122
PI-RADS score 4–5 versus 2–3	5.57(2.53–12.27)	< 0.001	4.81(2.07–11.18)	< 0.001
Cores obtained	–	–	–	–
12-23	1.00(Reference)	–	–	–
24	0.63(0.23–1.78)	0.385	–	–
25–30	0.42(0.10–1.72)	0.231	–	–
FPC	1.24(0.37–4.14)	0.731	–	–
GPC	5.34(1.98–14.39)	0.001	3.09(1.05–9.07)	0.040
Experience in biopsy, senior versus junior	1.04(0.59–1.85)	0.886	–	–

OR odds ratio, *CI* confidence interval, *MS* metabolic syndrome, *RP* radical prostatectomy, *BMI* body mass index, *PV* prostate volume, *PSA* prostate specific antigen, *PSAD* PSA density, *PI-RADS* Prostate Imaging Reporting and Data System, *FPC* fraction of positive cores, *GPC* the greatest percentage of cancer

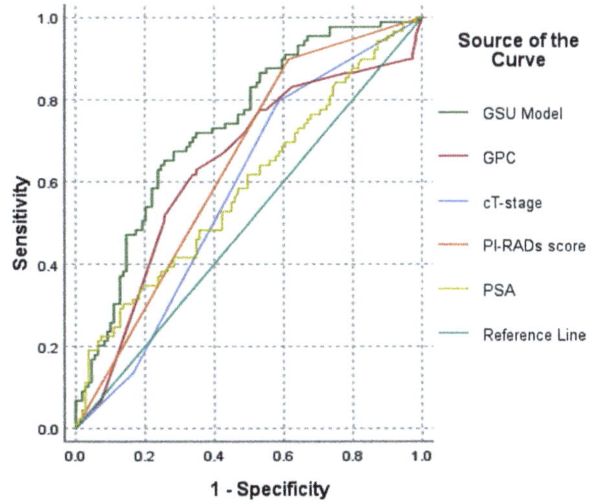

Fig. 2 ROC of Gleason sum upgrading model and independent predictors. *GSU* Gleason sum upgrading, *GPC* the greatest percentage of cancer, *PSA* prostate specific antigen, *PI-RADS* Prostate Imaging Reporting and Data System

of Urological Surgeons (BAUS) Radical Prostatectomy Registry database, a study of 17,598 patients [10] demonstrated that concordance rate was 58.9%, whilst upgrading rate was 25.5%. Our study showed that the concordance rate was 41.4%, while GSU was 44.4%. Concordance rates and upgrading rates vary from study to study which might be attributed to reasons as follows: different demographic characteristics of study cohorts, sampling error of biopsy approach, different biopsy techniques, variability of pathologic assignment and non-uniform interpretation of pathology reports.

PSA is a widely used indicator for both risk stratification and prognosis evaluation, and it also plays a role in predicting Gleason sum upgrading [11–19]. High level of serum PSA was partially attributed to large prostate glands in elder patients. However, Davis et al. [18] found that PSA was still an independent predictor after adjusting for PV. In the current study, we found that PSA was also predictive and increasing PSA level was strongly correlated with GSU. For every increasing PSA unit, there was a 2% increased risk of upgrading. Hence, urologists

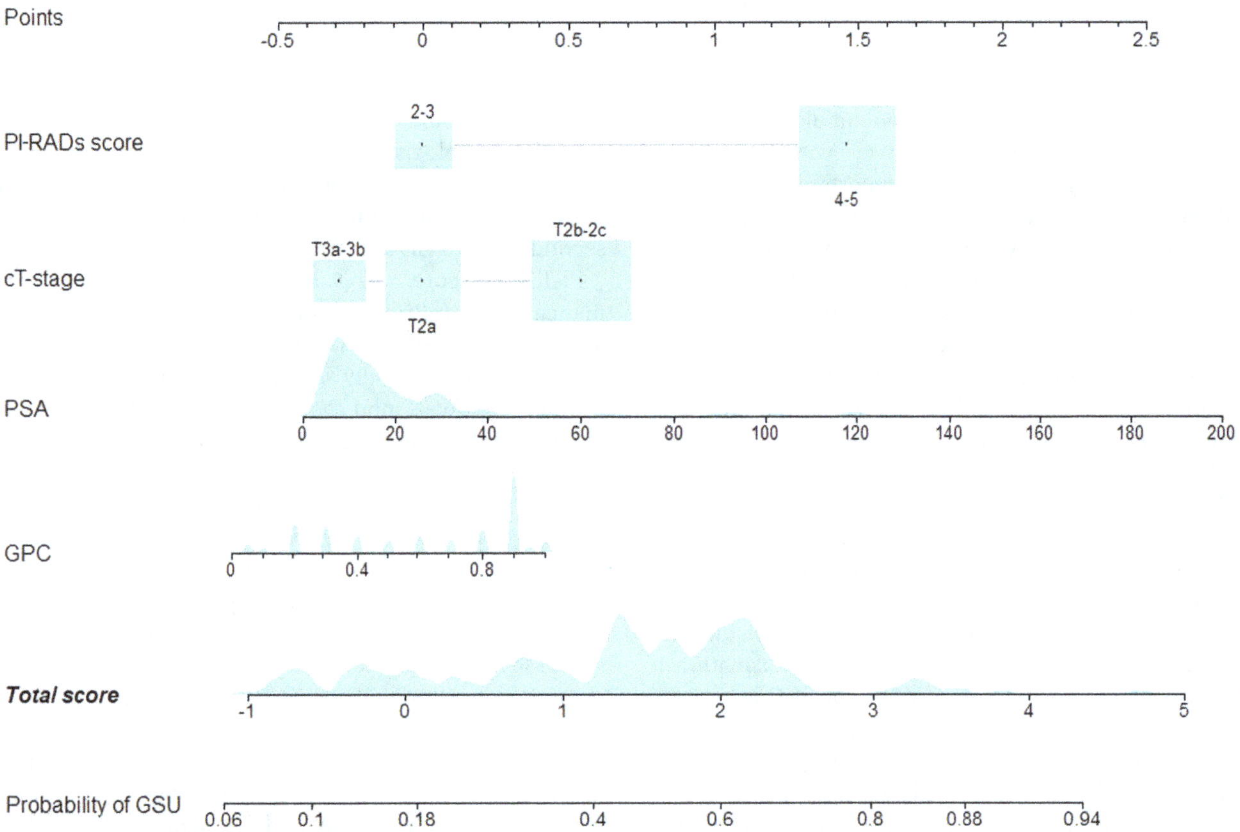

Fig. 3 Nomogram of predicting the probability of Gleason sum upgrading. To obtain the predicted probability of GSU, locate each variable of one patient at corresponding axis. Draw a vertical line to the "Points" axis to determine how many points are attributed for each variables. Sum the points of all variables. Locate the sum point on the "Total Points" line to determine the individual probability of GSU on the "Probability of GSU" line. *GSU* Gleason sum upgrading, *GPC* the greatest percentage of cancer, *PSA* prostate specific antigen, *PI-RADS* Prostate Imaging Reporting and Data System

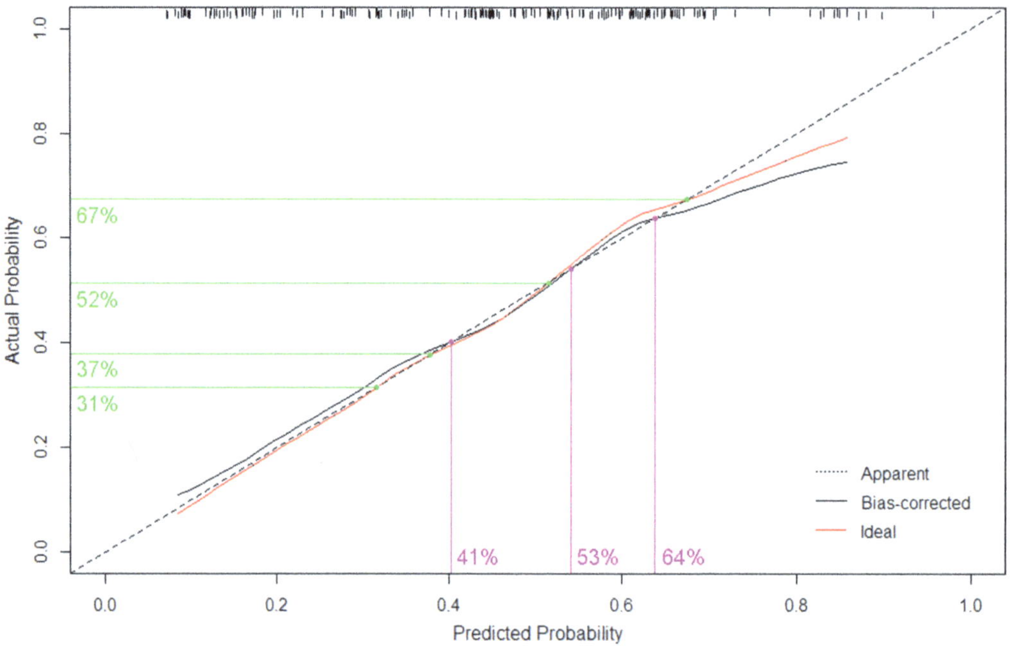

Fig. 4 Calibration curve of the Gleason sum upgrading model. The nomogram-predicted probabilities are comparable to the actual probabilities of GSU. Perfect prediction would correspond to a slope of 1 (diagonal 45° broken line). The solid red line indicates the original predictive ability. The solid black line indicates the bootstrap-corrected model performance

should raise concern about the cumulative effect in patients with high level of PSA.

Clinical T-stage is another important preoperative indicator as for guiding treatment decisions and evaluating prognosis, and it was also found to be predictive of upgrading in several studies [11, 12, 15–17]. Advanced T-stage is in general correlated with large tumor volume and sampling error trends to appear when biopsies are performed in patients with large tumor focus. However, T_2 tumors were associated with more upgrading compared to T_3 tumors in the study of Chun et al. [12], the finding of which was consistent with the current study. PCa occurs mainly in the PZ which is compressed by hyperplastic TZ tissue in elder patients. Under this circumstance, small tumor volume and tumor extracapsular extension might coexist. Additionally, diagnostic accuracy of predicting RP Gleason sum varied in different prostate zones which might give another explanation to this phenomenon [20]. However, the correlation between GSU and clinical T-stage needs further investigations.

GPC which was commonly used by pathologists to determine TTE was reported to be correlated with upgrading [13, 18, 19, 21]. In the current study, this pathologic variable was an independent predictor of GSU. High maximum percentage of cancer reflects larger tumor volume which might increase sampling error. Under this circumstance, high-grade masses in large tumor foci would be less detected. Even if small GPC provides pathologists with inadequate information which could increase the possibilities of incorrect scoring, it seems that impacts on the assignment of primary and secondary patterns are slight.

PI-RADS score was validated to have good performance for both PCa detection and foci localization [22]. The utilization of mpMRI was confirmed the value of differentiating clinically significant PCa from indolent tumors [23]. We found that PI-RADS score was also an independent predictor of GSU, which is consistent with the findings of Song et al. [24]. Gleason sum were more likely to be upgraded among patients with PI-RADS 4–5 (54.4% compared with 17.6% for PI-RADS 2–3). High-grade patterns with MRI manifestation of PI-RADS 4–5 which are not identified in biopsy cores result in GSU. Gondo et al. [25] found that Gleason sum downgrading was associated with negative MRI findings, which demonstrated that mpMRI might have favorable diagnostic performance in predicting Gleason sum change.

We successfully developed and validated a model predicting Gleason sum upgrading from biopsy to RP utilizing clinical variables (PSA and T-stage) combined with imaging variable (PI-RADS) and pathological variable (GPC). Our model is 73.5% accurate and its predictions closely approximate the observed rate. Our study was not the first one to construct models or nomograms.

Chun et al. [12] built a model including PSA, clinical stage and biopsy Gleason score and yielded accuracy of 0.804 based on a large scale of population. The number of biopsy cores ranged from 6 to 12 in their study. However, excluding the number of cores from multivariable analysis would affect the stability of their model. Moussa et al. [16] incorporated manifold variables especially pathologic parameters into their model. However, including statistically insignificant variables leaded to their model becoming unstable. Therefore, their model yielded a C-index of 0.68. Both Kulkarni et al. [14] and Capitanio et al. [26] have built models for patients with Gleason sum 6, which yielded accuracy of 0.71 and 0.66 respectively. These two models fit low-risk population well, however, which could not represent the real situation of overall GSU. Both Wang et al. [17] and He et al. [27] developed models based on Chinese population. The model of Wang et al. [17] included only PSA, clinical stage and biopsy Gleason score which showed favorable statistical performance with C-index of 0.795. Wang et al. also externally validated Chun's model in the set of Chinese population and the results showed poor concordance between the predicted and observed probabilities. What Wang et al. have found demonstrated that new models need to be constructed to fit specific population and should be further validated with large patient cohorts. He et al. [27] built models predicting upgrading for both overall patients and patients with GS=6. Two models including variables such as BMI and FPC showed good performance and yielded the AUC of 0.753 and 0.727 respectively. Our model incorporated not only basic clinical features such as PSA and clinical stage, but also pathologic and imaging parameters, which is more suitable for clinical practice. Including independent predictors leaded to our model becoming more stable and the predicted probabilities closely approximated to the actual risk in calibration plot. When probabilities ranged from 53 to 64% and below 41%, underestimation of the risk occurred, while overestimation of risk ranged from 42 to 52% and above 64%.

According to our present study, several clinical implications might be taken into consideration. Patients who have low-risk PCa but high probabilities of GSU could consider curative therapies instead of active surveillance in case of delayed treatment. For these patients who are under active surveillance could adhere to more active follow-up policies. On the contrary, patients with low probabilities of GSU who are unwilling to receive aggressive treatment or have contraindications of operation or radiotherapy are more confidence to undergo the active surveillance. According to the probabilities of GSU, extended periods of close clinical follow-up could be warranted. Moreover, patients might benefit from resection of neurovascular bundle or lymph node dissection who are at high risk of GSU. Similarly, the hormonal therapy as ancillary treatment to radiotherapy might be considered in patients with high probabilities of GSU. These clinical recommendations might give urologists more confidence in clinical decision-making. New model might provide urologists not only precise and comprehensive assessment of PCa risk but also personalized and optimal treatment options for PCa patients. However, there is still far to go before robust evidence emerges.

There are limitations of the present study. First of all, information from database included potential inaccuracy due to the retrospective nature. Secondly, our study was lack of large population because of our strict indications to perform RP and monocentric design. Thus, we need further prospective large-scale studies with selective patients for validation. Thirdly, external validation for our model would be furtherly necessitated, even if our model served as a statistically well-performed tool. Fourthly, only patients undergone RP were selected into cohort which might not represent the reality. Finally, the accuracy of our model could potentially be improved by integrating findings of genetic and molecular biomarker analysis.

Conclusions

Utilization of basic clinical variables (PSA and T-stage) combined with imaging variable (PI-RADS) and pathological variable (GPC) could improve performance in predicting actual probabilities of GSU in the 24-core biopsy scheme. Our nomogram could help to assess the true risk and make optimal treatment decisions for PCa patients. However, our nomogram needs to be tested for the performance in an external dataset or other study cohorts.

Abbreviations

GSU: Gleason sum upgrading; PCa: Prostate cancer; RP: Radical prostatectomy; MS: Metabolic syndrome; BMI: Body mass index; PV: Prostate volume; PSA: Prostate specific antigen; PSAD: PSA density; PI-RADS: Prostate Imaging Reporting and Data System; mpMRI: Multiparametric magnetic resonance imaging; GSU: Gleason sum upgrade; GPC: Greatest percentage of cancer; FPC: Fraction of positive cores; TTE: Tissue tumor extent; ROC: Receiver operating curve; AUC: Area under the curve.

Acknowledgements

Not applicable.

Authors' contributions

XW was a major contributor in conception and writing the manuscript. XW and YZ analyzed and interpreted the patient data. ZJ and FZ drafted and supervised the work and PY and YT substantively revised it. All authors read and approved the final manuscript and have agreed both to be personally accountable for the author's own contributions and to ensure that questions related to the accuracy or integrity of any part of the work, even ones in which the author was not personally involved, are appropriately investigated, resolved, and the resolution documented in the literature. All authors read and approved the final manuscript.

Competing interests

The authors declare that they have no competing interests.

References

1. Cohen MS, Hanley RS, Kurteva T, et al. Comparing the Gleason prostate biopsy and Gleason prostatectomy grading system: the Lahey Clinic Medical Center experience and an international meta-analysis. Eur Urol. 2008;54:371–81.
2. Thomsen FB, Brasso K, Klotz LH, et al. Active surveillance for clinically localized prostate cancer–a systematic review. J Surg Oncol. 2014;109:830–5.
3. Briganti A, Larcher A, Abdollah F, et al. Updated nomogram predicting lymph node invasion in patients with prostate cancer undergoing extended pelvic lymph node dissection: the essential importance of percentage of positive cores. Eur Urol. 2012;61:480–7.
4. D'Amico AV, Chen MH, Renshaw AA, et al. Androgen suppression and radiation vs radiation alone for prostate cancer: a randomized trial. JAMA. 2008;299:289–95.
5. Bakavicius A, Drevinskaite M, Daniunaite K, et al. The impact of prostate cancer upgrading and upstaging on biochemical recurrence and cancer-specific survival. Medicina (Kaunas). 2020;56:61.
6. Kovac E, Vertosick EA, Sjoberg DD, et al. Effects of pathological upstaging or upgrading on metastasis and cancer-specific mortality in men with clinical low-risk prostate cancer. BJU Int. 2018;122:1003–9.
7. Barentsz JO, Weinreb JC, Verma S, et al. Synopsis of the PI-RADS v2 guidelines for multiparametric prostate magnetic resonance imaging and recommendations for use. Eur Urol. 2016;69:41–9.
8. Varma M, Narahari K, Mason M, et al. Contemporary prostate biopsy reporting: insights from a survey of clinicians' use of pathology data. J Clin Pathol. 2018;71:874–8.
9. Brimo F, Vollmer RT, Corcos J, et al. Prognostic value of various morphometric measurements of tumour extent in prostate needle core tissue. Histopathology. 2008;53:177–83.
10. Bullock N, Simpkin A, Fowler S, et al. Pathological upgrading in prostate cancer treated with surgery in the United Kingdom: trends and risk factors from the British Association of Urological Surgeons Radical Prostatectomy Registry. BMC Urol. 2019;19:94.
11. Budaus L, Graefen M, Salomon G, et al. The novel nomogram of Gleason sum upgrade: possible application for the eligible criteria of low dose rate brachytherapy. Int J Urol. 2010;17:862–8.
12. Chun FK, Steuber T, Erbersdobler A, et al. Development and internal validation of a nomogram predicting the probability of prostate cancer Gleason sum upgrading between biopsy and radical prostatectomy pathology. Eur Urol. 2006;49:820–6.
13. Epstein JI, Feng Z, Trock BJ, et al. Upgrading and downgrading of prostate cancer from biopsy to radical prostatectomy: incidence and predictive factors using the modified Gleason grading system and factoring in tertiary grades. Eur Urol. 2012;61:1019–24.
14. Kulkarni GS, Lockwood G, Evans A, et al. Clinical predictors of Gleason score upgrading: implications for patients considering watchful waiting, active surveillance, or brachytherapy. Cancer. 2007;109:2432–8.
15. Kvale R, Moller B, Wahlqvist R, et al. Concordance between Gleason scores of needle biopsies and radical prostatectomy specimens: a population-based study. BJU Int. 2009;103:1647–54.
16. Moussa AS, Kattan MW, Berglund R, et al. A nomogram for predicting upgrading in patients with low- and intermediate-grade prostate cancer in the era of extended prostate sampling. BJU Int. 2010;105:352–8.
17. Wang JY, Zhu Y, Wang CF, et al. A nomogram to predict Gleason sum upgrading of clinically diagnosed localized prostate cancer among Chinese patients. Chin J Cancer. 2014;33:241–8.
18. Davies JD, Aghazadeh MA, Phillips S, et al. Prostate size as a predictor of Gleason score upgrading in patients with low risk prostate cancer. J Urol. 2011;186:2221–7.
19. Gofrit ON, Zorn KC, Taxy JB, et al. Predicting the risk of patients with biopsy Gleason score 6 to harbor a higher grade cancer. J Urol. 2007;178:1925–8.
20. Huo AS, Hossack T, Symons JL, et al. Accuracy of primary systematic template guided transperineal biopsy of the prostate for locating prostate cancer: a comparison with radical prostatectomy specimens. J Urol. 2012;187:2044–9.
21. Truong M, Slezak JA, Lin CP, et al. Development and multi-institutional validation of an upgrading risk tool for Gleason 6 prostate cancer. Cancer. 2013;119:3992–4002.
22. Le JD, Tan N, Shkolyar E, et al. Multifocality and prostate cancer detection by multiparametric magnetic resonance imaging: correlation with whole-mount histopathology. Eur Urol. 2015;67:569–76.
23. Park SY, Jung DC, Oh YT, et al. Prostate cancer: PI-RADS version 2 helps preoperatively predict clinically significant cancers. Radiology. 2016;280:108–16.
24. Song W, Bang SH, Jeon HG, et al. Role of PI-RADS version 2 for prediction of upgrading in biopsy-proven prostate cancer with Gleason score 6. Clin Genitourin Cancer. 2018;16:281–7.
25. Gondo T, Hricak H, Sala E, et al. Multiparametric 3T MRI for the prediction of pathological downgrading after radical prostatectomy in patients with biopsy-proven Gleason score 3 + 4 prostate cancer. Eur Radiol. 2014;24:3161–70.
26. Capitanio U, Karakiewicz PI, Valiquette L, et al. Biopsy core number represents one of foremost predictors of clinically significant gleason sum upgrading in patients with low-risk prostate cancer. Urology. 2009;73:1087–91.
27. He B, Chen R, Gao X, et al. Nomograms for predicting Gleason upgrading in a contemporary Chinese cohort receiving radical prostatectomy after extended prostate biopsy: development and internal validation. Oncotarget. 2016;7:17275–85.

24

Surgical benchmarks, mid-term oncological outcomes and impact of surgical team composition on simultaneous enbloc robot-assisted radical cystectomy and nephroureterectomy

Stephan Buse[1,2*†], Assen Alexandrov[3†], Elio Mazzone[4,5], Alexandre Mottrie[6,7] and Axel Haferkamp[2]

Abstract

Background: Simultaneous urothelial cancer manifestation in the lower and upper urinary tract affects approximately 2% of patients. Data on the surgical benchmarks and mid-term oncological outcomes of enbloc robot-assisted radical cystectomy and nephro-ureterectomy are scarce.

Methods: After written informed consent was obtained, we prospectively enrolled consecutive patients undergoing enbloc radical cystectomy and nephro-ureterectomy with robotic assistance from the DaVinci Si-HD® system in a prospective institutional database and collected surgical benchmarks and oncological outcomes. Furthermore, as one console surgeon conducted all the procedures, whereas the team providing bedside assistance was composed ad hoc, we assessed the impact of this approach on the operative duration.

Results: Nineteen patients (9 women), with a mean age of 73 (SD: 7.5) years, underwent simultaneous enbloc robot-assisted radical cystectomy and nephro-ureterectomy. There were no cases of conversion to open surgery. In the postoperative period, we registered 2 Clavien-Dindo class 2 complications (transfusions) and 1 Clavien-Dindo class 3b complication (port hernia). After a median follow-up of 23 months, there were 3 cases of mortality and 1 case of metachronous urothelial cancer (contralateral kidney).The total operative duration did not decrease with increasing experience ($r=0.174$, $p=0.534$). In contrast, there was a significant, inverse, strong correlation between the console time relative to the total operative duration and the number of conducted procedures after adjusting for the degree of adhesions and the type of urinary diversion($r=-0.593$, $p=0.02$).

Conclusions: These data suggest that en bloc simultaneous robot-assisted radical cystectomy and nephro-ureterectomy can be safely conducted with satisfactory mid-term oncological outcomes. With increasing experience, improved performance was detectable for the console surgeon but not in terms of the total operative duration.

*Correspondence: stephan.buse@krupp-krankenhaus.de; stephan.buse@gmx.ch

†Shared first authorship: Stephan Buse and Assen Alexandrov

[1] Department of Urology, Alfried Krupp Krankenhaus, Hellweg 100, 45276 Essen, Germany

Simulation training of all team members for highly complex procedures might be a suitable approach for improving team performance.

Trial registration: Not applicable.

Keywords: Minimally invasive surgery, Radical cystectomy, Radical nephroureterectomy

Background

The guideline-adherent treatment of bladder and upper urinary tract malignancies implies radical cystectomy and nephroureterectomy [1, 2]. While metachronous urothelial cancer in the lower and upper urinary tract has been reported in a relevant proportion of patients initially diagnosed with urothelial cancer in the upper urinary tract [3] and to a lesser extent in patients initially diagnosed with urothelial cancer in the bladder [4], simultaneous urothelial cancer manifestation in the lower and upper urinary tract affects 2% of patients [5]. Combined lower and upper urinary tract resection is warranted in these patients. While data describing the surgical benchmarks of simultaneous enbloc robot-assisted radical cystectomy and nephro-ureterectomy [6–11] have been reported, information on mid-term oncological outcomes is lacking.

Without the proper training of the whole surgical team (not only console surgeons), the operative duration will unavoidably be prolonged, particularly for complex procedures. A prolonged operative duration has been associated with an increased incidence of postoperative complications in laparoscopic and robotic procedures [12, 13]. In addition, a predictable operative duration is crucial for the efficient scheduling of operating room utilization, as both under- and overscheduling have major economic impacts. Among other factors, the team composition plays a relevant role in the operative duration beyond the learning curve [14–18]. To date, the impact of the surgical team composition on the duration of enbloc robot-assisted radical cystectomy and nephro-ureterectomy, a complex, multistep procedure, has not been explored.

The aims of this manuscript were as follows: (1) to report the surgical benchmarks and postoperative complications; (2) to report mid-term oncological outcomes of simultaneous enbloc robot-assisted radical cystectomy and nephro-ureterectomy at a single centre; and (3) to assess the impact of the team composition (console surgeon vs patient-side surgeon) on the duration of this procedure.

Methods

Patient population and study design

After written informed consent was obtained, we enrolled 19 consecutive patients undergoing simultaneous enbloc robot-assisted radical cystectomy and nephro-ureterectomy between 2010 and 2019 at Alfried Krupp Hospital, Essen, Germany, in a prospective institutional database; routine clinical data, including surgical benchmarks, postoperative complications and oncological outcomes of patients on follow-up at our institution, were prospectively entered into the institutional database. This was a retrospective analysis of the data collected in the institutional database. The need for ethics approval for the retrospective analysis of routine clinical data was waived by the local ethics board (Ethik-Kommission, Ärztekammer Nordrhein).

Surgical team and technique

A single, experienced (over 3000 robot-assisted procedures) console surgeon (SB) performed all procedures. Patient-side surgical assistance was provided by various urology residents based on availability (ad hoc composition). All residents were exposed daily to routine robotic surgery. The surgical nurse team was also assigned ad hoc from a dedicated robotic surgery team of 5 nurses.

We performed all procedures with robotic assistance from the DaVinci Si-HD® system (Intuitive Surgical, Inc., Sunnyvale, US), a four-arm robotic system. We have previously described in detail our technique for simultaneous enbloc robot-assisted radical cystectomy and nephro-ureterectomy [6]. Briefly, with the patient in a 60-degree flank position, we introduced 5 ports for transperitoneal nephro-ureterectomy preparation and prepared the ureter and the renal hilum. Next, the renal vessels were clipped, and the kidney was completely mobilized while maintaining ureter continuity. Cystectomy was then completed with the patient in a supine position using 5 ports, i.e., the system had to be undocked/redocked, and new ports had to be inserted. The patient was positioned in a Trendelenburg position for mobilization and preparation of the seminal vesicles, the base of the prostate and the bladder or the uterus, the ovaries and the bladder. The enbloc specimen (kidney, ureter, bladder, prostate or uterus/ovaries) was removed using a specimen bag through expansion to 6–8 cm of the previous port incision in the lower abdomen in men or transvaginally in women. After reduction of the Trendelenburg position to a tilt of 10 degrees, we performed urinary diversion using an ileal conduit or ureterocutaneostomy (UCST).

The video in the online supplements (Additional file 1) shows the surgical technique step by step and provides a video abstract of the results.

UCST was conducted in palliative situations, in patients with severe comorbidities either to limit the operative duration or to avoid bowel resection in patients at high risk for anastomotic complications, or based on patient-specific considerations [6] after a detailed discussion of the benefits and risks with the individual patients prior to surgery.

Endpoints and data collection

Surgical benchmarks of interest included the total operative duration (incision to skin suture) and console time, blood loss, surgical margins, conversion to open surgery, and postoperative complications ≥ class 2 according to the Clavien-Dindo classification [19]. The endpoints for mid-term outcomes, defined as a follow-up duration > = 1 year [20], were all-cause death and cancer recurrence.

Preoperatively, we collected data on age, body mass index (BMI), American Society of Anesthesiologists (ASA) classification, and tumour stage. The degree of intrabdominal adhesions was extracted from the surgical reports, where it was recorded as "none", "minor to moderate" or "extensive" by the surgeon. The institutional convention is to describe the degree of adhesions in the surgical report as "minor to moderate" if adhesiolysis required less than 30 min or as "extensive" if adhesiolysis required more than 30 min.

Statistical analysis

We described frequency data as counts and percentages and continuous data as the median (interquartile range Q1–Q3) or the mean (standard deviation, SD), as appropriate. Surgical benchmarks, postoperative complications, and mid-term oncological outcomes are reported descriptively.

To assess the impact of the experience of the console surgeon vs that of the patient-side team, we used a partial correlation to quantify the relationship between each console and non-console time by the number of conducted simultaneous enbloc robot-assisted radical cystectomy and nephro-ureterectomy (main independent variable) procedures, controlling by the degree of intraperitoneal adhesions and the type of urinary diversion (UCST vs ileal conduit) as covariables.The console and non-console times are both expressed as percentages of the total operative duration. The limited number of cases prevented the entry of additional covariables, e.g., BMI. SPSS 25 was used for all analyses.

Results

Surgical benchmarks and postoperative complications

Nineteen patients (9 women), with a mean age of 73 (SD: 7.5) years and a mean BMI of 27.5 (SD: 5), underwent simultaneous enbloc robot-assisted radical cystectomy and nephroureterectomy. The ASA class was ≥ 3 in 13 patients (68.4%), i.e., indicating a major comorbidity burden. Ten (52.6%) patients had a history of previous abdominal procedures: 5 (26.3%) patients presented minor to moderate intraperitoneal adhesions, and 5 (26.3%) patients presented extensive intraperitoneal adhesions. The bladder tumour stage was pTa/pTis, pT1, and pT2a and prostate pT4a in one patient each, pT3a/b in 6 (31.6%) patients, and pT4a/b in 9 (47.4%) patients. Upper urinary tract tumours consisted of 1 renal oncocytoma and urothelial cancer pTa in 3, pT1 in one, and pT3 in 2 patients. In 12 patients, the indication for the combined procedure was a functionless kidney. Urinary diversion consisted of an ileal conduit in 5 patients and of a UCST in 14 patients in the presence of severe comorbidities, advanced age, or a palliative approach.

Overall, surgery lasted 324 min (SD: 65), with 208 min (SD: 57) of console time. The median estimated blood loss was 220 mL (Q1–Q3: 200–250). There were no cases of conversion to open surgery. The bladder resection margins were positive in 3 patients (1 pT4a and 2 pT4b), and the ureteral resection margins were positive in 1 patient (pT3).

In the postoperative period, 2 patients required transfusion (Clavien-Dindo class 2) and one patient suffered from a port hernia (Clavien-Dindo class 3b).

Mid-term oncological outcomes

During a median follow-up of 23 months (IQR: 9–42), 1 patient developed metachronous urothelial cancer (contralateral kidney) at 24 months, 1 patient died at 1 month from pulmonary embolism, and 2 patients died from tumour progression, one at 4 and one at 62 months.

At the mid-term, the median estimated creatinine clearance was 44 mL/min (IQR: 36–50), which did not significantly differ from the preoperative clearance (median: 45 mL/min, IQR: 32–62).

Impact of team composition on operative duration

UCST surgery lasted a mean of 310 min (SD: 68), with a console duration of 204 min (SD: 58). Surgery in patients receiving ileal conduit lasted a mean of 355 min (SD: 69), with a mean console duration of 217 min (SD: 59). The total operative duration did not change with the progression of surgical experience ($r = 0.174$, $p = 0.534$). On average, the console duration represented 65% (SD:10) of the total operative duration in UCST patients and 60%

(SD 10%) in ileal conduit patients. In contrast to the total duration, there was a significant, inverse, strong correlation between the console time relative to the total operative duration and surgical experience ($r = -0.593$, $p = 0.02$) after controlling for the degree of adhesions and the type of urinary diversion. Blood loss was not correlated with the progression of surgical experience (Spearman r: -0.150, $p = 0.593$). The low number of complications prevented any assessment in this regard.

Discussion

This series of consecutive patients undergoing enbloc robot-assisted radical cystectomy and nephro-ureterectomy suggests that this complex procedure can be conducted with an acceptable operative duration and limited blood loss by an experienced robotic surgeon. Furthermore, the procedure resulted in a limited postoperative complication rate. The mid-term oncological outcomes were in line with the survival estimates for urothelial bladder cancer [21, 22]. As such, these findings support the findings from previous reports [6–11] regarding surgical safety while adding information in terms of mid-term oncological outcomes.

With regard to the team composition, the data suggested a steep improvement in console surgeon performance (expressed as the console duration) with the progression of surgical experience after taking into account the degree of abdominal adhesions. This is in line with previous data reporting that experienced console surgeons have a steep learning curve even for technically demanding procedures, e.g., 20–30 cases for radical cystectomy [23, 24]. As such, these data seem to expand the applicability of a steep learning curve in experienced surgeons to include very rarely performed procedures.

In contrast to the console duration, the total operative duration did not decrease with increasing centre experience with this specific procedure, even after taking into account the degree of adhesions. This fact suggests that while the console surgeon improved his performance, for the patient-side part of the procedure, i.e., positioning, pneumoperitoneum, port insertion, docking and undocking, there was stagnation. We interpret this observation as the result of an ad hoc composition of the surgical team (patient-side surgeon and nurses). Indeed, while the same console surgeon performed all procedures, the patient-side surgeon and surgical nurses were assigned ad hoc from a pool of urology residents and specialized robotic surgical nurses. While exposed daily to routine robot-assisted procedures, such as prostatectomy, the rare confrontation of the team composed ad hoc with this infrequent procedure might have, in our interpretation, prevented increases in the efficiency of the surgical team as a whole and therefore might have negatively affected the total operative duration. Because the total operative duration is a crucial variable for resource utilization and for patient outcomes [12, 13], this issue is of clinical relevance. Simulation training research [25–32] often focuses on the console surgeon, and only recently have virtual simulators integrating the console surgeon and bedside assistants become available. However, considering that a non-negligible part of the operative duration (on average, approximately 1/3 in this cohort) seems to be driven by the patient-side steps of the procedure, training including positioning and port placement/replacement and docking/undocking specific to the procedure [27] might be helpful to improve performance in terms of the total operative duration.

Previous studies have addressed the impact of the team composition regarding the experience of the patient-side assistant [33–35] for different robot-assisted urological procedures. After adjusting for prostate size, the seniority of the bedside assistant did not affect the total operative duration in a retrospective cohort of 106 patients undergoing robot-assisted prostatectomy [33]. We consider that the divergence to our findings is the result of a very different type of procedure: on the one hand, RALP is acommon and routine intervention; on the other hand, en bloc cystectomy and nephro-ureterectomy is a rarely performed, extensive procedure requiring different patient positions, port locations and repeated docking/undocking. Furthermore, the classification of residency by year used in that study might not optimally reflect the actual proficiency level of residents in procedural assistance. In the context of a more complex routine procedure, such as robot-assisted partial nephrectomy, there was a significant association [34] or a strong trend ($p = 0.051$) [35] for an impact of the level of experience of the bedside assistant on the operative duration. Other perioperative benchmarks, e.g., blood loss, warm ischaemia time, and surgical margin status, did not differ [35].

Limitations

At our centre, we conduct over 400 robot-assisted procedures per year; however, since 2010, a limited number of patients have required simultaneous enbloc robot-assisted radical cystectomy and nephro-ureterectomy. As such, the main limitation of this study is the limited sample size. However, due to the low prevalence of simultaneous urothelial cancer [5], this might reflect the clinical reality even for high-volume centres. The limited sample size prevented adjustment for multiple potentially relevant variables (e.g., T-stage, BMI), and we limited adjustment to the degree of adhesions and the type of urinary diversion. The small sample size also resulted in high variability. We addressed this issue by using relative (percentage of the total operative duration) rather than absolute console and non-console durations. Furthermore, during the study period, the console surgeon had performed a large number of other robot-assisted procedures that may have influenced the reported outcomes on console time improvement; however, this was also the case for the bedside assistants, so this fact is first, reflective of the clinical reality and second, was not differential, i.e., it applied to all members of the surgical team.

Conclusions

These data suggest that en bloc simultaneous robot-assisted radical cystectomy and nephro-ureterectomy can be safely conducted with satisfactory mid-term oncological outcomes. With increasing experience, improved performance was detectable for the console surgeon but not in terms of the total operative duration. Simulation training of all team members for highly complex procedures might be a suitable approach for improving team performance.

Abbreviations

ASA: American society of anesthesiologists; BMI: Body mass index; Q1-Q3: Interquartile range; SD: Standard deviation; UCST: Ureterocutaneostomy.

Acknowledgements

Not applicable.

Authors' contributions

SB: Conception and design of the work; data acquisition; data analysis; data interpretation; manuscript drafting; approval of the final version (and any substantially modified version that involves the author's contribution to the study); and agreement both to be personally accountable for the author's own contributions and to ensure that questions related to the accuracy or integrity of any part of the work, even those in which the author was not personally involved, are appropriately investigated and resolved, with the resolution documented in the literature. AA: Data acquisition; data interpretation; substantial revision and approval of the final version (and any substantially modified version that involves the author's contribution to the study); and agreement both to be personally accountable for the author's own contributions and to ensure that questions related to the accuracy or integrity of any part of the work, even those in which the author was not personally involved, are appropriately investigated and resolved, with the resolution documented in the literature. EM: Substantial revision and approval of the final version (and any substantially modified version that involves the author's contribution to the study); and agreement both to be personally accountable for the author's own contributions and to ensure that questions related to the accuracy or integrity of any part of the work, even those in which the author was not personally involved, are appropriately investigated and resolved, with the resolution documented in the literature. AM: Substantial revision and approval of the final version (and any substantially modified version that involves the author's contribution to the study); and agreement both to be personally accountable for the author's own contributions and to ensure that questions related to the accuracy or integrity of any part of the work, even those in which the author was not personally involved, are appropriately investigated and resolved, with the resolution documented in the literature. AH: Substantial revision and approval of the final version (and any substantially modified version that involves the author's contribution to the study); and agreement both to be personally accountable for the author's own contributions and to ensure that questions related to the accuracy or integrity of any part of the work, even those in which the author was not personally involved, are appropriately investigated and resolved, with the resolution documented in the literature.

Competing interests

Stephan Buse acts as a proctor for the DaVinci Si-HD® system, Intuitive Surgical Inc., Sunnyvale, US. All other authors do not report any competing interests.

Author details

[1]Department of Urology, Alfried Krupp Krankenhaus, Hellweg 100, 45276 Essen, Germany. [2]Department of Urology and Paediatric Urology, University Medical Center, Johannes-Gutenberg-University, Mainz, Germany. [3]Landesklinikum Wiener Neustadt, Vienna, Austria. [4]Division of Oncology/Unit of Urology, URI, IRCCS Ospedale San Raffaele, Milan, Italy. [5]Vita-Salute San Raffaele University, Milan, Italy. [6]Department of Urology, OLV Aalst, Aalst, Belgium. [7]ORSI Academy, Melle, Belgium.

References

1. Oosterlinck W, Solsona E, van der Meijden AP, Sylvester R, Bohle A, Rintala E, et al. EAU guidelines on diagnosis and treatment of upper urinary tract transitional cell carcinoma. Eur Urol. 2004;46(2):147–54.
2. Witjes JA, Comperat E, Cowan NC, De Santis M, Gakis G, Lebret T, et al. EAU guidelines on muscle-invasive and metastatic bladder cancer: summary of the 2013 guidelines. Eur Urol. 2014;65(4):778–92.
3. Novara G, De Marco V, Dalpiaz O, Gottardo F, Bouygues V, Galfano A, et al. Independent predictors of metachronous bladder transitional cell carcinoma (TCC) after nephroureterectomy for TCC of the upper urinary tract. BJU Int. 2008;101(11):1368–74.
4. Picozzi S, Ricci C, Gaeta M, Ratti D, Macchi A, Casellato S, et al. Upper urinary tract recurrence following radical cystectomy for bladder cancer: a meta-analysis on 13,185 patients. J Urol. 2012;188(6):2046–54.
5. Palou J, Rodriguez-Rubio F, Huguet J, Segarra J, Ribal MJ, Alcaraz A, et al. Multivariate analysis of clinical parameters of synchronous primary superficial bladder cancer and upper urinary tract tumor. J Urol. 2005;174(3):859–61.
6. Buse S, Hach CE, Alexandrov A, Mager R, Haferkamp A. Simultaneous en-bloc robot-assisted radical cystectomy and nephro-ureterectomy: technique description, outcomes, and literature summary. J Robot Surg. 2016;10(4):315–22.
7. Barros R, Frota R, Stein RJ, Turna B, Gill IS, Desai MM. Simultaneous laparoscopic nephroureterectomy and cystectomy: a preliminary report. Int Braz J Urol. 2008;34(4):413–21.
8. Deng DY, Meng MV, Grossfeld GD, Stoller ML. Simultaneous laparoscopic management of 3 urological malignancies. J Urol. 2002;167(5):2125–6.
9. Ou YC, Yang CR, Yang CK, Cheng CL, Hemal AK. Simultaneous robot-assisted nephroureterectomy and cystectomy in patients with uremia and multifocal urothelial carcinoma. J Endourol Endourol Soc. 2011;25(6):979–84.
10. Perez-Utrilla Perez M, Aguilera Bazan A, Alonso Dorrego JM, Viton Herrero R, Cisneros Ledo J, de la Pena BJ. Simultaneous cystectomy and nephroureterectomy due to synchronous upper urinary tract tumors and invasive bladder cancer: open and laparoscopic approaches. Curr Urol. 2012;6(2):76–81.
11. Peter J, May M, Ahmed AM, Ahmed A, Gilfrich C. Simultaneous robot-assisted laparoscopic cystectomy and laparoscopic nephrectomy: first experience on 3 patients with short-term follow-up. Aktuelle Urol. 2012;43(4):255–61.
12. Catanzarite T, Saha S, Pilecki MA, Kim JY, Milad MP. Longer operative time during benign laparoscopic and robotic hysterectomy is associated with increased 30-day perioperative complications. J Minim Invasive Gynecol. 2015;22(6):1049–58.

8. Deng DY, Meng MV, Grossfeld GD, Stoller ML. Simultaneous laparoscopic management of 3 urological malignancies. J Urol. 2002;167(5):2125–6.
9. Ou YC, Yang CR, Yang CK, Cheng CL, Hemal AK. Simultaneous robot-assisted nephroureterectomy and cystectomy in patients with uremia and multifocal urothelial carcinoma. J Endourol Endourol Soc. 2011;25(6):979–84.
10. Perez-Utrilla Perez M, Aguilera Bazan A, Alonso Dorrego JM, Viton Herrero R, Cisneros Ledo J, de la Pena BJ. Simultaneous cystectomy and nephroureterectomy due to synchronous upper urinary tract tumors and invasive bladder cancer: open and laparoscopic approaches. Curr Urol. 2012;6(2):76–81.
11. Peter J, May M, Ahmed AM, Ahmed A, Gilfrich C. Simultaneous robot-assisted laparoscopic cystectomy and laparoscopic nephrectomy: first experience on 3 patients with short-term follow-up. Aktuelle Urol. 2012;43(4):255–61.
12. Catanzarite T, Saha S, Pilecki MA, Kim JY, Milad MP. Longer operative time during benign laparoscopic and robotic hysterectomy is associated with increased 30-day perioperative complications. J Minim Invasive Gynecol. 2015;22(6):1049–58.
13. Jackson TD, Wannares JJ, Lancaster RT, Rattner DW, Hutter MM. Does speed matter? The impact of operative time on outcome in laparoscopic surgery. Surg Endosc. 2011;25(7):2288–95.
14. Eijkemans MJ, van Houdenhoven M, Nguyen T, Boersma E, Steyerberg EW, Kazemier G. Predicting the unpredictable: a new prediction model for operating room times using individual characteristics and the surgeon's estimate. Anesthesiology. 2010;112(1):41–9.
15. Gillespie BM, Chaboyer W, Fairweather N. Factors that influence the expected length of operation: results of a prospective study. BMJ Qual Saf. 2012;21(1):3–12.
16. Levine WC, Dunn PF. Optimizing operating room scheduling. Anesthesiol Clin. 2015;33(4):697–711.
17. Pike TW, Mushtaq F, Mann RP, Chambers P, Hall G, Tomlinson JE, et al. Operating list composition and surgical performance. Br J Surg. 2018;105(8):1061–9.
18. Stepaniak PS, Heij C, Mannaerts GH, de Quelerij M, de Vries G. Modeling procedure and surgical times for current procedural terminology-anesthesia-surgeon combinations and evaluation in terms of case-duration prediction and operating room efficiency: a multicenter study. Anesth Analg. 2009;109(4):1232–45.
19. Dindo D, Demartines N, Clavien PA. Classification of surgical complications: a new proposal with evaluation in a cohort of 6336 patients and results of a survey. Ann Surg. 2004;240(2):205–13.
20. UK CR. https://www.cancerresearchuk.org/health-professional/cancer-statistics/statistics-by-cancer-type/bladder-cancer/survival London, UK
21. Abdollah F, Gandaglia G, Thuret R, Schmitges J, Tian Z, Jeldres C, et al. Incidence, survival and mortality rates of stage-specific bladder cancer in United States: a trend analysis. Cancer Epidemiol. 2013;37(3):219–25.
22. Zhai M, Tang C, Li M, Chen X, Jin Y, Ying X, et al. Short-term mortality risks among patients with non-metastatic bladder cancer. BMC Cancer. 2020;20(1):1148.
23. Mazzon G, Sridhar A, Busuttil G, Thompson J, Nathan S, Briggs T, et al. Learning curves for robotic surgery: a review of the recent literature. Curr Urol Rep. 2017;18(11):89.
24. Dell'Oglio P, Mazzone E, Lambert E, Vollemaere J, Goossens M, Larcher A, Mottrie A. The effect of surgical experience on perioperative and oncological outcomes after robot-assisted radical cystectomy with intracorporeal urinary diversion: evidence from a referral centre with extensive experience in robotic surgery. EUr Urol Focus. 2020. https://doi.org/10.1016/j.euf.2020.01.016.
25. Bric JD, Lumbard DC, Frelich MJ, Gould JC. Current state of virtual reality simulation in robotic surgery training: a review. Surg Endosc. 2016;30(6):2169–78.
26. Moglia A, Ferrari V, Morelli L, Ferrari M, Mosca F, Cuschieri A. A systematic review of virtual reality simulators for robot-assisted surgery. Eur Urol. 2016;69(6):1065–80.
27. Sridhar AN, Briggs TP, Kelly JD, Nathan S. Training in robotic surgery-an overview. Curr Urol Rep. 2017;18(8):58.
28. Hung AJ, Chen J, Gill IS. Automated performance metrics and machine learning algorithms to measure surgeon performance and anticipate clinical outcomes in robotic surgery. JAMA Surg. 2018;153(8):770–1.
29. Raison N, Ahmed K, Abe T, Brunckhorst O, Novara G, Buffi N, et al. Cognitive training for technical and non-technical skills in robotic surgery: a randomised controlled trial. BJU international. 2018.
30. Bertolo R, Garisto J, Dagenais J, Sagalovich D, Kaouk JH. Single session of robotic human cadaver training: the immediate impact on urology residents in a teaching hospital. J Laparoendosc Adv Surg Tech Part A. 2018.
31. Hertz AM, George EI, Vaccaro CM, Brand TC. Head-to-head comparison of three virtual-reality robotic surgery simulators. JSLS. 2018;22(1).
32. van der Poel H, Brinkman W, van Cleynenbreugel B, Kallidonis P, Stolzenburg JU, Liatsikos E, et al. Training in minimally invasive surgery in urology: european association of urology/international consultation of urological diseases consultation. BJU Int. 2016;117(3):515–30.
33. Abu-Ghanem Y, Erlich T, Ramon J, Dotan Z, Zilberman DE. Robot assisted laparoscopic radical prostatectomy: assistant's seniority has no influence on perioperative course. J Robot Surg. 2017;11(3):305–9.
34. Mitsinikos E, Abdelsayed GA, Bider Z, Kilday PS, Elliott PA, Banapour P, et al. Does the level of assistant experience impact operative outcomes for robot-assisted partial nephrectomy? J Endourol Endourol Soc. 2017;31(1):38–42.
35. Potretzke AM, Knight BA, Brockman JA, Vetter J, Figenshau RS, Bhayani SB, et al. The role of the assistant during robot-assisted partial nephrectomy: does experience matter? J Robot Surg. 2016;10(2):129–34.

25

Buccal mucosal graft urethroplasty for anterior urethral stricture: Experience from a low-income country

Sami Mahjoub Taha Awad[1,2*], Musab Abdalla M. Ahmed[2,3], Yassin Mohamed Osman Abdalla[2], Mohammed El Imam M. Ahmed[1,2] and Mohamed Daffalla-Awadalla Gismalla[1]

Abstract

Background/purpose: This study was conducted to present our experience in urethral mucosal graft urethroplasty to repair urethral stricture, as the first experience in our context.

Methods: This is a prospective hospital-based study that had been designed to review management outcomes of buccal mucosal graft urethroplasty for anterior urethral stricture from January 2017 to January 2019.

Results: The total number of involved patients was 60. The success rate was found to be 90% (n = 54), while 6 (10%) had a recurrence of stricture. Pain and pain combined bleeding from internal suture lines were the only early complication encountered in 50 (83.3%) and 2 (3.3%) patients, respectively. late complications occurred as follows 14 (23.3%) patients had UTI, 12 (20%) had wound infections, 8 (13.3%) had changes in ejaculation, and decrease in intensity of orgasm, and 6 (10%) had erectile dysfunction. One of the long-term complications was graft diverticulum in one case and was treated conservatively (in ventral on lay BMG).

Conclusion: Improvement of the service in limited resources countries like Sudan and was reflected in the excellent outcome of BMG urethroplasty as treatment of anterior urethral stricture (success rate 90%).

Keywords: Urethroplasty, Anterior urethral stricture, Buccal mucosal graft urethroplasty, Urine retention

Backgrounds

Urethral stricture disease is a condition that affects 300 per 100,000 males and its surgical treatment can represent a challenge [1]. Several approaches including direct visual internal urethrotomy (DVIU) and anastomotic or augmentation urethroplasty based on the use of flaps and graft have been reported [2]. Barbagli described the dorsal onlay free graft urethroplasty in 1996 and since then graft urethroplasty has gained worldwide application for the treatment of penile and bulbar urethra strictures [3, 4].

Urethral reconstruction using a buccal mucosal graft (BMG) to substitute the urethral mucosa has become a well-established modality in the management of bulbar and penile urethral strictures, not amenable for excision and anastomosis. The various configurations of BMG urethroplasty have included ventral onlay, dorsal onlay, dorsal inlay via a ventral sagittal urethrotomy approach, dorsolateral onlay with one-sided mobilization of the urethra, combined dorsal plus ventral double mucosal grafts, two-stage repairs, and augmented anastomotic urethroplasty [5].

Although surgical short-term visits tend to be the most predominant approach for overseas surgical assistance,

*Correspondence: samimahj@gmail.com
[1] Department of Surgery, Faculty of Medicine, University of Gezira, Wad Medani, Gezira State, Sudan

workshops were a common method of overseas surgical support and if designed with a clear aim and locally relevant objectives, can be an excellent platform to augment surgical skills and meet specific learning needs [6].

Urethral stricture is one of the commonest obstructive uropthy which occur in urethra and presented to urologist in Sudan [7]. This is the first time to adopt BMG urethroplasty for management of anterior urethral stricture in our facility and this will affect the further outcome for patients and it will change the training and experience of the young surgeon and treatments provider. Further more, according to our data, this is the first written scientific work regarding BMG urethroplasty in Sudan. Previously it was managed with frequent DVIU and serial dilatation, whatever the stricture site and the length of the stricture, which was reflected in the poor outcomes [8].

In this study, we aimed to study the outcomes and complications for patients who underwent BMG urethroplasty at Gezira Hospital for Renal Disease and Surgery (GHRDS).

Materials and methods

Study design

This is a prospective hospital-based study designed to review the outcomes of buccal mucosal graft urethroplasty while treating anterior urethral stricture. The study was conducted from January 2017 to January 2019. The inclusion criteria in this study were: males patients above 15 years of age diagnosed with anterior urethral stricture (penile and bulbar), who underwent BMG with regular follow-up.

Study area

Gezira Hospital for renal disease and Surgery is a governmental hospital located in Wad Medani city the Capital of Gezira state. It is the only referral hospital for the nearby state, Senar state, Blue Nile state, White Nile state, Gadarif state, and Kassala state. The total population cover is around 15 million. The hospital has a dialysis unit, nephrology department, surgical department, emergency department, operations room, radiological center, and laboratory center. The total number of beds is 100.

Sudan has been withered with the great devaluation of its currency and super inflation of its economy plus the four decades of civil wars. It was classify as low-income country.

The training of the health professionals was done by The SIU, IVUmed groups from India and Egypt conducted three training workshops in urethral strictures management including on hand surgery specially BMG in the hospital where four urologists are trained to shoulder these services in this hospital. They proved to have the sound capability and perfect skills.

Perioperative care

Patients had been diagnosed with anterior urethral stricture after proper history, detailed examination, and urethrogram outpatient clinic visits. The operation was performed under spinal anesthesia until the time of graft harvesting then general anesthesia with nasal intubation for bilateral cheek graft or oral intubation for unilateral cheek graft, then the patient was put in a lithotomy position. Urethroscopy was done by semi-rigid ureteroscope (URS) size 6.5 FR tip to assess site, complete or partial obstruction, and the length of the stricture if only the guidewire was passed considered a complete obstruction, and if passable by URS considered as partial and then can be augmented. While the guidewire was placed in the urethra longitudinal incision was made along the subscrotal raphe and the bulbar urethral was explored, but the penile urethra usually invaginated below the scrotum in penile stricture.

The bulbospongiosum muscle was cut in the middle (nerve preservation), then the corpus spongiosum was mobilized and separated from the corpus cavernosum. The urethra was opened dorsally (the attached part of corpus cavernosum to corpus spongiosum) from a healthy-to-healthy urethral area under direct vision, then the BMG harvested by the following technique:

1. Using mouth retractor (Steinhauser retractor).
2. Identification of the parotid duct and marking the edges of the graft by povidone-iodine (marker pen is not available).
3. Hydro dissection by submucosal injection of saline mixed with adrenaline (every 2 ml diluted with 200 ml saline).
4. Then harvesting the BMG followed by de fating of the graft. The harvested graft was fixed dorsally to the corpus cavernosum by quilting stitch then the edges of the graft were sutured continuously to the urethra, corpus spongiosum, and corpus cavernosum bilaterally using 4/0 vicyl over silicon catheter of adequate size (14 or 16 FR). Then the harvested site most of the time is not sutured. Bleeding controlled only by external ice pack and coagulation. Lastly, the wound closed in layers. No drain was fixed in all operations.

Post-operative follow-up

For perineal wound: removal of covering gauze on the second day and application of fusidic acid ointment for 1 week. For harvested BMG site: in the first day: internal packing and external ice packing, in the second day: non-spicy oral fluid, and the third day: soft diet.

Patient discharged from 4th to the 7th postoperative day on injectable third-generation cephalosporin and oral metronidazole for 7 days. The removal of the urethral catheter depends on the absence of extravasation on the per catheter urethrogram after 28 days.

Note: a suprapubic catheter is fixed as routine, then the urethral catheter was removed and the suprapubic catheter was tight for 3 days. After good micturition, for 3 days the suprapubic catheter was removed.

Long-term follow-up: after 3 months, the clinical assessment was conducted, and ascending urethrogram was performed. After 1 year, follow up also with clinical assessment and ascending urethrogram. Uroflowmetry was not functioning at the time of the study.

Ethical approval was obtained from approval acceptance to the hospital authority. Written and verbal consent were obtained from patients. Data used anonymously by using identity numbers instead of names is ordered to protect the patient's identity and kept securely and in a separate file.

Data collection

Data were collected from hospital records and patient's file through structured questionnaires was used to collect data. Success and failure in terms of stricture recurrence, patient demographics, stricture etiology and anatomy, and the adverse outcomes and complications were recorded to determine risk factors for recurrent stricture and complications.

Data were analyzed by using a computer program Statistical Package for Social Sciences (SPSS V. 21.0). The analyzed data presented in tables and figures designed by Microsoft Excel 2007. Chi-square used as a significance test for categorical data respectively. The *P* value considered significant if < 0.05.

Ethical approval to conduct the study was obtained from the ethical committee of Faculty of Medicine, University of Gezira, all methods were carried out in accordance with relevant guidelines and regulations" in the methods section. A written consent was obtained from all subjects (under 18 years the concent obtained from a parent) to participate in the study and publish the data.

Results

A total number of 60 patients was involved in the study. All of them underwent buccal mucosal graft (BMG) urethroplasty for anterior urethral stricture. Their mean age was 47 ± 15.3 years. Regarding the presenting complains, all the patients (n = 60; 100%) has weak stream, 40 (66.7%) patients had straining, 36 (60%) had burning micturition, 26 (43.3%) had acute urine retention and 16 (26.7%) patients had dribbling. Hypertension was the most common comorbidity presented in 26 (43.3%) of the patients and Diabetes Miletus in 16 (26.7%) patients. Mainly previous procedures were the main etiology of strictures as catheterization (n = 46; 76.7%). On the other hand, perineal pelvic injury was encountered in 14 (23.3%) patients and sexual transmitted disease (STDs) or non-gonococcal urethritis in 8 (13.3%) patients (Table 1). In the history of pervious surgery management, 22 (36.7%) patients underwent visual internal urethrotomy (DVIU) and 6 (10%) patients underwent urethral dilatation. Fifty-four (90%) of the patients underwent BMG urethroplasty for first time and 6 (10%) redo the operation (previous surgery was anastomotic or BMG).

Regarding the stricture features, in majority of the patients 48 (80%) had stricture in bulbar site and 46 (76.7%) had stricture with more than 5 cm in length. Concerning to the operation characteristics, most of the cases underwent dorsal onlay operation (n = 54; 90%), had blood loss volume less than 500 ml (n = 58; 96.7%), had operation time from 1 to 2 h (n = 52; 86.7%) and used 16 FR catheter size (n = 44; 73.3%) (Table 2). Buccal mucosa harvesting site was mainly unilateral in 50 (83.3%) patients and bilateral in 10 (16.7%) patients (Table 2).

The success rate was found to be 90% (n = 54), while 6 (10%) had recurrence of stricture (Fig. 1). Pain and pain combined bleeding from internal suture lines were the only early complication encountered in 50 (83.3%) and 2 (3.3%) patients, respectively. Late complications occurrence was found as follow, 14 (23.3%) patients had UTI, 12 (20%) had wound infections, 8 (13.3%) had changes in ejaculation, and decrease in intensity of orgasm, and 6 (10%) had erectile dysfunction (Fig. 1). One of the long-term complication was graft diverticulum in one case and was treated conservatively (in ventral onlay BMG).

According to the perioperative complications in harvesting site, pain presented in all patients (n = 60; 100%), 32 (53.3%) as moderate and 28 (46.7%) as minimal. Also, all the patients (n = 60; 100%) were normally able to drink, 40 (66.7%) patients were not able to eat initially, 6 (10%) had tightness and 4 (6.7%) patients had numbness.

Table 1 The stricture etiologies among patient's anterior urethral stricture who underwent buccal mucosal graft (BMG) urethroplasty (N = 60)

Catheterization	46	76.7
Cystoscopy	16	26.7
Pelvic surgery	8	13.3
Transurethral resection of the prostate (TURP)	6	10
Perineal pelvic injury	14	23.3
STDs or non-gonococcal urethritis	8	13.3

Table 2 Predictors for the outcome among patients of anterior urethral stricture who underwent buccal mucosal graft (BMG) urethroplasty (N = 60)

Variables	Success [n = 54]	Stricture recurrence [n = 6]	*P* value
Age			
< 20	2 (3.7%)	0 (0%)	0.857*
20–40	22 (40.7%)	2 (33.3%)	
41–60	24 (44.4%)	4 (66.7%)	
> 60	6 (11.1%)	0 (0%)	
Operation frequency			
First	52 (96.3%)	2 (3.7%)	0.020*
Redo	2 (33.3%)	4 (66.7%)	
Site of stricture			
Bulbar	48	0	0.000*
Penile	5	5	
Pan stricture	1	1	
Types of BMG urethroplasty			
Dorsal onlay	51 (94.4%)	3 (5.6%)	0.001**
Ventral onlay	2 (50%)	2 (50%)	
Anastomotic augmented dorsal onlay	1 (50%)	1 (50%)	
Expected blood loss			
< 500 ml	54 (93.1%)	4 (6.9%)	0.000**
> 500 ml	0 (0%)	2 (100%)	
Time of operation			
1–2 h	50 (96.2%)	2 (3.8%)	0.039**
> 2 h	4 (50%)	4 (50%)	
Size of catheter used			
14 FR	14 (85.7%)	2 (12.5%)	0.679*
16 FR	40 (90.9%)	4 (9.1%)	

**P* value is not statistically significant

***P* value is statistically significant

The median duration of pain relieving was 5 days, ranged from 3 to 14 days. Tightness was relieved after 2 days in 2 (33.3%) patients and after 3 days in 4 (66.7%) patients. numbness was relieved after one month in the 4 patients.

Peri-catheter urethrogram showed no extravasations in 56 (93.3%) patients and extravasations in 4 (6.7%) patients, so the catheter was kept for another 2 weeks. also, post-operative ascending urethrogram (3rd and 12th month) was normal 53 (88.3%), abnormal (filing defect) in 6 (10%) patients and one patient (1.7%) had diverticulum.

The volume of blood loss was significantly affected the outcomes (*P* value = 0.000) as the success rate was 93.1% in those lost less than 500 ml of blood compared to no patients of those lost more than 500 ml of blood. The time of operation was significantly affected the outcomes (*P* value = 0.039) as the success rate was high in patients with operation time from 1 to 2 h (96.2%) more than those with operation time more than 2 h (50%). The success or outcomes of BMG urethroplasty was not significantly affected by the sizes of catheter used (*P* value = 0.679).

Discussion

Humby was the first to use buccal mucosa for urethral reconstruction in 1941 for hypospadias repair [9]. Because buccal mucosal grafts have advantages over other grafts, they have been popular since the 1990s. Open urethroplasty is the gold standard treatment for urethral strictures, but it is not a routine operation for a general urologist. Since 1993 El-Kasaby et al. reported the first experience with buccal mucosa urethroplasty for treatment of penile and bulbar urethral strictures [10].

In the present study, most of the patients 48 (80%) had a stricture in the bulbar site. This is in concordance with literature as up to 90% of urethral strictures were in the anterior urethra, and approximately two-thirds (75%) of them occur in the bulbar urethra [1, 11, 12]. The common etiologies of urethral strictures in this study was catheterization (76.7%), while, perineal pelvic injury found in 14 (23.3%) patients and STDs or non-gonococcal urethritis in 8 (13.3%) patients. However, in the study of Mohamed et al.; the cause of stricture was idiopathic in 47, inflammatory in 15, lichen-sclerosis in 26, and post failed hypospadias repair in 35 patients [13]. In the study of Kamyar et al., the etiology of the urethral stricture was sexually transmitted disease (STD) in (14.53%), lichen sclerosis in (12.82%), a trauma in (12.82%), catheterization in (11.11%), transurethral resection (TUR) in (5.13%), and unknown in (43.59%) [14].

In this study, the vast majority of the patients underwent dorsal onlay operation (n = 54; 90%). And this can be explained by the dorsal onlay procedure are a more stable and reliably well-vascularized graft bed, and less possibility of sacculation our results were similar to Figler et al. [15]. The time of catheter removal was fewer than 4 weeks (22–26 days) in 12 patients (20%) due to uncontrolled infection, fortunately, post operatively was good. The current study reported, the overall success rate was 90% (n = 54 patients). This rate was similar to the studies of Tarun et al. who reported the rate of 91% [6], Mohamed et al. who reported a success rate of 91.1% [11], Kamyar et al. who reported the tare of 93.3% [14]. And the lowest success rates reported by Marco et al. (81%) [16] and Yalcinkaya et al. (70%) [17] and Guido et al. (80%) [18]. Barbagli described the dorsal onlay graft urethroplasty in 1996 in 12 patients, reporting a successful outcome in all patients [19]. Morey and McAninch reported similar results in 13 patients who underwent ventral onlay BMG urethroplasty for anterior urethral

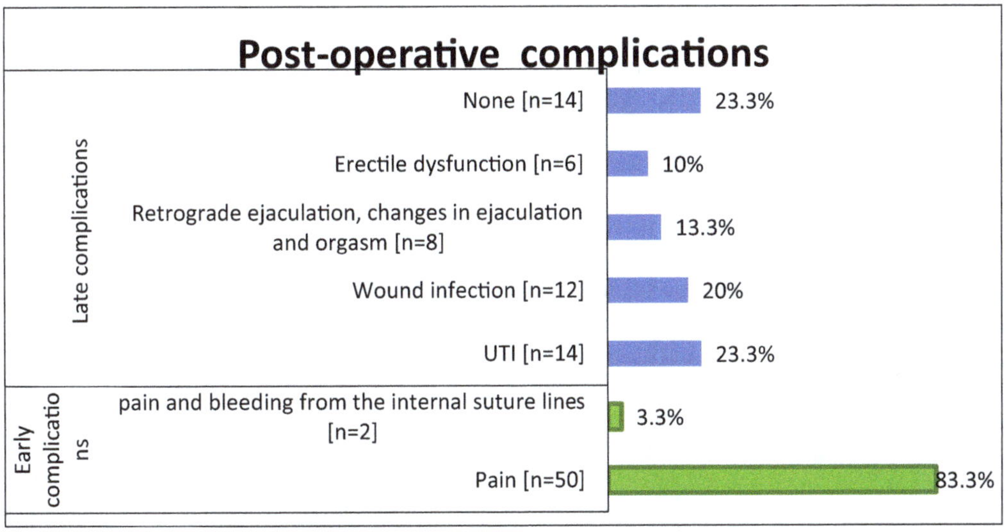

Fig. 1 The postoperative complications among patients of anterior urethral stricture who underwent buccal mucosal graft (BMG) urethroplasty (N = 60)

stricture [20]. Barbagli more recently reported the 80.2% long-term success rate for dorsal onlay bulbar urethroplasty using BMG [19]. Variations to this approach have been reported by Kulkarni, with success rates up to 92% [21]. Asopa described the dorsal inlay free graft urethroplasty and with this technique, excellent results up to 87% of success rate have been reported [22]. The variations in the success rates might be attributed to the difference in geographical areas, sampling as well as the types of BMG urethroplasty.

Not surprisingly, the pain was presented in all the patients' post-operation, in addition to urinary tract infection (23.3%) and superficial wound infection (20%) were the major late complications, the high incidence of infection (UTI and superficial wound infection) can be explained by the absence of urine culture and sensitivity test in this study as a prerequisite before surgery, which might reduce this rate especially most of the patients had an increase in post voiding residual urine volume, which predispose to UTI. In the study of Marco et al., the most frequent complications recorded were urinary fistula (3.1%), graft contracture (3.1%), and graft failure (3.1%) [16]. While Tarun et al. reported wound infection was the main postoperative complication [6]. The study of Mohamed et al. reported patients complicated by fistula (5.7%), wound infection (1.9%), and meatal stenosis (2.9%) [13].

Regarding the complication in the harvesting site, all the patients (n = 60) had pain, and two-thirds (66.7%) were unable to eat initially, 6 (10%) had tightness and 4 (6.7%) patients had numbness. This compatible with the findings of Wood et al. study [23]. The results showed the age of the patients was not significantly affected the outcomes of BMG urethroplasty. This finding was in agreement with the study of Yalcinkaya et al. [17] and Biswajit et al. [24]. Interestingly, the success rate of BMG urethroplasty was significantly high among the patients who underwent the procedure for the first time (93.3%) more than those with redo (33.3%) (P value = 0.020) because of less fibrous tissue in comparison with redo urethroplasty. This was in agreement with a review of Lindsay et al. who reported the failure rate of urethroplasty increases substantially with repeated procedures [25].

Also, showed the success rate was 100% among the patients with stricture in bulbar, 50% in a pan, and penile stricture (P value = 0.000). These findings were comparable to the study of Marco et al. [16] and Yalcinkaya [17]. The success rate was 100% among the patients with stricture length less than 5 cm whilst in those with stricture length more than 5 cm the success rate was 87% (P value = 0.043) the restructure was found in the proximal and distal end of the graft anastomosis. The current results were consistent with the studies of Marco et al. (14) [16] and Yalcinkaya et al. [17]. The type of operation has significantly affected the outcomes (P value = 0.001) as the success rate was high in dorsal onlay (92.9%) more than ventral onlay (50%). A recent review described the outcome of 35 studies of the success rate of the dorsal onlay urethroplasty in a total of 934 patients and reported that with an average follow-up of 42.2 months the average success rate was 88.4% [26].

The volume of blood loss has significantly affected the outcomes (*P* value = 0.000) as the success rate was 93.1% in those who lost less than 500 ml of blood compared to no patients of those who lost more than 500 ml of blood. The time of operation has significantly affected the outcomes (*P* value = 0.039) as the success rate was high in patients with operation time from 1 to 2 h (96.2%) more than those with operation time of more than 2 h (50%). And remarkably, this study showed the success rate was 100% among the patients with unilateral buccal mucosal sites whilst in those with bilateral buccal mucosal sites the success rate was 40% (*P* value = 0.002). This observation was comparable to the study of Irekpita et al. [27].

Conclusion

Inside training by expert international trainers is an excellent method of improvement of the service in limited resources countries like Sudan and that was reflected on the excellent outcome of BMG urethroplasty as treatment of anterior urethral stricture (success rate 90%).

Abbreviations

BMG: Buccal mucosal graft; STDs: Sexual transmitted diseases; GHKDS: Gezira Hospital for Kidney Disease and Surgery.

Acknowledgements

Authors would like to grateful the the patients' record staff of GHKDS Gezira hospital for kidney disease and Urology

Authors' contributions

Conceptualisation of the study, data acquisition, analysis and interpretation, and writing: SMT, MAMA and MDAG. Conceptualisation of the study, interpretation, and writing: SMT MAMA YMO. Interpretation and critical revision: YMO, MEM and MDAG. All authors agree with the submission. All authors read and approved the final manuscript.

Competing interests

The authors declare that they have no competing interests.

Author details

[1]Department of Surgery, Faculty of Medicine, University of Gezira, Wad Medani, Gezira State, Sudan. [2]Department of Urology, Gezira Hospital for Kidney Disease and Surgery, Wad Medani, Gezira State, Sudan. [3]Sudan Medical Specialization Board, Khartoum, Sudan.

References

1. Stein DM, Thum DJ, Barbagli G, et al. A geographic analysis of male urethral stricture aetiology and location. BJU Int. 2013;112:830–4.
2. Mangera A, Osman N, Chapple C. Evaluation and management of anterior urethral strictre disease. F1000Res. 2016;5:153.
3. Barbagli G, Selli C, Tosto A, et al. Dorsal free graft urethroplasty. J Urol. 1996;155:123–6. https://doi.org/10.1016/S0022-5347(01)66566-2.
4. Chapple C, Andrich D, Atala A, et al. SIU/ICUD consultation on urethral strictures: the management of anterior urethral stricture disease using substitution urethroplasty. Urology. 2014;83:S31-47.
5. Tarun D, Amit K, Harohalli K. Management of recurrent anterior urethral strictures following buccal mucosal graft-urethroplasty: a single center experience. Urol Ann. 2016;8(1):31–5.
6. Shrime MG, Sleemi A, Ravilla TD. Charitable platforms in global surgery: a systematic review of their effectiveness, cost-effectiveness, sustainability, and role training. World J Surg. 2015;39:10–20.
7. El Imam M, Omran M, Nugud F, Elsabiq M, Saad K, Taha O. Obstructive uropathy in Sudanese patients. Saudi J Kidney Dis Transplant. 2006;17(3):415.
8. Mansour MO, Aboagla YA, Taha SM, Khalid KE. Urethral stricture; etiology, presentation, complications, and outcome of management at Gezira State, Central Sudan. Gezira J Health Sci. 2013;9(2):1–10.
9. Humby G. A one-stage operation for hypospadias. Br J Surg. 1941;29:84–92.
10. El-Kasaby AW, Fath-Alla M, Noweir AM, El-Halaby MR, Zakaria W, El-Beialy MH. The use of buccal mucosa patch graft in the management of anterior urethral strictures. J Urol. 1993;149:276–8.
11. Fenton AS, Morey AF, Aviles R, Garcia CR. Anterior urethral strictures: etiology and characteristics. Urology. 2005;65:1055–8.
12. Palminteri E, Berdondini E, Verze P, De Nunzio C, Vitarelli A, Carmignani L. Contemporary urethral stricture characteristics in the developed world. Urology. 2013;81:191–6.
13. Mohamed S, Shady S, Eid E, Atef B. Outcome of staged buccal mucosal graft for repair of long segment anterior urethral stricture. BMC Urol. 2019;19:38.
14. Kamyar T, Alireza G. Dorsally placed buccal mucosal graft urethroplasty in treatment of long urethral strictures using one-stage transperineal approach. Int Sch Res Not. 2014;2014:792982.
15. Figler BD, Malaeb BS, Dy GW, Voelzke BB, Wessells H. Impact of graft position on failure of single-stage bulbar urethroplasties with buccal mucosa graft. Urology. 2013;82:1166–70.
16. Marco S, Neha S, Sachin M, Mahreen H. Buccal mucosal graft urethroplasty in men—risk factors for recurrence and complications: a third referral centre experience in anterior urethroplasty using buccal mucosal graft. Transl Androl Urol. 2017;6(3):510–6.
17. Yalcinkaya F, Zengin K, Sertcelik N, Yigitbasi O. Dorsal onlay buccal mucosal graft urethroplasty in the treatment of urethral strictures—does the stricture length affect success? Adv Clin Exp Med. 2015;24(2):297–300.
18. Guido B, Giorgio G, Enzo P. Anastomotic fibrous ring as cause of stricture recurrence after bulbar onlay graft urethroplasty. J Urol. 2006;176:614–9.
19. Barbagli G, Kulkarni SB, Fossati N, et al. Long-term followup and deterioration rate of anterior substitution urethroplasty. J Urol. 2014;192:808–13.
20. Morey AF, McAninch JW. Technique of harvesting buccal mucosa for urethral reconstruction. J Urol. 1996;155:1696–7.
21. Kulkarni S, Barbagli G, Sansalone S, et al. One-sided anterior urethroplasty: a new dorsal onlay graft technique. BJU Int. 2009;104:1150–5.
22. Asopa HS, Garg M, Singhal GG, et al. Dorsal free graft urethroplasty for urethral stricture by ventral sagittal urethrotomy approach. Urology. 2001;58:657–9.
23. Wood D, Allen S, Andrich D. The morbidity of buccal mucosal graft harvest for urethroplasty and the effect of nonclosure of the graft harvest site on postoperative pain. J Urol. 2004;172(2):580–3.
24. Biswajit DM, Rao RP, Acharya L. Dorsal onlay buccal mucosal graft urethroplasty in long anterior urethral stricture. Int Braz J Urol. 2007;33(2):181–7.
25. Lindsay A, Jack W, Benjamin N. Male urethral strictures and their management. Nat Rev Urol. 2014;11(1):43–50.
26. Mangera A, Patterson JM, Chapple CR. A systematic review of graft augmentation urethroplasty techniques for the treatment of anterior urethral strictures. Eur Urol. 2011;59:797–814.
27. Irekpita E, Esezobor E. Buccal mucosal graft urethroplasty for proximal bulbar urethral stricture: a revisit of the surgical technique and analysis of eleven consecutive cases. Niger Med J. 2016;57(5):266–71.

26

Staged transverse preputial island flap urethroplasty for some proximal hypospadias with moderate-to-severe chordee

Hai Lin*, Yu-Yun Wang, Shi-Bing Li, Ze-Ting Chen and Liang-Ju Su

Abstract

Background: We aimed to assess the outcome of staged transverse preputial island flap (TPIF) urethroplasty for repairing certain cases of primary proximal hypospadias with moderate-to-severe chordee in children.

Methods: Nighty-two consecutive boys who underwent either one-stage or staged TPIF urethroplasty for the repair of proximal hypospadias with moderate-to-severe chordee between August 2015 and December 2019 were evaluated retrospectively. Patients were divided into two groups: one-stage TPIF urethroplasty group (n = 44) and staged TPIF urethroplasty group (n = 48). We noted and compared the postoperative complications, including urethrocutaneous fistula, urethral diverticula, residual penile curvature, and urethral stricture in both groups.

Results: Both groups were followed up for 1–5 years, with an average of 3 years. No cases of residual or recurrence of penile chordee were reported in either group. In Group A, 9 patients (9/44, 20.4%) had postoperative urethrocutaneous fistula, and all patients underwent urinary fistula repair or urethroplasty. In Group B, postoperative urethrocutaneous fistula occurred in 2 cases (2/48, 4.1%), and one patient developed a urethrocutaneous fistula after the first operation, which was successfully repaired during the second operation. A urethrocutaneous fistula occurred in 1 case after completion of the second-stage operation; urethral fistula repair was performed successfully 6 months later. There were 2 cases of urethral stricture in Group A (2/44, 4.5%) and none in Group B. There were 6 cases of urethral diverticulum in Group A (6/44, 13.6%) and no cases of urethral diverticulum in Group B. The operative success rates were 61.3% and 95.8% in Group A and Group B, respectively ($P < 0.001$).

Conclusions: Compared with one-stage TPIF urethroplasty, staged TPIF urethroplasty in the treatment of certain cases of primary proximal hypospadias with moderate-to-severe chordee resulted in fewer postoperative fistulas, urethral strictures and urethral diverticula. The staged TPIF urethroplasty procedure was effective in reducing the operation difficulty and complication rate of hypospadias, improving the curative effect of complex hypospadias and having good clinical application value.

Keywords: Proximal hypospadias, Staged, Urethroplasty, Surgical outcome

Background

Which operative technique can we choose to repair severe hypospadias? It depends on the severity of hypospadias and the experience of the surgeon. Severe hypospadias is often accompanied by severe malformations and limited repair materials, which will lead to more postoperative complications. Proximal hypospadias [1] is

*Correspondence: linhai2317@163.com
Department of Pediatric Surgery, Hainan General Hospital (Hainan Affiliated Hospital of Hainan Medical University), Xiuying District, Haikou 570311, Hainan, People's Republic of China

defined by an external orifice of the urethra located on the proximal penile shaft to perineum at the beginning of urethroplasty after the chordee is corrected. "Severe" hypospadias specifically refers to cases with $\geq 30°$ chordee after degloving. Staged surgery is often required, and satisfactory efficacy and good cosmesis still cannot be achieved. Therefore, the treatment of severe hypospadias is a great challenge for pediatric urologists. There are different opinions on the choice of single-stage versus staged operations [2, 3]. We believe that the experience of the surgeon and the severity of hypospadias are the main determinants. We aimed to assess the outcome of staged transverse preputial island flap (TPIF) urethroplasty for repairing certain cases of primary proximal hypospadias with moderate-to-severe chordee in children. We have performed one-stage and two-stage urethroplasty combining transected urethral plate and TPIF to treat initially severe hypospadias in our hospital since 2015, with two-stage procedures producing desirable effects.

Methods

The study was conducted in accordance with the Declaration of Helsinki (as revised in 2013). The study was approved by the ethics board of Hainan General Hospital (2021-005) and informed consent was obtained from a parent or guardian for participants under 16 years old.

Patient criteria

Ninety-two children underwent their first surgery at the average age of 18 months. All were penoscrotal hypospadias or perineal hypospadias. Forty-four patients underwent one-stage TPIF urethroplasty (Group A), including 10 patients with penoscrotal hypospadias and 34 patients with perineal hypospadias. Forty-eight patients underwent staged TPIF urethroplasty (Group B), including 20 patients with penoscrotal hypospadias (Fig. 1a–c) and 28 patients with perineal hypospadias, and the interval between the two stages was at least 6 months. The preoperative data of the patients are summarized in Table 1.

Operative technique

The same surgical team performed all the operations. The procedure was divided into two phases. The first phase was performed with chordee correction and partial urethroplasty with a dorsal transverse pedicled island flap, leaving a fistula at the scrotum. The second phase was performed with urethral fistula repair at least 6 months later.

Single-stage repair

Chordee correction

In the first stage, 5/0 polypropylene was sutured longitudinally through the tip of the glans for traction, and a circumferential incision was made 3 mm below the corona, preserving the urethral plate. Then, we excised the whole ventral bands by degloving the penile skin to the root. Next, an artificial erection test (a tourniquet was bonded at the root of the penis, and a butterfly needle was inserted into the tip of the penis. Normal saline solution was intermittently injected into the corpus cavernosum during the operation to evaluate the degree of penile chordee.) was performed. The urethral plate was transected at the corona if the penis could not be straightened. Then, the artificial erection test was repeated. Dorsal plication using 5–0 polypropylene was performed to gain a straight penis when residual chordee remained. The artificial erection test was performed again.

Urethroplasty

Next, the free residual urethral plate with a length of approximately 1.0–1.5 cm was fixed on the cavernosal body without tension. The dorsal prepuce inner plate of the penis was cut horizontally, and the vascular pedicle of the island flap was separated to the prepuce root. The length of the island flap was consistent with the length of the urethra, and the width was approximately 1.0–1.2 cm. The pedicled island skin flap was wrapped around a 6–8 F silicone catheter to form a tubular urethra, and 6/0 monofilaments were sutured continuously and transposed ventrally.

Meatoplasty and glanuloplasty

The ventral side of the glans was split longitudinally in the midline from the subcoronal sulcus to the tip, and both sides of the glanular wings were dissociated. The distal end of the neourethra was sutured with the penile head, and the two wings of the penile head were closed (Fig. 1d). The proximal end of the neourethra was sutured with the urethral plate. The dorsal prepuce was transferred to cover the ventral defect.

Scrotoplasty

The extra skin of the penile scrotum was cut to form the penile scrotum, and a Y-shaped incision at the junction of the penile scrotum was made to correct the transposition of the penile scrotum.

Postoperative management

The child was discharged home with a catheter on the fifth day after surgery, and the catheter remained in place for 21 days after the operation. Intravenous antibiotics were administered for 3 days and then changed to oral antibiotics until the catheter was removed.

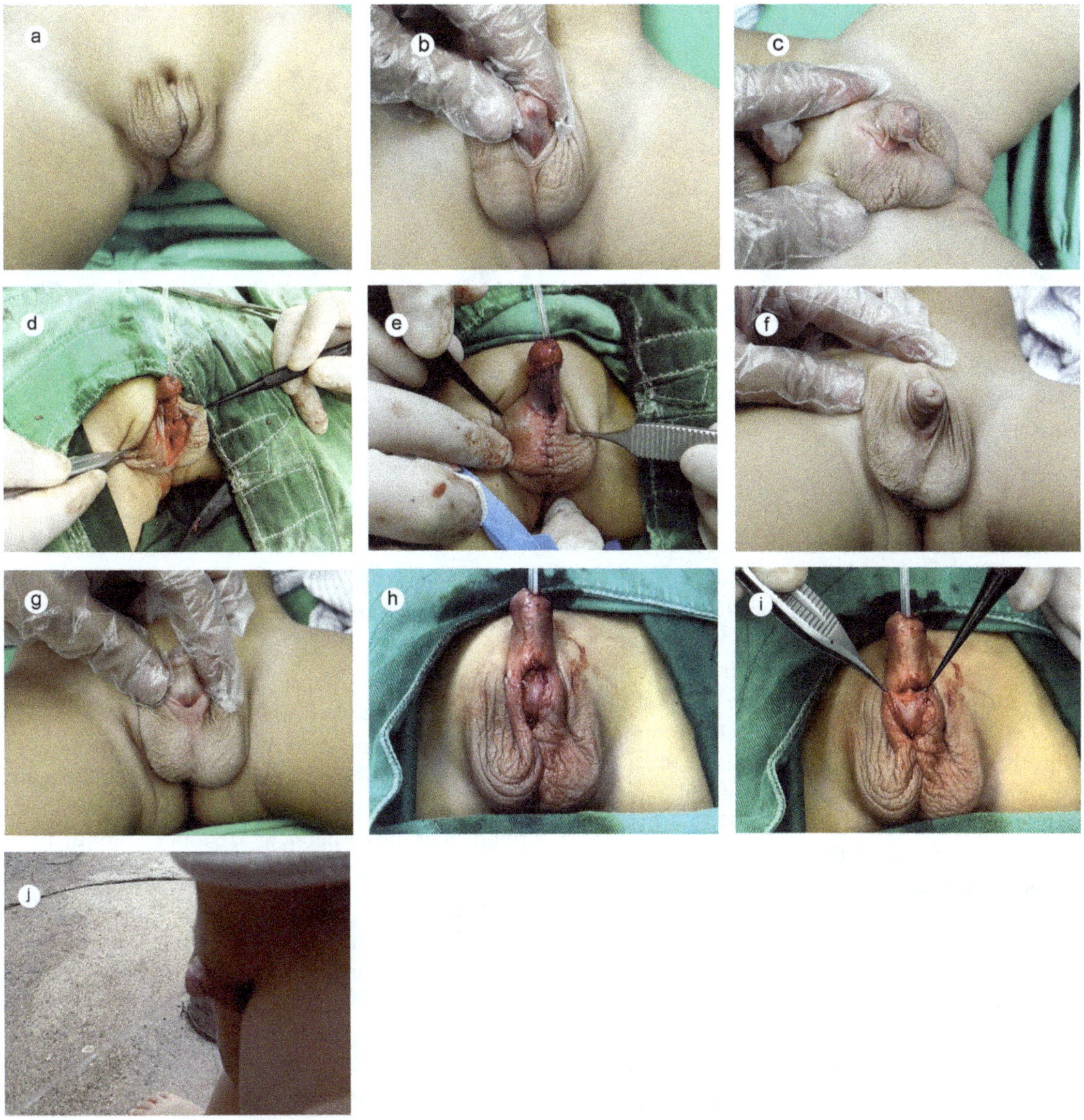

Fig. 1 **a–c** Front and lateral views before stage I repair. Bilateral scrotal separation, severe chordee of the penis, urethra external orifices located at the penile scrotal junction. **d** The island flap was sutured to form a tube and transposed ventrally. The distal end of the neourethra was sutured with the penile head, and the two wings of the penile head were closed. The proximal end of the formed urethral tube was anastomosed with the urethral plate. **e** Appearance immediately after stage I repair. Byar's flaps were created and swung ventrally to cover the ventral defect, and the ventral side of the anastomosis was sutured with the skin around the scrotum to form the stoma. **f, g** Appearance before stage II repair. The penis was straightened satisfactorily, and the fistula was located at the junction of the penis and scrotum. **h** The urethral stoma formed in the first stage was dissociated, and the urethra was sutured. **i** Ventrally transposed thick and healthy dartos tissue near the fistula was used to cover the neourethra. **j** State during urination 3 months after stage II repair. The patient achieved an apical slit-like meatus at the tip of the glans penis, a single forward stream, unimpeded voiding, and good cosmesis

Two-stage repair

Partial urethroplasty and urethrostomy

The procedure of the first stage was almost the same as that of single-stage urethroplasty. After the proximal end of the formed urethral tube was anastomosed with the urethral plate, the ventral side of the anastomosis was sutured with the skin around the scrotum to form the stoma (Fig. 1e). The stoma was placed as far as possible into the scrotum.

Table 1 Basic characteristics of patient

	One-stage (n = 44)	Two-stage (n = 48)
Location of the meatus (n)		
Penoscrotal	10	20
Perineal	34	28
Chordee (n)		
Severe angulation (> 45°)	30	38
Moderate angulation (> 10°, < 45°)	14	10
Surgical ages (months, median [IQR])		
Age at the first stage	18	18
Age at the second stage	–	24
Time between stages	–	10

Data are expressed as number of patients

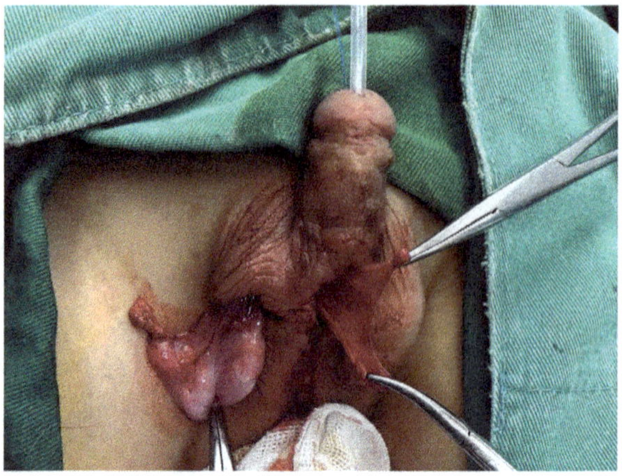

Fig. 2 In cases of insufficient or thin dartos tissue, a healthy and thick tunica vaginalis flap was used as a second layer of coverage for the neourethra (another patient)

Urethral fistula repair/urethroplasty

We performed the second-stage surgery at least 6 months after the initial operation, after edema subsided and healing was adequate. A 5/0 polypropylene was sutured longitudinally through the tip of the glans for traction. Artificial erection was performed as the first step to ensure that there was no residual chordee. The second step was to detect urethrocutaneous fistulae and urethral diverticulum in the distal urethra by water injection and to investigate urethral strictures with a urethral probe. The stoma was closed by annular incision, and the skin of the fistula was sutured by double-layer varus (Fig. 1h).

Protective intermediate layer

A ventrally transposed thick and healthy dartos tissue near the fistula was used to cover the neourethra (Fig. 1i). In cases of insufficient or thin dartos tissue, a healthy and thick tunica vaginalis flap was used as a second layer of coverage (Fig. 2).

Postoperative management

The child was discharged home with a catheter on the fifth day after surgery, and the catheter was withdrawn 21 days postoperatively. Intravenous antibiotics were administered for 3 days and then changed to oral antibiotics until the catheter was removed.

Statistical analysis

Statistical differences in the detection rates of postoperative incidences of penile chordee, urethrocutaneous fistula, urethral stricture, and urethral diverticulum between the two groups were compared using the chi-squared test. SPSS software (Version 25.0, Chicago, IL) was used for the statistical analysis. Data were considered significant if the p-value < 0.05.

Follow-up

Postoperative follow-up included answering inquiries about the voiding pattern from parents by phone calls or WeChat; physical examination of the genitalia; and direct observation of the voiding stream by the doctor (after removal of the catheter, at 3, 6 and 12 months).

Results

A total of 92 patients who underwent either one-stage or staged TPIF urethroplasty were identified. All patients were followed up for more than 12 months after the operation. Both groups were followed up for 1 to 5 years, with an average of 3 years. No cases of residual or recurrence of penile chordee were reported in the two groups. All patients achieved good cosmesis and normal urination.

During the follow-up period, the postoperative complication rates were 38.6% and 4.2% in Group A and Group B, respectively. 9 patients (9/44, 20.4%) in Group A developed postoperative urethrocutaneous fistula, which was located at the anastomosis of the old and new urethra. Fistula repair was performed 1 year after the first operation, and no recurrence of fistula occurred. In Group B, postoperative urethrocutaneous fistula occurred in 2 cases (2/48, 4.1%), and one patient developed a urethrocutaneous fistula after the first operation, which was successfully repaired during the second operation. A urethrocutaneous fistula occurred in 1 case after completion of the second-stage operation, and urethral fistula repair was performed successfully 6 months later.There was statistical significance in the incidence of urethrocutaneous fistula between the two groups ($P = 0.016$).

There were 2 cases of urethral stricture in Group A (2/44, 4.5%) and none in Group B. Urethral dilation was not routinely performed between two surgeries in Group B. There was no significant difference between the two groups ($p = 0.226$). In Group A, 2 cases of urethral stricture appeared 1–2 months after the operation. One case achieved good results in urination 1 month after urethral dilation and an indwelling urethral catheter was performed. One patient underwent urethrostomy and two-stage urethroplasty due to failure of urethral dilation, and 1 was cured. No recurrent urethral stricture occurred.

There were 6 cases of urethral diverticulum in Group A (6/44, 13.6%) and no cases of urethral diverticulum in Group B. There was statistical significance in the incidence of urethral diverticulum between the two groups ($P = 0.026$). Six cases of urethral diverticulum in Group A underwent diverticulectomy and urethroplasty 6 months after the operation. Five cases healed. One patient had a urethrocutaneous fistula after surgery and was cured by fistula repair 1 year later. The operative success rates were 61.4% and 95.8% in Group A and Group B, respectively ($P < 0.001$) (Table 2).

Discussion

The debate over repair of proximal hypospadias continues, two-stage or single-stage, and neither method is accepted universally. In terms of the current technical level, the vast majority of severe hypospadias operations can be performed in one stage [4, 5], and Duckett [6] and Koyanagi [7] urethroplasties are currently the most commonly used one-stage procedures. For patients with severe hypospadias (treated initially) and failed hypospadias, a staged operation may be a wise choice. There are many two-stage operations, such as Byar's operation [8], Bracka's operation [9, 10], staging Duckett surgery [11], and free graft roll tube surgery [12, 13]. At present, in the first stage of staged surgery, the penis should be fully extended, and part of the urethra should be reconstructed; this approach is different from previous staging surgeries. The choice of surgical treatment for severe hypospadias should be different from person to person, emphasizing individual treatment and objectively choosing a one-stage or two-stage operation to achieve the best therapeutic effect.

Table 2 Comparison of postoperative complications and success rate

Treatment	Success	Failure			
		Penis curvature	Fistula	Stricture	Diverticulum
One-stage	27 (44)	0	9	2	6
Two-stage	46 (48)	0	2	0	0
P value	<.001	NS	.016	.226	.026

Data are expressed as the number of patients, and *P* values were calculated for the comparison of postoperative complications and success rates between one-stage and two-stage treatment

We have performed one-stage and two-stage urethroplasty combining transected urethral plate and TPIF to treat initial severe hypospadias in our hospital since 2015. We observed a success rate of 61.3% for one-stage TPIF urethroplasty and 95.8% for staged TPIF urethroplasty from August 2015 to December 2019, and there was statistical significance in the incidence of success rate between the two groups. The incidence of urinary fistula and urethral diverticulum after staging operation was significantly decreased compared with that of one-stage operation, and the differences between the two groups were statistically significant.

Almost all severe hypospadias cases have different degrees of chordee [14, 15], especially the Donnahoo IV type form [16], which has been described as a developmental defect in the distal urethra of fibrous shortening. The difficulty of correction involves not only cutting off the developmental defects of the fibrous urethra to fully correct the bending deformity but also selecting the appropriate self-tissue to reconstruct the urethra. Therefore, when we treat severe hypospadias, the urethral plate should be transected after the fibrous cord on the ventral surface of the cavernous body of the penis is released [17], and dorsal plications should be used to straighten the penis and completely correct the ventral penile curvature. Schlomer [18] proposed that mild-to-moderate residual ventral curvature of the penis after transection of the urethral plate should be corrected with dorsal plication, while severe ventral penile curvature should be corrected with ventral lengthening. In the two groups of patients, dorsal plication was used to correct residual chordee after transection of the urethral plate, with satisfactory results, and no ventral lengthening of the penis was used. No cases of residual or recurrence of penile chordee were reported in the two groups.

Urethrocutaneous fistula easily occurs after hypospadias repair. The occurrence of a urethrocutaneous fistula is closely related to the blood supply of the urethral flap and the quality of the waterproof layer between the urethra and the skin. Since the length of the urethroplasty at the first stage of Group B has no strict requirement, the surgeon can select the part with the best vascular conditions of the island flap to form the urethra, which is conducive to the healing of the urethra and thus reduces the incidence of urinary fistulas. In addition, the urethral tube should be formed at the first stage with one end opening at the scaphoid fossa to create an external urethral orifice and the other end opening between the scrotum. Both ends of the urethral tube have openings, forming a good drainage channel. Even if the wound produces postoperative secretions, they can flow out from both ends of the formed urethra relatively easily, avoiding the accumulation of secretions in the wound and affecting wound healing, which is conducive to reducing the occurrence of a urinary fistula. In the present study, during the second operation, the operative site was located in the scrotum, and the formed urethra was covered with rich dartos tissue or a tunica vaginalis flap, which greatly reduced the incidence of urethral fistula. In agreement with the findings of Pescheloche et al., using the tunica vaginalis flap as an intermediate layer to cover the neourethra can effectively reduce postoperative complications [19].

Inconsistent with the findings of Tiryaki et al., modification of the Bracka technique using a flap for the urethral plate resulted in a high incidence of diverticulum formation [20]. No urethral diverticula occurred in Group B (how to reduce or avoid complications is the goal we pursue). One reason is that the pedicled island flap was taken from the relatively flat prepuce portion, and the width of the flap was appropriate for preventing the new urine tube from being too loose or too tight; another reason is that staged TPIF urethroplasty enables voiding through the stoma after the first stage, which can effectively reduce the impact of high pressure flow on the distal newly formed urethra in the early postoperative period. This procedure provided at least 6 months for the reconstructed neourethra to gradually adhere to the corpora and surrounding fascial tissue, and the outer wall of the urethra was well supported, avoiding the above risk factors for the formation of urethral diverticula.

Urethral stricture is a serious complication after proximal hypospadias repair and commonly occurs at the urethra anastomosis site in one-stage TPIF urethroplasty. In recent years, some scholars [21] have advocated that a three-week instead of one-week catheterization and an age below 6 months at hypospadias repair are associated with a better outcome and fewer complications. Urethral stricture often occurs 2–4 weeks after removal of the catheter. Prolonging the dwelling time of the urinary catheter is beneficial for the subsidence of inflammatory reactions and edema in the operative area, reduction in the occurrence of urinary extravasation, and passage through the urethral scar period. At the same time, the catheter provides better support for the newly formed urethra, which can avoid urethral angulation and distortion and reduce the occurrence of urethral strictures. In addition, expansion of the glans during the first stage of the operation can also effectively prevent the risk of postoperative metal stenosis or glans dehiscence. In the two groups, the urethral catheter was removed 3 weeks after the operation, and none of the patients developed narrowing of the new urethra in Group B.

The limitations of our study were the absence of urodynamic tests and the absence of an objective scoring system to evaluate postoperative urination.

Conclusions

In summary, staged surgery should be considered for the correction of severe hypospadias, especially when repair materials are insufficient, penile dysplasia combined with many deformities is present, and surgical experience is inadequate. Staged TPIF urethroplasty has a low incidence of total complications compared with one-stage TPIF urethroplasty. The staged TPIF urethroplasty procedure was effective in reducing the operation difficulty and complication rate of severe hypospadias, improving the curative effect of complex hypospadias and having good clinical application value.

Abbreviation

TPIF: Transverse preputial island flap.

Acknowledgements

Not applicable.

Authors' contributions

Conception and manuscript writing: HL, provision of study materials or patients: YYW, SBL, collection and assembly of data: ZTC, LJS. All authors final approval of manuscript.

Competing interests

The authors declare that they have no competing interests.

References

1. Cilento BG Jr, Atala A. Proximal hypospadias. Urol Clin North Am. 2002;29(2):311–28.
2. Babu R, Chandrasekharam VVS. Meta-analysis comparing the outcomes of single stage (foreskin pedicled tube) versus two stage (foreskin free graft & foreskin pedicled flap) repair for proximal hypospadias in the last decade. J Pediatr Urol. 2021;17(5):681–9.
3. Castañón M, Prat-Ortells J, García-Aparicio L, et al. Single-repair for primary proximal hypospadias. Lessons learned after 196 primary repairs. Cir Pediatr. 2019;32(4):201–6.
4. Cui X, He Y, Huang W, et al. Clinical efficacy of transverse preputial island flap urethroplasty for single-stage correction of proximal hypospadias: a single-centre experience in Chinese patients. BMC Urol. 2020;20(1):118.
5. Misra D, Elbourne C, Vareli A, et al. Challenges in managing proximal hypospadias: a 17-year single-center experience. J Pediatr Surg. 2019;54(10):2125–9.
6. Duckett JW Jr. Transverse preputial island flap technique for repair of severe hypospadias. Urol Clin North Am. 1980;7:423–30.
7. Vu TH, Viet Nguyen H, Quy Hong Q, et al. Results of the one-stage proximal hypospadias repair with modified Koyanagi technique: a prospective cohort study in a single Vietnam centre. Ann Med Surg Lond. 2021;71:103012.
8. Wani SA, Baba AA, Mufti GN, et al. Bracka verses Byar's two-stage repair in proximal hypospadias associated with severe chordee: a randomized comparative study. Pediatr Surg Int. 2020;36(8):965–70.
9. Manasherova D, Kozyrev G, Nikolaev V, et al. Bracka's method of proximal hypospadias repair: preputial skin or buccal mucosa? Urology. 2020;138:138–43.

10. Kozyrev GV, Manasherova DT, Abdulkarimov GA, et al. Comparative histological analysis of different materials used for urethroplasty in children with proximal forms of hypospadias: preputial skin vs buccal mucosa. Urologiia. 2019;6:87–91.
11. Wang C, Song H, Zhang W, et al. Staged transverse preputial island flap urethroplasty for proximal hypospadias: a single-center experience. Pediatr Surg Int. 2019;35(7):823–7.
12. Tijani KH, Idiodi-Thomas E, Elebute AO, et al. Two-stage flap repair of severe hypospadias: usefulness of the tubularized incised plate urethroplasty. J Pediatr Urol. 2017;13(5):483.e1-483.e5.
13. Snodgrass W, Bush N. Staged tubularized autograft repair for primary proximal hypospadias with 30-degree or greater ventral curvature. J Urol. 2017;198(3):680–6.
14. Bandini M, Sekulović S, Dangi AD, et al. Corporeal penile curvature (CPC) and surgical complications in hypospadias repairs: associations and outcomes. Eur Urol Suppl. 2019;18:e752.
15. Sekulović S, Bandini M, Spiridonescu B, et al. Real prevalence and severity of penile curvature in diferent types of hypospadias. Eur Urol Suppl. 2019;18:e750–1.
16. Donnahoo KK, Cain MP, Pope JC, et al. Etiology, management andsurgical complications of congenital chordee without hypospadias. J Urol. 1998;160(3 Pt 2):1120–2.
17. Acimi S, Acimi MA. Can we preserve the urethral plate in proximal hypospadias repair? Ann Plast Surg. 2017;79(1):68–72.
18. Schlomer BJ. Correction of residual ventral penile curvature after division of the urethral plate in the first stage of a 2- stage proximal hypospadias repair. Curr Urol Rep. 2017;18(2):13.
19. Pescheloche P, Parmentier B, Hor T, et al. Tunica vaginalis flap for urethrocutaneous fistula repair after proximal and mid-shaft hypospadias surgery: a 12-year experience. J Pediatr Urol. 2018;14(5):421.e1.
20. Tiryaki S, Ələkbərova V, Dokumcu Z, et al. Unexpected outcome of a modification of Bracka repair for proximal hypospadias: High incidence of diverticula with flaps. J Pediatr Urol. 2016;12(6):395.e1-395.e6.
21. Daher P, Khoury A, Riachy E, et al. Three-week or one-week bladder catheterization for hypospadias repair? A retrospective-prospective observational study of 189 patients. J Pediatr Surg. 2015;50(6):1063–6.

27

Comparative assessment of biodegradable-antireflux heparine coated ureteral stent: Animal model study

Federico Soria[1*], Julia E. de La Cruz[2], Juan Pablo Caballero-Romeu[3], Manuel Pamplona[4], Daniel Pérez-Fentes[5], Luis Resel-Folskerma[6] and Francisco M. Sanchez-Margallo[7]

Abstract

Background: Double J ureteral stents are widely used on urological patients to provide drainage of the upper urinary tract. Unfourtunately, ureteral stents are not free from complications, as bacterial colonization and require a second procedure for removal. The purpose of the current comparative experimental study is to evaluate a new heparin-coated biodegradable antireflux ureteral stent (BraidStent®-H) to prevent urinary bacterial colonization.

Methods: A total of 24 female pigs were underwent determination of bacteriuria and nephrosonographic, endoscopic and contrast fluoroscopy assessment of the urinary tract. Afterward, were randomly assigned animals to Group-I, in which a 5Fr double-pigtail ureteral stent was placed for 6 weeks, or Group-II, in which a BraidStent®-H was placed. Follow-up assessments were performed at 1, 3, 6, 8, 12 weeks. The final follow-up includes the above methods and an exhaustive pathological study of the urinary tract was accomplished after 20 weeks.

Results: Bacteriuria findings in the first 48 h were significant between groups at 6 h and 12 h. Asymptomatic bacteriuria does not reach 100% of the animals in Group-II until 48 h versus Group-I where it appears at 6 h. The weekly bacteriuria mean rate was 27.7% and 44.4% in Group I and II respectively, without statistical significance. In Group II there were no animals with vesicoureteral reflux, with statistical significance at 3 and 6 weeks with Group-I. The 91.2% of stents in Group-II were degraded between 3 and 6 weeks, without obstructive fragments. Distal ureteral peristalsis was maintained in 66.6–75% in Group-II at 1–6 weeks.

Conclusions: The heparin coating of BraidStent® allows an early decrease of bacterial colonization, but its effectiveness is low at the long term. Heparin coating did not affect scheduled degradation rate or size of stents fragments. BraidStent®-H avoids the side effects associated with current ureteral stents, thus should cause less discomfort to patients.

Keywords: Biodegradable ureteral stent, Heparin coated, Biofilm, Antireflux stents, Morbidity

Background

Double J ureteral stents are widely used on urological patients to provide drainage of the upper urinary tract [1]. However, these stents are not free from complications and side effects. These mainly include vesicoureteral reflux (VUR), a high rate of bacterial colonisation, incrustation and lower urinary tract symptoms [1, 2]. Furthermore, current ureteral stents require a second procedure for removal. This causes anxiety, an increase in healthcare costs and additional anaesthesia requirements in paediatric patients.

*Correspondence: fsoria@ccmijesususon.com
[1] Endoscopy-Endourology Department, Jesús Usón Minimally Invasive Surgery Centre Foundation, Carretera N-521, Km. 41.8, C.P.10071 Cáceres, Spain

The development of biodegradable ureteral stents (BUS) aims to avoid stent removal and forgotten stent syndrome [3]. In recent years there has been an increase in translational research into biodegradable stents. BUSs are made of several natural and synthetic polymers, with hydrolysis being the main biodegradation process [3–5]. One of the recently described BUS is BraidStent®, which has shown a controlled, predictable biodegradation rate in the porcine model. This stent design is anti-reflux, as it does not interfere with the ureterovesical junction after placement [3, 6]. This represents an important development in the search for the ideal ureteral stent, together with its biodegradable characteristic. However, one of the weaknesses of the BraidStent® was its high asymptomatic bacteriuria rate at 3 weeks of stenting: up to 41%. Heparin coating has shown an ability to reduce bacterial adhesion and incrustation on stent surfaces in previous studies [7, 8], although several authors have disagreed on the ability of the heparin coating to decrease bacterial adhesion [9].

The endpoint of this comparative study was to assess the short- and long-term inhibitory capacity of the novel biodegradable ureteral stent BraidStent®-H in a pig model. This new stent is provided with a heparin coating to avoid the main source of bacterial colonization that occurs at the time of retrograde placement by the introduction of bacteria through the transurethral route in the urinary tract [10] and aims to improve the results achieved with the BraidStent® biodegradable bare stent [3]. Secondary endopoints are related to the evaluation the effect of the heparin coating on the degradation rate, the fragmentation size and excretion of the BraidStent®-H.

Methods

Twenty-four healthy female pigs were used in this study. The experimental protocol was approved by the Minimally Invasive Surgery Centre´s Ethical Committee for Animal Research (Reference:003/13). This Committee also certifies that the above-mentioned research study was carried out following the guidelines of the of the Animals used for scientific purposes (Directive 2010/63/EU-European Commision). The study was carried out in compliance with the ARRIVE guidelines.

Phase I: Baseline studies and ureteral stenting

Blood and urine samples were collected to assess blood and biochemical parameters and confirm urine sterility. The urine sample is collected by ultrasound-guided cystocentesis before administration of antibiotic prophylaxis. Next, nephrosonography was performed to assess the degree of upper collecting system dilatation [11] and alterations in the ureteral orifices and bladder trigone [12]. The urothelial alterations at the ureteral orifice and bladder trigone were assessed endoscopically, and categorised according to a validated UOScore (UO_0: normal ureteral orifice; UO_1: enlarged ureteral orifice with light surrounding inflammatory reaction; UO_2: enlarged ureteral orifice with moderate surrounding inflammatory reaction; UO_3: enlarged ureteral orifice with severe surrounding inflammatory and cystic reaction) [3, 6, 12]. Serum urea and creatinine levels were measured during all study phases.

Simulated voiding cystourethrography (SVCUG) was performed to evaluate VUR at baseline, and at 1, 3, 6, 8 and 12 weeks after ureteral stenting, with a final follow-up at 20 weeks. To perform SVCUG, a Foley catheter was inserted into the urinary bladder and filled. To simulate micturition, the bladder was manually compressed until the pressure reached 50 cm H_2O for 60 s [3, 6, 12].

Afterwards, excretory urography (EU) was performed to assess upper urinary tract morphology and evaluate ureteral peristalsis under fluoroscopic control (the frequency of ureteral peristalsis from renal pelvis to urinary bladder was evaluated for each animal; waves/min). Finally, the internal lumen of the right ureteropelvic junction (UPJ) was measured by retrograde ureteropyelography to accurately determine the UPJ diameter.

Animals were simple randomization distributed into two homogeneous groups:

Group-I: A 5Fr, 22 cm polymeric ureteral double pigtail stent was placed during a 6-week period (Universa® Soft, 22 cm, Cook® Medical). (Control group).
Group-II: A new self-retaining, anti-reflux and biodegradable stent, BraidStent-H, was placed using the transurethral approach by sliding over a guide under fluoroscopy control. The placement technique is the same as for conventional stents, with the exception that the pusher is pushed into the ureter. BraidStent®-H is an intra-ureteral stent (14 cm length) designed as follows: proximal end with a 3 cm pigtail with an internal channel; a 9 cm-long central section; a four-thread braided section that was 3Fr in diameter; and a distal anchoring system with a rounded edge four-thread basket that measures 2 cm in length and is 36Fr when expanded [3, 6]. Two biodegradable copolymers with different degradation times were used. Polymer-I was Glycomer-631 and polymer-II was pure polyglycolic acid (PGA) [3, 6]. Polymer-II was only used for the central section and was braided with polymer-I. The distal and proximal anchoring systems were manufactured exclusively with polymer-I because it has better biomechanical characteristics and a slower degradation time. This feature allows the stent to remain in place

for 3–6 weeks. The BraidStent®-H was designed to avoid passing through the ureterovesical junction (UVJ) to prevent bladder trigone irritation and VUR [3, 6] (Fig. 1).

The Heparin coating of the BraidStent®-H is carried out using the "dip coating" technique. The stents are completely immersed in aluminium containers with sodium heparin with a concentration of 5000 UI/ml (Heparin Hospira 5%, Pfizer Inc, NY, US), in order to be dried afterwards in an oven at 60°C for 2 h. After this process, each BraidStent®-H has 233 mg of heparin coating. In in vitro studies, we were able to determine the release over time of heparin by the BraidStent-H. The presence and concentration of heparin were analysed by means of an ELISA kit: Human Heparin Sodium ELISA kit MBS3802043MYBIOSOURCE. The heparin coating of the BraidStent®-H starts its release at the beginning of the contact with the urine and is released mainly in the first 72 h.

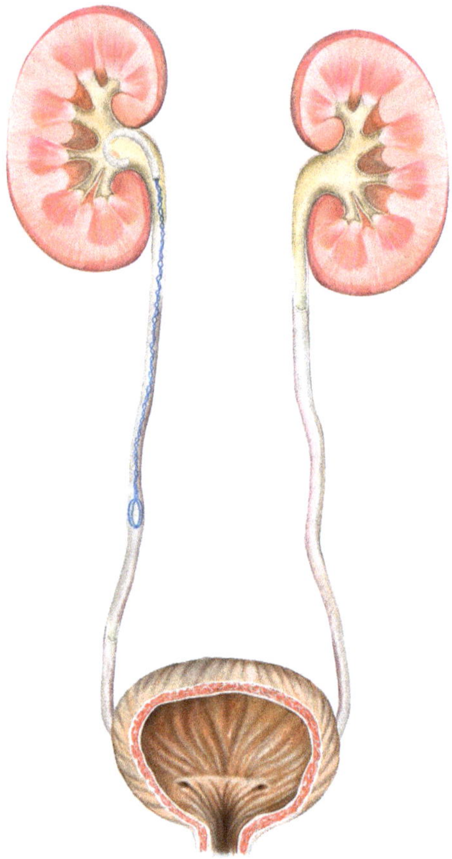

Fig. 1 Illustration of the BraidStent®-H in upper urinary tract

The onset of asymptomatic bacteriuria was assessed during the first 48 h post-stenting in both study groups in order to evaluate the heparin coating's ability to inhibit early bacterial colonisation. A urine sample was therefore obtained from the animals by ultrasound-guided cystocentesis at the 0, 3, 6, 12, 24 and 48-h study points. The CFU/ml number of the sample was determined and samples were considered positive for bacteriuria if there was growth ($>10^5$ cfu/ml) (Table 1). All study animals received antibiotic prophylactic treatment with enrofloxacin on the previous day and 2 days after every study phase.

Follow-ups

Follow-ups were performed at 1 (Phase-II), 3 (Phase-III) and 6 weeks (Phase-IV), which correspond to ureteral stent removal in Group-I, and at 8 (Phase-V) and 12 weeks (Phase-VI), using the same diagnostic procedures described above (Table 2).

Phase VII: Final follow-up: imaging and pathological assessment

The final follow-up was performed at 20 weeks and included ultrasonography, cystoscopy, ureteroscopy and contrast fluoroscopy assessment. The animal study was completed by removing the urinary tract *en bloc* for blind pathological analysis. Histological slices were obtained from proximal ureters, the ureteral segment where the distal end of BraidStent®-H was placed, and ureteral orifices/bladder trigone. A validated healing score was used, and each parameter was graded according to the following scores: 0: no histopathological changes; 1: mild; 2: moderate; 3: severe [3, 6, 12] (Table 3).

Statistical analysis

SPSS 22.0 program was used for statistical analysis. To determine the sample size, a hypothesis contrast was performed (the means were compared); a total of 12

Table 1 Early bacteriuria

Group/% animals with bacteriuria	0 h	1 h	3 h	6 h	12 h	24 h	48 h
Group-I	0	50	58.3	100*	100*	100	100
Group-II	0	41.6	50	50*	50*	66.6	100

*$p<0.05$, Group-I versus Group-II. 6 h and 12 h

Table 2 Results summary

	Groups	Baseline	1 weeks	3 weeks	6 weeks	8 weeks	12 weeks	20 weeks	Significant
Ultrasound Mode B (SFU score) (G_0-G_4)	G-I	G_0-12	G_0-1 G_1-4 G_2-5 G_3-2	G_0-0 G_1-5 G_2-7	G_0-1 G_1-6 G_2-2 G_3-3	G_0-6 G_1-5 G_2-1	G_0-12	G_0-11 G_1-1	3 weeks*
	G-II	G_0-12	G_0-2 G_1-5 G_2-4 G_3-1	G_0-3 G_1-7 G_2-2	G_0-3 G_1-7 G_2-2	G_0-12	G_0-10 G_1-2	G_0-12	
Proximal ureter (diameter. mm)	G-I	6.7±0.5	24.6±3.0	20.8±1.4	16.3±1.2	13.1±1.8	10.9±0.7	8.8±1.2	
	G-II	5.9±0.6	13.7±3.0	16.1±1.3	17.6±1.3	14.7±1.8	12.5±0.7	10.1±1.2	
Bacteriuria (Animals)	G-I	0	2	2	6	N.A	N.A	N.A	
	G-II	0	3	5	8	N.A	N.A	N.A	
Migration	G-I	N.A	2	2	0	N.A	N.A	N.A	
	G-II	N.A	2	3	0	N.A	N.A	N.A	
VUR Score	G-I	G_0-12	G_0-10 G_1-2	G_0-7 G_1-5	G_0-4 G_1-6 G_2-2	G_0-10 G_1-2	G_0-10 G_1-2	G_0-11 G_1-1	3–6 weeks*
	G-II	G_0-12	G_0-12	G_0-12	G_0-12	G_0-12	G_0-12	G_0-12	
Ureteral orifice Score (UOScore)	G-I	UO_0-12	UO_0-1 UO_1-4 UO_2-5 UO_3-2	UO_0-0 UO_1-2 UO_2-8 UO_3-2	UO_0-0 UO_1-4 UO_2-5 UO_3-3	UO_0-3 UO_1-5 UO_2-3 UO_3-1	UO_0-8 UO_1-2 UO_2-2 UO_3-0	UO_0-10 UO_1-2 UO_2-0 UO_3-0	1–3–6–8 weeks*
	G-II	UO_0-12	UO_0-11 UO_1-1	UO_0-11 UO_1-1	UO_0-12	UO_0-12	UO_0-12	UO_0-12	
Ureteral peristalsis (% animals)	G-I	100	0	0	0	100	100	100	1–3–6 weeks*
	G-II	100	66.6	58.3	75	100	100	100	

*$p < 0.005$

Table 3 Histological score

Group/ureteral segment	Urothelial resurfacing	Mural inflammation	Lamina propia fibrosis	Integrity of muscular layer	Serosal alterations	0–3
Group-I-Upper ureter	0.85	0.77	0.31	1.31	0.15	0.67±0.41
Group-II-Upper ureter	0.85	0.54	0.08	1.08	0	0.51±0.42
Group-I-UVJ	2.00	1.38*	0.85	0.69	0	0.98±0.67
Group-II-UVJ	1.01	0.62*	0.77	0.46	0	0.57±0.33

*$p < 0.05$, Group-I-UVJ versus Group-II-UVJ. Mural inflammation

animals per group were obtained (0.05 level of significance and 90% statistical power). Normal distribution of variables was confirmed using the Kolmogorov–Smirnov test. Parametric variables were assessed using repeated measures analysis of variance. Categorical variables are expressed as percentages. Comparison between groups of categorical variables were analysed using Fisher's exact test, and evolution over the course of the study was analysed with McNemar's test.

Results

Phase I: Baseline studies and ureteral stenting

Bacteriuria determinations during the first 48 h shown statistical significance between groups was found at 6 and

12 h, which shows a bacteriuria delaying effect in Group-II caused by the heparin coating. Positive bacteriuria did not reach 100% of animals in Group-II until 48 h, compared with Group-I, in which it appeared at 6 h (Table 1).

No animals showed alterations in the urinary tract or bacteriuria in basal studies. No complications arose during stent placement in any of the groups (Table 2).

Phase II

A ureteral non-obstructive polypoid growth at the distal end of BraidStent®-H was found in 100% of Group-II animals. Ureteral peristalsis was inhibited in Group-I, and 66.6% of animals in Group-II maintained peristalsis at the distal ureter with statistical significance. Significance was also observed in the evolution of tissue damage at the bladder trigone between groups assessed by UOScore. The most severe damage was found in Group-I (Table 2).

Phase III

Mild urothelial polypoid growth remained in 100% of animals in Group-II at the distal end of the stent. Overall, 27% of BraidStent®-H showed macroscopic partial degradation, especially of the PGA polymer. Small fragments in the urinary bladder and decolouration of BraidStent®-H components were observed. A higher degree of hydroureteronephrosis in Group-I was noted in this follow-up. No statistical significance regarding stent migration between groups was found; however, this was observed regarding UOScore assessment, and greater damage was found in Group-I.

Phase IV

Overall, 91.7% of BraidStent®-H were completely degraded (Fig. 2). Non-obstructive polypoid growth associated with the BraidStent®-H distal end disappeared. The only exception was the stent, which had not yet fully degraded, 8.3%.

Phase V

The only partially degraded BraidStent®-H completed degradation and its fragments were eliminated in urine. All study animals recovered ureteral peristalsis. No ureteroscopic evidence of the polypoid growth, found during the early phases in Group-II, was observed. Overall, 100% of animals in Group-II and 50% in Group-I did not show any dilatation of the upper urinary tract after nephrosonographic assessment. Although 2 weeks passed after double pigtail stent removal, statistical significance between groups was observed; with Group-I showed greater macroscopic vesical damage.

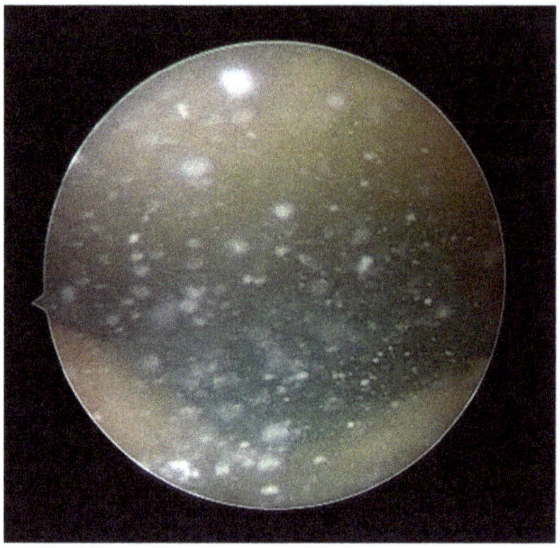

Fig. 2 Cystoscopic view of the floating tiny BraidStent®-H fragments at 6 weeks

Phase VI

Ureteral internal diameters, hydronephrosis degree and ureteral peristalsis did not show any statistical significance after 12 weeks in both groups versus baselines values. Nevertheless, statistical significance regarding the assessment of urothelial damage at vesical level between groups was still observed.

End-of-study evaluation

The final follow-up showed the recovery of basal values in all parameters assessed, except for one animal in Group-I, which showed low degree VUR. Statistical significance was only found in lamina propria inflammation of UVJ between groups, after pathological assessment of the ureteral wall and UVJ; Group-I showed greater histological damage (Table 3). The evaluation of the location of the distal end of the BraidStent®-H showed no changes in the ureteral wall.

Discussion

In the search for an ideal ureteral stent, its biodegradation ability to avoid a new procedure for removal is one of the requirements which have not yet been achieved. BUS not only avoid removal, but also have a series of important advantages, such as the reduction of patient anxiety, since they know they will not need further outpatient cystoscopy stent removal; being cost-saving for the health system; avoiding anaesthetic procedures in paediatric patients; and, last but not least, avoiding the syndrome of forgotten stent [3, 13, 14].

Therefore, several research groups have assessed different BUS prototypes in animal model in the last decade

[4, 5, 15, 16]. This research obtained encouraging, but inconclusive results, mainly due to the limitations of experimental studies and the scarce number of animals involved in the studies. A research group with a higher number of BUS-assessed animal models, 36 stents, and with a longer follow-up period (5 months) evaluated the BraidStent® [3, 6, 12]. This biodegradable intraureteral stent shows a limitation due to its high asymptomatic bacteriuria rate, which is up to 41.6%. However, it has shown a predictable degradation rate and non-obstructive stent fragmentation.

The use of heparin for stent coating and to prevent bacterial adhesion, avoiding biofilm and incrustation formation, was previously assessed in depth [7, 8, 17]. Heparin is useful because it has a high negative charge which provides it an important bacterial anti-adhesive effect. However, in an in vitro study, Lange et al. [9] found that the heparin coating did not decrease bacterial adhesion, although they initially obtained encouraging results.

Comparative results of the current experimental study confirm that the heparin coating shows statistical significance regarding bacteriuria between groups, from the sixth hour post-stenting. Asymptomatic bacteriuria did not affect 100% of animals in the BraidStent®-H group until 48 h compared with standard ureteral stents, which showed positive bacteriuria at 6 h. Therefore, heparin coating shows differences compared to a standard stent, although it does not have a significant antibacterial effect, and it also fulfils the purpose for which it was used in this study: to avoid bacterial colonisation at stent placement. BraidStent®-H, unlike other heparin-coated stents, is designed so that the coating disappears within the first 72 h and does not affect the stent degradation rate [7, 8]. In previous in vitro and in in vivo studies by other researchers' evaluated stents incorporate heparin inside of the polyurethane matrix rather than a heparin coating [7, 8, 17]. Consequently, heparin release is scarce and may hamper the prevention of bacterial adhesion [17]. This is an important difference to our coating technique, as our heparin coating is designed to be released in the early days of stenting. Research into a coating that prevents bacterial adhesion is extremely complicated, since bacteria utilise a multitude of mechanisms for surfaces attaching, which are specific to bacterial species [9].

The intermediate follow-ups in Group-II at 1, 3 and 6 weeks were disappointed (25% in the first week, 41.6% in the third week and 66.6% in the sixth week, with a 44.4% study average), despite the initial bacteriuria rate decreasing. This means a setback of the heparin coating in this formulation to reduce bacteriuria in the long-term. Different factors need to be considered in order to discuss these results. Firstly, it is necessary to compare them with other results described in clinical trials evaluating 30–60 days of standard ureteral stenting: 21.9% [18], 24.3% [10], 23.6% [19], 28% [20], 45.8% [21]. In this regard, our positive asymptomatic bacteriuria rate was within an elevated range: BraidStent®-H values were 1.5–2 times higher than the bacteriuria rate, except for in the study by Shabeena (45.8%) [21]. Nevertheless, a second, very important factor must be considered in order to critically assess these unsatisfactory results. When assessing a BUS, stent fragments carry the biofilm which covers all ureteral stents and causes the bacteria embedded in the biofilm to become free or results in planktonic bacteria in the urine by breaking the integrity of the biofilm. Consequently, if our results are compared with scientific literature on the bacterial colonisation of ureteral stents with a similar stenting time (29.4% [22], 42% [20], 46.2% [21], 58.6% [23], 82.9% [10], 98.5% [20], 100% [24]), experimental values are not as high as they initially seemed to be, since they take into account the continuous fragmentation of the biofilm layer. One final factor could explain these disappointing, asymptomatic bacteriuria results: all study animals were females. Several authors have reported that women can double the likelihood of ureteral stent colonisation, due to the length of their urethra [25]. Gender is not considered in any of the percentages described in the above-mentioned clinical trials.

However, is obviously necessary to study the control of asymptomatic bacteriuria in BUS in greater depth, in order to avoid possible urinary tract infections (UTI) with these new ureteral stent designs. In previous experimental studies assessing other BUS designs, high variability and methodologies were found. Thus, there are BUS in which bacteriuria is not evaluated [4], or others in which the placement of the stent is by cystotomy, which produces a great bias to evaluate the bacterial colonization of the BUS [5, 15, 26]. Others assess urinary infection only by determining WBCs in urine, but this assesment is not comparable to the appropriate protocol for assessing colonisation, such as measurement of bacteriuria, urine culture or stent culture [5, 27, 28]. In two studies of the same research group, researchers found that after evaluating their BUS, Uriprene®, in a pig model, different results were found with higher positive urine cultures in biostable stents in one study and in the other slightly higher positive cultures in BUS [16, 29]. Therefore, at present, due to high variability in the studies and designs evaluated, it is not possible to conclude whether BUSs favour urinary bacterial contamination.

With regard to the other properties evaluated in the comparative study, BraidStent®-H shows a similar passive dilatation at the proximal ureter, although there is a less hydronephrotic effect, with significance noted after 3 weeks. We have shown that BraidStent®-H will predictably decrease patient discomfort due to its design, as it keeps ureteral peristalsis below the stent, with significance in the first, third and sixth weeks. Other factors that predict less discomfort in patients are the absence of VUR and less macroscopic damage at the bladder trigone (UOScore), as shown by the statistical significance of the study [2]. The preservation of peristalsis, absence of VUR and absence of ureteral stent in the distal ureter should avoid the onset of ureteral spasms in patients at the ureteral segment with a higher density of nerve fibers [30]. On the other hand, as shown by the results of UOScore and pathological UVJ assessment between groups, and as also demonstrated by Yoshida et al. [31] in a study of patients, an intra-ureteral stent was associated with less bladder discomfort than a standard ureteral stent.

Degradation rate control is one of the major challenges to the clinical use of BUS. Our study shows the BraidStent®-H unlike other evaluated BUS showed a predictable degradation rate despite its heparin coating [4, 5, 27, 29]. Furthermore, degradation fragments were easily eliminated, finding that in others BUS experimental studies triggered problems, with small fragments in the upper tract and embedded in the ureteral wall [5, 26]. The positive results of BraidStent®-H in this regard are due to its braided design, which produced very small fragments, as well as the choice of polymers with different degradation rates, which allowed the progressive stent hydrolysis.

The current weaknesses of the BraidStent®-H are linked to asymptomatic bacteriuria rates and migration rates. We only found a slight dislodgement of the proximal end. However, this provided information on a small structural weakness in the BraidStent®-H proximal tip. Since BraidStent®-H is an intraureteral stent, dislodgment in placement or early migration implies a technical challenge for urologists.

Study limitations are intrinsic to the animal model, as it is obviously not possible to develop any kind of USSQ questionnaire in order to assess degree of discomfort in study subjects. On the other hand, SVCUG was used for VUR assessment instead of voiding cystourethrography. Finally, it is difficult to evaluate whether daily changes of pH in humans can modify the BraidStent-H degradation rate, as animals follow a controlled diet. Despite the encouraging results, further studies will be required to determine whether the use and safety of BUS with changing urinary pH conditions in patients allows adequate control in the rate of BUS degradation.

Conclusions

The heparin coating of BraidStent® allows an early decrease in urinary bacterial colonization, but its effectiveness is low at the long term. The heparin coating did not affect the scheduled degradation rate or the size of the stent fragments. The BraidStent®-H avoids the side effects associated with current ureteral stents, and should therefore cause less discomfort to patients. However, further studies will be needed to improve the anchoring system and reduce the risk of bacterial colonisation.

Abbreviations

VUR: Vesico-ureteral reflux; BUS: Biodegradable ureteral stent; UOScore: Ureteral orifice score; SVCUG: Simulated voiding cystourethrography; EU: Excretory urography; UPJ: Ureteropelvic junction; UVJ: Ureterovesical junction; PGA: Poliglicolic acid; CFU: Colony forming unit; UTI: Urinary tract infection; WBCs: White blood cells.

Acknowledgements

Special gratefulness to Fernanda Carrizosa for her generous support during the performance of this manuscript and Paula Martín Rodríguez and María Pérez Vela for the BraidStent illustrations.

Authors' contributions

FS: project development, data collection, data analysis, manuscript writing, and editing. Principal Investigator; JEdLC: data collection, data analysis, manuscript writing; JPC-R: data collection, data analysis; MP: data collection, data analysis; DP-F: data collection, data analysis; LR-F: data collection, data analysis; FMS-M: data collection. All authors read and approved the final manuscript.

Competing interests

The authors declare that they have no competing interests.

Author details

[1] Endoscopy-Endourology Department, Jesús Usón Minimally Invasive Surgery Centre Foundation, Carretera N-521, Km. 41.8, C.P.10071 Cáceres, Spain. [2] Endoscopy-Endourology Department, Jesús Usón Minimally Invasive Surgery Centre Foundation, Cáceres, Spain. [3] Urology Department, Alicante University General Hospital, Alicante Institute for Health and Biomedical Research (ISABIAL Foundation), Alicante, Spain. [4] Urology Department, 12 de Octubre University Hospital, Madrid, Spain. [5] University Hospital Santiago de Compostela, Santiago de Compostela, Spain. [6] Urology Department, University Hospital Clínico San Carlos, Madrid, Spain. [7] Jesús Usón Minimally Invasive Surgery Centre Foundation, Cáceres, Spain.

References

1. Sali GM, Joshi HB. Ureteric stents: overview of current clinical applications and economic implications. Int J Urol. 2020;27:7–15.
2. Giannarini G, Keeley FX Jr, Valent F, Manassero F, Mogorovich A, Autorino R, Selli C. Predictors of morbidity in patients with indwelling ureteric stents: results of a prospective study using the validated ureteric stent symptoms questionnaire. BJU Int. 2011;107:648–54.
3. Soria F, de la Cruz JE, Budia A, Serrano A, Galán-Llopis JA, Sánchez-Margallo FM. Experimental assessment of new generation of ureteral stents: biodegradable and antireflux properties. J Endourol. 2020;34:359–65.
4. Barros AA, Oliveira C, Ribeiro AJ, Autorino R, Reis RL, Duarte ARC, Lima E. In vivo assessment of a novel biodegradable ureteral stent. World J Urol. 2018;36:277–83.
5. Jin L, Yao L, Zhou Y, Dai G, Zhang W, Xue B. Investigation of a novel gradient degradable ureteral stent in a beagle dog model. J Biomater Appl. 2018;33:466–73.
6. Soria F, Morcillo E, Serrano A, Budia A, Fernández I, Fernández-Aparicio T, Sánchez-Margallo FM. Evaluation of a novel design of antireflux-biodegradable ureteral stent in animal model. Urology. 2018;115:59–64.
7. Ruggieri MR, Hanno PM, Levin RM. Reduction of bacterial adherence to catheter surface with heparin. J Urol. 1987;138:423–6.
8. Cauda F, Cauda V, Fiori C, Onida B, Garrone E. Heparin coating on ureteral double J stents prevents encrustations: an in vivo case study. J Endourol. 2008;22:465–72.
9. Lange D, Elwood CN, Choi K, Hendlin K, Monga M, Chew BH. Uropathogen interaction with the surface of urological stents using different surface properties. J Urol. 2009;182:1194–200.

10. Zhang JM, Liu J, Wang K, Zhang X, Zhao T, Luo HM. Observations of bacterial biofilm on ureteral stent and studies on the distribution of pathogenic bacteria and drug resistance. Urol Int. 2018;101:320–6.
11. Fernbach SK, Maizels M, Conway JJ. Ultrasound grading of hydronephrosis: introduction to the system used by the Society for fetal Urology. Pediatr Radiol. 1993;23:478–80.
12. Soria F, Morcillo E, de la Cruz JE, Serrano A, Estebanez J, Sanz JL, Chicharro J, Pamplona M, Sánchez FM. Antireflux ureteral stent proof of concept assessment after minimally invasive treatment of obstructive uropathy in animal model. Arch Esp Urol. 2018;71:607–13.
13. Acosta-Miranda AM, Milner J, Turk TM. The FECal double-J: a simplified approach in the management of encrustated and retained ureteral stents. J Endourol. 2009;23:409–15.
14. Sancaktutar AA, Söylemez H, Bozkurt Y, Penbegül N, Atar M. Treatment of forgotten ureteral stents: how much does it really cost? A cost-effective study in 27 patients. Urol Res. 2012;40:317–25.
15. Zhang MQ, Zou T, Huang YC, Shang YF, Yang GG, Wang WZ, Zhou JM, Wang L, Chen F, Xie H. Braided thin-walled biodegradable ureteral stent: preliminary evaluation in a canine model. Int J Urol. 2014;21:401–7.
16. Chew BH, Paterson RF, Clinkscales KW, Levine BS, Shalaby SW, Lange D. In vivo evaluation of the third generation biodegradable stent: a novel approach to avaoiding the forgotten stent syndrome. J Urol. 2013;189:719–25.
17. Riedl CR, Witkowski M, Plas E, Pfluefer H. Heparin coating reduces encrustation of ureteral stents: a preliminary report. Int J Antimicrob Agents. 2002;19:507–10.
18. Weber A, Zumstein V, Betschart P, Nolte O, Engeler DS, Schmid HP, Güsewell S, Abt D. Prediction of bacteriuria based on clinical or laboratory parameters in patients with indwelling ureteral stents before ureterorenoscopy should not substitute for urine cultures. J Endourol. 2018;32:739–45.
19. Klis R, Korczak-Kozakiewicz E, Denys A, Sosnowski M, Rozanski W. Relationship between urinary tract infection and self-retaining double-J catheter colonization. J Endourol. 2009;23:1015–9.
20. Kehinde EO, Rotimi VO, Al-Hunayan A, Abdul-Halim H, Boland Al-Awadi KA. Bacteriology of urinary tract infection associated with indwelling J ureteral stents. J Endourol. 2004;18:891–6.
21. Shabeena KS, Bhargava R, Manzoor MAP, Mujeeburahiman M. Characteristics of a bacterial colonization after indwelling double-J ureteral stents for different time duration. Urol Ann. 2018;10:71–5.
22. Akay AF, Aflay U, Gedik A, Sahin H, Bircan MK. Risks factors for lower urinary tract infection and bacterial stent colonization in patients with a double J ureteral stent. Int Urol Nephrol. 2007;39:95–8.
23. Farsih HM, Mosli HA, Al-Zemaity MF, Bahnassy AA, Álvarez M. Bacteriuria and colonization of double-pigtail ureteral stens. Long-term experience with 237 patients. J Endourol. 1995;9:469–72.
24. Riedl CR, Plas E, Hübner WA, Zimmerl H, Ulrich W, Pflüger H. Bacterial colonization of ureteral stents. Eur Urol. 1999;36:53–9.
25. Kehinde EO, Rotimi VO, Al-Awadi KA, Abdul-Halim H, Boland F, Al-Hunayan A, Pazhoor A. Factors predisposing to urinary tract infection after J ureteral stent insertion. J Urol. 2002;167:1334–7.
26. Lumiaho J, Heino A, Kauppinen T, Talja M, Alhava E, Valima T, Tormala P. Drainage and antireflux characteristics of a biodegradable self-reinforced, self-expanding X-ray-positive poly-L, D-lactide spiral partial ureteral stent: an experimental study. J Endourol. 2007;21:1559–64.
27. Wang X, Shan H, Wang J, Ding J, Chen Q, Guan J, Wang C, Chen X. Characterization of nanostructured ureteral stent with gradient degradation in a porcine model. Int J Nanomed. 2015;10:3055–64.
28. Jin L, Yao L, Yuan F, Dai G, Xue B. Evaluation of a novel biodegradable ureteral stent produced from polyurethane and magnesium alloys. J Biomed Mater Res B Appl Biomater. 2020. https://doi.org/10.1002/jbm.b.34730.
29. Hadaschik BA, Paterson RF, Fazli L, Clinkscales KW, Shalaby SW, Chew BH. Investigation of a novel degradable ureterl stent in a porcine model. J Urol. 2008;180:1161–6.
30. Vernez SL, Okhunov Z, Wikenheiser J, Khoyilar C, Dutta R, Osann K, Kaler K, Lee TK, Clayman RV, Landmand J. Precise characterization and three-dimensional reconstruction of the autonomic nerve distribution of the human ureter. J Urol. 2017;197:723–9.
31. Yoshida T, Inoue T, Taguchi M, Matsuzaki T, Murota T, Kinoshita H, Matsuda T. Efficacy and safety of complete intraureteral stent placement versus conventional stent placement in relieving ureteral stent related symp toms: a randomized, prospective, single blind, multicenter clinical trial. J Urol. 2019;202:164–70.

28

Bulbar urethrocavernous fistula in setting of inflatable penile prosthesis

Hannah Botkin*, Brian Barnes and Amy Pearlman

Abstract

Background: Urethral injury or erosion of an inflatable penile prosthetic (IPP) cylinder is a rare complication of IPP placement. It can present with varying symptoms and management can be difficult with risk for future complications.

We present a patient with an eroded IPP who developed a secondary contralateral urethrocavernous fistula requiring repeat urethroplasty. We also describe the literature surrounding these complications and strategies to prevent them.

Case presentation: A 69-year-old man with poorly controlled diabetes presented to our clinic with 6 months of intermittent white urethral discharge first noted after IPP removal and replacement by an outside urologist for device malfunction. Office cystoscopy revealed an eroded right-sided prosthetic cylinder in the bulbar urethra. The patient was taken to the operating room for IPP explantation with closure of right corporal defect, left sided malleable prosthesis placement, and primary excision with anastomosis of his bulbar urethra. A catheter was left in place for two weeks postoperatively, at which time a peri-catheter retrograde urethrogram was performed which showed no evidence of contrast extravasation and his catheter was subsequently removed. Several months later, he presented with recurrent urethral discharge without evidence of recurrent erosion on cystoscopy with development of scrotal abscesses following office cystoscopy, concerning for an unidentified urethral defect. He returned to the operating room for scrotal exploration and was noted on cystoscopy to have a pinpoint fistula between his left corporal body and his bulbar urethra. He underwent left sided malleable prosthetic explant, and non-transecting bulbar urethroplasty. Peri-catheter retrograde urethrogram two weeks later showed no contrast extravasation and he has had no recurrence of urethral discharge or scrotal abscesses since.

Conclusions: Urethral erosion and urethrocavernous fistula formation are rare complications of penile prosthesis placement. Risks are elevated in patients with corporal fibrosis, diabetes, those undergoing penile implant revision surgery, and those requiring prolonged urethral catheterization.

Keywords: Urethrocavernous fistula, Inflatable penile prosthesis, Urethroplasty

Background

Surgical placement of inflatable (IPP) or malleable penile prostheses (MPP) continue to be a viable option for the definitive management of erectile dysfunction (ED). The long-term reliability, as well as patient satisfaction, of these devices is generally high [1], but are not without risk of intraoperative or postoperative complication. Intraoperatively, the urethra may be injured at time of corporotomy or corporal dilation [2]. Post-operatively, risks include infection, device malfunction, and/or erosion. Risk of surgical complications are elevated in those with prior procedures, diabetes, smoking, and/or prior radiation [3].

Urethrocavernous fistula has been reported in patients with a history of proximal corporospongiosal shunt for priapism [4], injury during sexual activity [5], blunt penile trauma [6], or even spontaneously presenting

*Correspondence: hannah-botkin@uiowa.edu
University of Iowa Hospitals and Clinics, 200 Hawkins Drive, Iowa City, IA 52242, USA

with urethral bleeding [7], but has most commonly been reported after penile prosthetic surgery [3].

Here, we present a patient who experienced a rare complication of urethrocavernous fistula involving his bulbar urethra after prior IPP revision surgery.

Case presentation

A 69-year-old African American male with hypertension, hyperlipidemia, chronic obstructive pulmonary disease, type 2 diabetes (hemoglobin A1C 8.4%) presented to our clinic with approximately six months of intermittent white urethral discharge which began shortly after penoscrotal IPP removal and replacement by an outside urologist for prior IPP malfunction. No operative note was available for review. The discharge did not change in quantity after ejaculation or intercourse and was not associated with any urinary symptoms. Testing for sexually transmitted diseases by local urologist was negative. Clinic cystoscopy revealed an eroded right sided IPP cylinder involving the bulbar urethra (Fig. 1).

The patient was taken to the operating room for removal of all IPP components through a penoscrotal incision. Erosion of the right IPP cylinder was confirmed by visualizing a 0.5 cm defect into the right lateral aspect of the bulbar urethra (Fig. 2). A transecting excision and primary anastomosis (EPA) urethroplasty was then performed in the area of urethral erosion through a perineal incision. The corporal defect was closed separately. A14 French foley catheter was left in place with plans to remain in place for two weeks postoperatively. A 21 cm malleable prosthesis was placed in the left corpora (purposely undersized by 1 cm to avoid distal erosion).

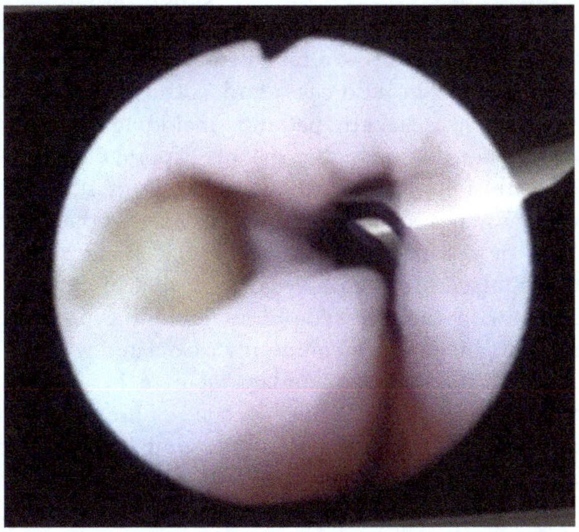

Fig. 1 Urethrocavernous fistula as seen via cystoscopy (inflatable penile implant cylinder seen eroding into bulbar urethra at time of initial surgery with our team)

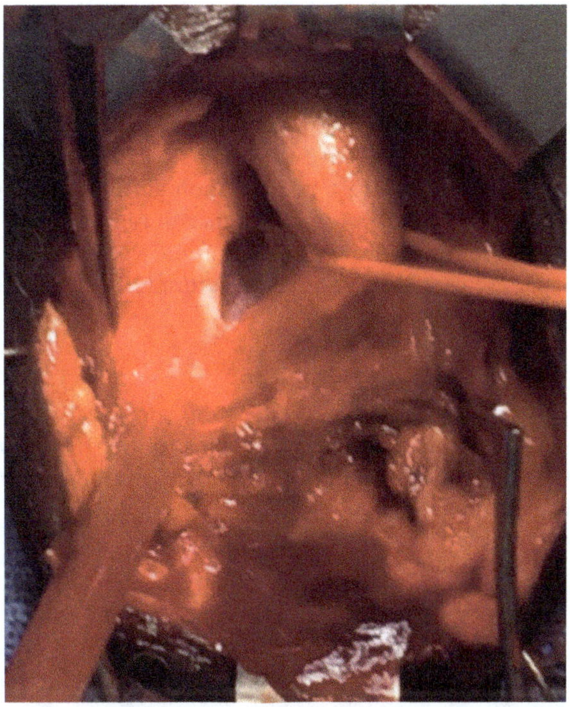

Fig. 2 Urethrocavernous fistula within perineal incision after removal of right inflatable penile implant cylinder at time of initial surgery with our team

A peri-catheter retrograde urethrogram (RUG) was performed 2 weeks postoperatively, which showed no evidence of contrast extravasation, and his catheter was removed. Six months postoperatively, he returned to clinic with continued urethral discharge and pain at the tip of his penis. Physical exam was concerning for impending MPP distal erosion. Office cystoscopy at that time showed a well-healed urethral anastomosis without visualization of the unilateral MPP cylinder, recurrent urethral erosion, or fistula. It was recommended that he undergo MPP explant (given concerns for impending distal erosion) but his surgery was delayed due to the COVID-19 pandemic in the context of his medical comorbidities.

Two weeks following office cystoscopy, the patient returned to clinic with new scrotal drainage and pain. Exam revealed an area of fluctuance concerning for scrotal abscess for which he underwent incision and drainage in clinic with evacuation of purulent material and clear fluid. He was prescribed antibiotics and scheduled for scrotal incision and drainage, MPP explant, and possible urethroplasty for presumed urethrocavernous fistula.

Intraoperative urethroscopy showed a pinpoint opening in the left bulbar urethra concerning for fistulous tract which was able to be cannulated with a wire (Fig. 3). Perineal exploration confirmed the wire exiting the bulbar urethra and entering the adjacent left corporal body (Fig. 4). The fistulous tract was excised and a non-transecting bulbar urethroplasty was performed. Two-week post-operative peri-catheter RUG showed no evidence of contrast extravasation and the catheter was removed. There was no evidence of recurrent scrotal abscess on exam. Despite multiple complications, the patient remains interested in future IPP placement.

Discussion and conclusions

This case illustrates multiple rare complications of penile prosthesis placement: bulbar urethral IPP cylinder erosion and secondary contralateral urethrocavernous fistula development.

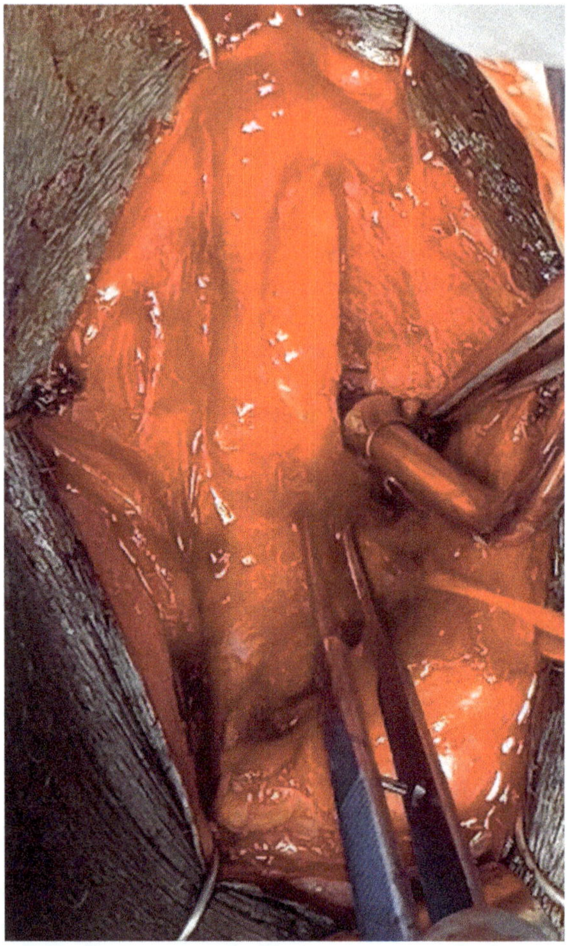

Fig. 3 Urethrocavernous fistula. Tip of suction tip denotes fistulous tract between the bulbar urethra and the left corporal body (at time of second surgery with our team)

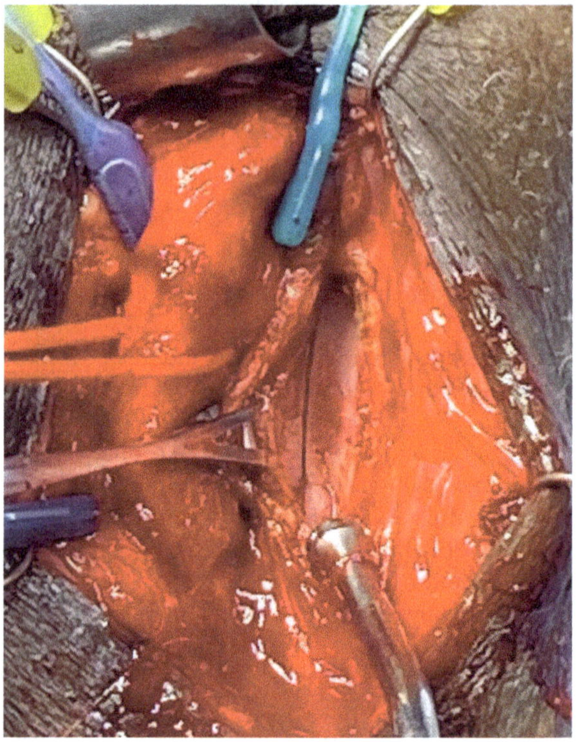

Fig. 4 Urethrocavernous fistula. Wire used to cannulate urethral fistula is noted entering left corporal body (as seen after left corporotomy is made) and left malleable implant has been removed (at time of second surgery with our team)

The overall rate of reoperation for penile prosthesis procedures approaches 15% after 10 years but is highest in the first year after surgery [8]. African-American, Hispanic, and younger men have a higher risk of reoperation. In regards to his first complication, device erosion more commonly involves the distal penile urethra. Rates of erosion range from 1 to 11% and are more common in redo cases and in those with corporal fibrosis [3]. Diabetic patients, including the patient reported here, are at higher risk of corporal fibrosis.

Urethral injury is a rare complication of IPP placement. When recognized intraoperatively, the injury should be repaired and prosthetic placement aborted. Unrecognized urethral injury can present months after surgery with variable symptoms, including prosthetic infection, and is more commonly associated with MPP than IPP. Though the standard of care in suspected intraoperative urethral injury is repair of urethral injury and aborting prosthesis placement, some have reported placing a prosthetic cylinder in the non-injured side [2]. Some have even performed suprapubic cystotomy to proceed with prosthesis placement after a urethral injury is detected [9] but these reports are rare.

One unique aspect of this case is that the complications occurred proximally in the bulbar urethra. Urethral erosion is more likely to occur at the distal penis near the glans, where the two cavernosal bodies converge, and the prosthetic cylinders create pressure on the distal penile urethra [2]. This further suggests that our patient sustained an unrecognized proximal corporal and/or bulbar urethral injury during corporal dilation, or less likely corporotomy at the time of his redo IPP placement leading to device erosion into the bulbar urethra. Other possibilities include peri-operative infection resulting in erosion or less likely, friction from simply using the device as directed.

Given that his second urethral complication involved the contralateral corpora, we chose to refer to this as a secondary, de novo urethrocavernous fistula since failure of the initial repair would present ipsilaterally. Our patient required extended 2-week catheter drainage for healing of his initial urethroplasty at the time of unilateral MPP placement. We suspect the pressure from MPP while the catheter remained in place contributed to poor wound healing and eventual secondary contralateral fistula formation. His risk of poor healing was further elevated by poorly controlled diabetes. This fistula led to persistent urinary extravasation causing recurrent scrotal abscesses and glanular pain even though the fistula was too small to identify on office cystoscopy.

Urethrocavernous fistula is a rare complication of penile prosthesis placement. Urethral erosion and/or fistula has been reported in up to 80 % of patients with chronic indwelling or intermittent catheterization secondary to friction and inflammation [10]. Though our patient was not catheter dependent, he did require a catheter for postoperative urethral healing which likely increased his risk for fistula formation. We intentionally chose a small-bore (14 French), catheter as a larger catheter would increase pressure on the urethral repair, and possibly increase the risk of this complication. Given the risk of fistula formation in catheter-dependent patients, some have reported performing perineal urethrostomy or suprapubic cystotomy at the time of penile prosthesis surgery [11]. Caraceni et al. reported a case of urethrocavernous fistula with successful IPP replacement, primary repair of urethral and cavernosal defects augmented by the use of a dry layer of the human coagulation factors fibrinogen and thrombin [12]. Given the paucity of cases of urethral erosion and urethrocavernous fistula secondary to penile prosthesis, no standard of care has been established.

Urethral erosion and urethrocavernous fistula formation are rare complications of penile prosthesis placement. It is important understand that patients with corporal fibrosis, diabetes, redo prosthesis surgeries, and those requiring catheterization will be at elevated risk of recurrent and de novo urethral complications. Presenting symptoms of these complications vary (in this case, only symptom was persistent urethral discharge) and may require careful consideration to successfully diagnose and repair.

Abbreviations

IPP: Inflatable penile prosthetic; MPP: Malleable penile prostheses; EPA: Excision and primary anastomosis; RUG: Retrograde urethrogram.

Acknowledgements

Not applicable.

Authors' contributions

HB analyzed the patient data and wrote the preliminary draft, BB and AP provided expertise and edited the manuscript. All authors read and approved the final manuscript.

Competing interests

Amy Pearlman is a consultant for and receives grant funding from Boston Scientific.

References

1. Jorissen C, De Bruyna H, Baten E, Van Renterghem K. Clinical outcome: patient and partner satisfaction after penile implant surgery. Curr Urol. 2019;13(2):94–100.
2. Carlos EC, Sexton SJ, Lentz AC. Urethral injury and the penile prosthesis. Sex Med Rev. 2019;7(2):360–8.
3. Sadeghi-Nejad H. Penile prosthesis surgery: a review of prosthetic devices and associated complications. J Sex Med. 2007;4(2):296–309.
4. Manjunath AS, Mazur DJ, Han JS, Gonzalez CM. Simultaneous urethrocutaneous and urethrocavernous fistula after proximal corporospongiosal shunt for priapism. Urology. 2015;85(3):e13-4.
5. Motiwala HG. Urethrocavernous fistula following sexual intercourse. J Urol. 1993;149(2):371.
6. Palaniswamy R, Rao MS, Bapna BC, Chary KS. Urethro-cavernous fistula from blunt penile trauma. J Trauma. 1981;21(3):242–3.
7. Pearlman AM, Rukstalis DB, Terlecki RP. Diagnosis and treatment of urethrocavernous fistula presenting as urethral bleeding. Urology. 2018;120:e5.
8. Mirheydar H, Zhou T, Chang DC, Hsieh TC. Reoperation rates for penile prosthetic surgery. J Sex Med. 2016;13(1):129–33.
9. Anele UA, Le BV, Burnett AL. Suprapubic cystostomy for the management of urethral injuries during penile prosthesis implantation. Sex Med. 2014;2(4):178–81.
10. Hisasue S, Sato Y, Horita H, Adachi H, Suzuki N, Kato R, et al. Erosion of a penile prosthesis due to an indwelling urethral catheter as a late complication. Int J Urol. 2002;9(9):525–7.
11. Steidle CP, Mulcahy JJ. Erosion of penile prostheses: a complication of urethral catheterization. J Urol. 1989;142(3):736–9.
12. Caraceni E, Marronaro A, Leone L. Salvage procedure in case of urethrocavernous fistula after revision surgery for malfunctioning three-piece penile prosthesis. Case Rep Urol. 2016;2016:4179862.

29

Autologous fascial slings remain viable at long-term follow-up: A post cystectomy case report

Jacopo Durante[1*], Francesca Manassero[1], Tiziana Fidecicchi[1], Alessio Tognarelli[1], Tommaso Di Vico[1], Pinuccia Faviana[2] and Cesare Selli[1]

Abstract

Background: Autologous fascial slings (AFS) have been used for a very long time in the treatment of female stress urinary incontinence, but the introduction of synthetic mesh slings placed either retropubicallyor trans-obturator has decreased the need to harvest the autologous rectus muscle fascia, thus reducing invasiveness and operative time. However AFS are still indicated in complicated cases and re-interventions, and the FDA has underlined safety concerns over the use of surgical meshes for the transvaginal repair of prolapsed pelvic organs.

Case presentation: A 76-year-old woman with muscle-invasivebladder cancer underwent radical cystectomy 16 years after retropubic positioning of an autologous rectus muscle fascial sling for SUI, with complete symptom resolution. The sling was easily identified and removed en bloc with the bladder and urethra, providing an opportunity to histologicallyevaluate the autologous fascial graft after its long permanence in the new position. Histopathological examination demonstrated increased fibroblastic proliferation and formation of capillaries. A slight separation and an increased waviness of the connective fibers were both evident. An increased vascularity was also apparent, including transverse vessels, with clusters of vessels. A relative inflammatory reaction was present in over 300 cells/10 HPF. All these characteristics indicated viable connective tissue.

Conclusions: AFS remain a valuable surgical option for both primary and recurrent SUI in women, showing high cure rates and low complications in the long-term. The present case, to the best of our knowledge, presents the longest follow-up period of an autologous rectus muscle fascia placed retropubically and its histological evaluation documents characteristics which support its mechanical strength and viability.

Keywords: Muscle fascia, Autologous fascial slings, Stress urinary incontinence, Suburethral slings, Case report

Background

Synthetic mid-urethral slings (MUS) have become the most frequently used surgical intervention for SUI for women [1, 2]

The original AFS technique was first described over a century ago and consisted in the placement of a strip of rectus muscle fascia at the bladder neck. This approach is durable and effective but may lead to the appearance of voiding problems and de novo storage symptoms [3]. A recent Cochrane review analyzed the outcomes between AFS and MUS finding similar effects in terms of continence but a higher rate of complications for the AFS. This review has two major weaknesses. The follow-up takes place after too short a period making it difficult to draw conclusions about the long-term safety

*Correspondence: jacopodurante@live.it
[1] Department of Translational Research and New Technologies in Medicine and Surgery, Section of Urology, University of Pisa, via Paradisa 2, 56126 Pisa, Italy

of MUS. The other major weakness is related to the patient groups which were not well randomized regarding the severity of symptoms [4].

However,of the FDA has recently reviewed the literature and has underlined serious safety and effectiveness concernover the use of surgical mesh for the transvaginal repair of pelvic organ prolapse (POP). Patients treated with syntheticmeshes are subject to mesh related complications and sequelae (10% erosion within 12 months of surgery) and re-operation,and, moreover,the use of synthetic tissue does not appear to provide any added benefit when compared to traditional surgery [5]. Within this lively panorama of literature that seeks to re-evaluate autologous slings with respect to synthetic meshes, we have decided to share the result of a case where an autologous sling has had an extremely long survival rate and long-term effectiveness.

Case presentation

In November 2016 a76-year-old woman underwent radical cystectomy for a muscle invasive bladder cancer (MIBC) in our urology unit. The patient had a history of SUI afterhysterectomy and adnexectomy for an ovarian carcinoma in 1997. SUI was treated with an autologous fascial sling from the rectus muscle in 2000according to McGuire [6] with a complete resolution of the urinary leakage up until September 2016, when the patient returned with urgency and urge incontinence. Cystoscopy was performed, showing multiple papillary lesions at the bladder neck and in the left bladder wall. In October 2016 the patient underwent transurethral bladder resection which revealed a muscle invasive bladder cancer. During the radical cystectomy, performing the section of the urethra, the autologous fascial sling was evidenced and macroscopically it appeared to be extremely well preserved. It was removed en bloc with the bladder and urethra.

The entire surgical specimen was fixed in 10% neutral-buffered formalin. The bladder neck, urethra and sling were isolated, embedded in paraffin and sectioned at 4–5 mm intervals, according to routine procedures. Histologic sections were stained with hematoxylin and eosin to evaluate fiber structure, the number of cells and vascularity. Increased fibroblastic proliferation was evident (Fig. 1), as well as a slight separation of fibers and increased waviness. There was increased vascularity, including transverse vessels relative to thefiber direction, with over 300 cells/10 HPF, with clusters of vessels (Fig. 2), and a modest increase in inflammatory infiltrate consisting mainly of lymphocytes and plasma cells.

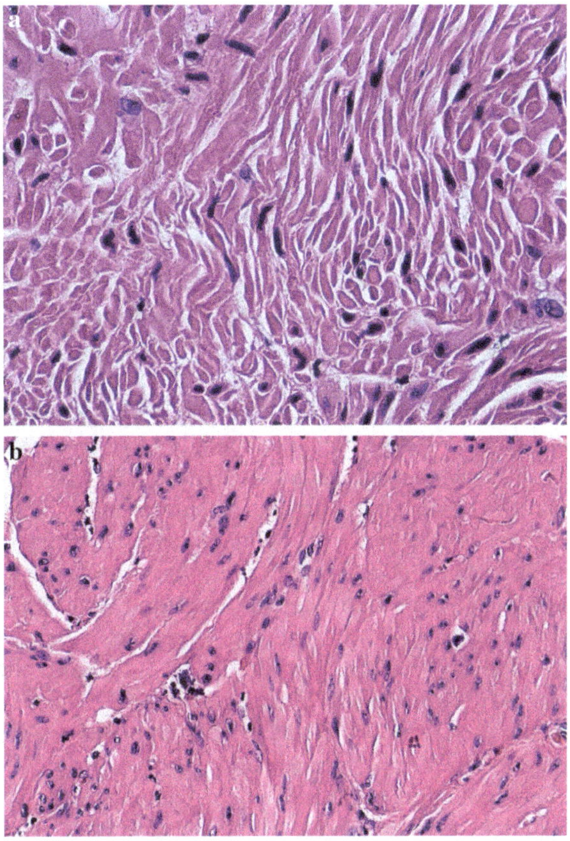

Fig. 1 **a** ×20Hematoxylin-eosin: increased fibroblastic proliferation. **b** ×40Hematoxylin-eosin:increased fibroblastic proliferation

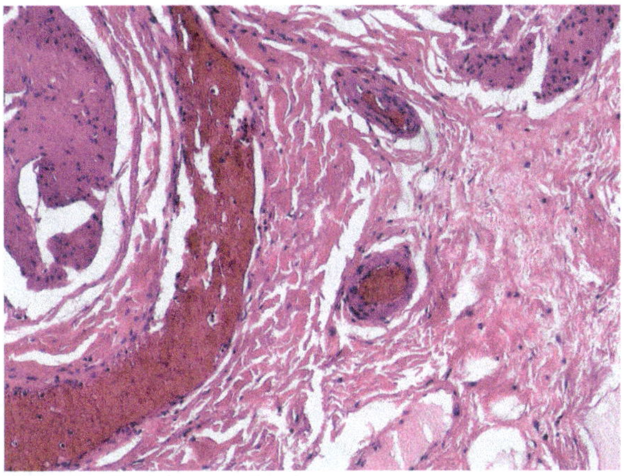

Fig. 2 ×10Hematoxylin-eosin: increased capillary formation and modest inflammatory reaction consisting mainly of lymphocytes and plasma cells

Discussion

Since their introduction, syntheticmid-urethral slings have become the most commonly used surgical intervention for the female SUI, since they require shorter intraoperative and hospitalization times as well a shorter learning curve [3–5]. A recent systematic review by Rehman et al. evaluated the difference between the traditional suburethral sling and other treatments for the mixed urinary incontinence. They found that rectus fascia slings have a better outcome in the first year of follow-up than other biological materials (porcine dermis, lyophilized dura mater, fascia lata and vaginal wall). However, in the review they reported more side effects with the traditional slings than the minivasiveones, when compared to a similar success rate (although the quality of the evidence was very variable in the various studies analyzed). The traditional sling seems to have a better cost-effective rate in comparison to other SUI treatments but not in comparison tosynthetics [7, 8].

Many studies analyzing the outcomes of synthetic mesh lack a long-term follow-up. A recent multicenter trial by Khan et al., however, found that even if there is not enough evidence to judge the long-term success rates between autologous and synthetic sling there is however some evidence that the "dry rate" for an autologous sling could be more durable. In the long term the AFS could be considered at least equivalent to TVT but with a higher success rate after mesh complication [9].

The histological evaluation of the sample taken from our patient demonstrates the scarcity of studies availableon the characteristics of the material used in autologous slings in the long-term. The behavior over time of biological tissues used for reconstructive treatment could be the basis for the success or failure of the application of an autologous sling. Fitzgerald et al. [10] removed non-functioning or obstructive suburethral AFS, between 5 and 18 weeks after placement, and removed only one after a period of 4 years. The latter showedincreased vascularityat histopathology, with connective tissue fibers organized longitudinally.

Animal models can provide useful information on how to integrate autologous tissues in the treatment of SUI or on which they can be most effective. McAdams et al. hypothesized that there may be a benefit in combining an autologous fascial graft and a deltoid flap into murine models [11].

Autologous fascial graft, according to Carvalho et al. seems not to cause inflammatory reaction response in the histologic evaluation on grafted fascia in vocal fold of dog harvested two months from its implantation [12].

The vitality of autologous grafted tissue many years after its implantation is not yet well known. Ahelen et al. hypothesized that there may be a regeneration and normalization, after a long period, of the semitendinosus tendon used for the reconstruction of the cruciate ligament. After an average of 8.4 years, they did not detect significant differences in the histological appearance between the regenerated tissues and those of the contralateral knee that had not been harvested [13].

The greater awareness of the side effects related to the use of synthetic mesh has also made way for stem cells in the treatment of SUI or other diseases in which autologous tissues or synthetic implants are used. In a phase-one clinical study, Choi et al. evaluated the efficacy of a periurethral injection of adipose-derived autologous stem cells. The assessment was based on questionnaires related to continence but also on more objective methods (the functional length of the urethra evaluated with MRI and the measure of maximum urethral closing pressure) and evidenced better continence without indicating serious side effects [14]. Orabi et al. managed to organize cells from the vaginal epithelium and vaginal stroma to form a neovagina that was guided to assemble on a three-dimensional matrix and then implanted in vivo. This study on mouse models shows how an autologous tissue can be used to create a vagina which is functionally and biologically similar to a natural one without using external materials [15].

What is interesting is the search for new surgical techniques which will be able to reduce the invasiveness of autologous slings. In a recent paper Osman et al. have illustrated a new andless invasive technique in which the autologous sling is positioned at the mid-level of the urethra and not at the level of the bladder neck. The midurethral placement of the graft is advantageous since it requires a lesser bladder neck dissection (thus avoiding the bladder base denervation and so lessening risk of detrusor overactivity and storage urinary symptoms), hematoma, bladder injury and fibrosis. This measure would allow patients with primary SUI to be treated with autologous material, thus extending the current indications which use the autologous sling mainly for patients with intrinsic sphincter deficiency or in the recurrences of SUI after a synthetic sling application. An additional benefit is that the learning curve of this technique is relatively short (approximately 20 procedures) [16].

Woodruff et al. evaluated 24 grafts of different origin (polypropylene mesh(PPM), autologous fascia, porcine dermis, cadaveric dermis, cadaveric fascia) removed between 2 and 34 months after implantation. They demonstrated a more marked graft degradation in autologous and cadaveric fascia grafts. The PPM had the greater number of fibroblastic infiltrations but neovascularity was mostly represented in AFS [17]. The histopathological analyses of our ASF highlighted the fibrotic and inflammatory reaction: peripheral infiltration of fibroblasts and the relative inflammatory response, consisting of lymphocytes and plasmacells. There were no signs of degradation. In our opinion, this is strongly linked to the clinical efficacy reported by the patient even after such a long interval after the implant. The AFS degradation finding in Woodruff's study could therefore be linked to the fact that these slings were no longer functional. Therefore a biological degradation of the autologous graft can correspond to a reduction of its efficacy from a clinical point of view. However, it is not known whether other well-functioning AFSs retain histological characteristics of integrity in the long-term. This data would be a useful tool for assessing the long-term reliability of this type of implant.

Discussion and conclusions

The renewed interest in autologous fascial slings in literature is supported both by its long-term efficacy on the symptoms and the reduced need for additional surgical adjustment and mesh-related compliances.

The present case report aims to sustain this new trend of thought and to focus the attention on the autologous sling.

In addition, an autologous fascial sling causes less fibrotic reaction than the synthetic, thus making future surgical treatments easier for SUI and other diseases.

For commercial reasons the evolution of synthetic meshes has been extremely rapid and, since they are associated with a simpler implant technique, they have become the most frequently adopted surgical solution in the treatment of SUI. As a result, this has hindered the evolution and study of autologous tissues and their properties as possible grafts.

The present histologic documentation of the preserved viability and strength of an autologous rectus fascia after being in use for 16 years provides further proof of the viability of this solution in the treatment of SIU.

Abbreviations

AFS: Autologous fascial slings; HPF: High power field; SIU: Stress urinary incontinence; TVT: Transvaginal.

Acknowledgements

Not applicable.

Authors' contributions

JD drafted the manuscript, FM was actively involved in surgical treatment, TF searched the literature, AT and TDV were involved in clinical management, PF performed histopathological studies, CS ideated and revised the manuscript. All Authors have read and approved the final manuscript.

Author details

[1]Department of Translational Research and New Technologies in Medicine and Surgery, Section of Urology, University of Pisa, via Paradisa 2, 56126 Pisa, Italy. [2]Department of Surgical, Medical, Molecular Pathology and Critical Area, Section of Pathology, University of Pisa, via Roma 67, 56124 Pisa, Italy.

References

1. Ogah J, Cody DJ, Rogerson L. Minimallyinvasivesyntheticsuburethral sling operations for stress urinary incontinence in women: a short version Cochrane review. Neurourol Urodyn. 2011;30:284–91. https://doi.org/10.1002/nau.20980.
2. Chughtai BL, Elterman DS, Vertosick E, et al. Midurethral sling is the dominant procedure for female stress urinary incontinence: analysis of case logs from certifying American urologists. J Urol. 2013;82:1267. https://doi.org/10.1016/j.urology.2013.07.040.
3. Ostergard DR. Primary slings for everyone with genuine stress incontinence? The argument against. Int Urogynecol J Pelvic Floor Dysfunct. 1997;8:321–2. https://doi.org/10.1007/BF02765588.
4. Plagakis S, Tse V. The autologous pubovaginal fascial sling: An update in 2019. Low Urin Tract Symptoms. 2020;12(1):2–7. https://doi.org/10.1111/luts.12281.
5. US Food and Drug Administration. UPDATE on serious complications associated with transvaginal placement of surgical mesh for pelvic organ prolapse. FDA Saf Commun. 2011. https://doi.org/10.1007/s00192-011-1581-2.
6. McGuire EJ, Bennet CJ, Konnak JA, Sonda LP, Savastano JA. Experience with pubovaginal slings for urinary incontinernce at the University of Michigan. J Urol. 1987;135:525–9. https://doi.org/10.1016/s0022-5347(17)43246-0.
7. Rodrigues P, Hering F. The role of a surgical learning curve in urethral obstruction following autologous fascial sling: a case-series study. Int Urogynecol J. 2012;23:211–6. https://doi.org/10.1007/s00192-011-1575-0.
8. Rehman H, Bezerra CA, Bruschini H, Cody JD, Aluko P. Traditionalsuburethral slingoperations for urinary incontinence in women. Cochrane Database Syst Rev. 2017;7:CD001754. https://doi.org/10.1002/14651858.
9. Khan ZA, Nambiar A, Morley R, Chapple CR, Emery SJ, Lucas MG. Long-termfollow-up of a multicentre randomised controlled trialcomparingtension-free vaginal tape, xenograft and autologousfascialslings for the treatment of stress urinary incontinence in women. BJU Int. 2015;115:968–77. https://doi.org/10.1111/bju.12851.
10. FitzGerald MP, Mollenhauer J, Brubaker L. The fate of rectus fascia suburethral slings. Am J ObstetGynecol. 2000;183:964–6. https://doi.org/10.1067/mob.2000.107091.
11. McAdams TR, Knudsen KR, Yalamanchi N, Chang J, Goodman SB. Deltoidflapcombined with fascia lata autograft for rotator cuff defects: a histologic study. Knee Surg Sports Traumatol Arthrosc. 2007;15:1144–9. https://doi.org/10.1007/s00167-006-0281-9.
12. Carvalho EGB, Pauna HF, Machado AJ Jr, Nicola EMD, Altemani AMAM, Crespo AN. Evaluation of the grafted fascia in the vocal fold of dogs: a histologic study. J Voice. 2017;31:605–9. https://doi.org/10.1016/j.jvoice.2016.12.022.
13. Åhlén M, Lidén M, Movin T, Papadogiannakis N, Rostgård-Christensen L, Kartus J. Histological evaluation of regenerated semitendinosus tendon a minimum of 6 years after harvest for anterior cruciate ligament reconstruction. Orthop J Sports Med. 2014. https://doi.org/10.1177/2325967114550274.
14. Choi JY, Kim TH, Yang JD, Suh JS, Kwon TG. Adipose-derived regenerative cell injection therapy for postprostatectomy incontinence: aphase I clinical study. Yonsei Med J. 2016;57:1152–8. https://doi.org/10.3349/ymj.2016.57.5.1152.
15. Orabi H, Saba I, Rousseau A, Bolduc S. Novel three-dimensional autologous tissue-engineered vaginal tissues using the self-assembly technique. Transl Res. 2017;180:22–36. https://doi.org/10.1016/j.trsl.2016.07.019.
16. Osman NI, Hillary CJ, Mangera A, Aldamanhoori R, Inman RD, Chapple CR. The midurethral fascial "sling on a string": an alternative to midurethral synthetic tapes in the era of mesh complications. Eur Urol. 2018;74:191–6. https://doi.org/10.1016/j.eururo.2018.04.031.7.
17. Woodruff AJ. Histologic comparison of pubovaginal sling graft materials: a comparative study. Urology. 2008;72(1):85–9. https://doi.org/10.1016/j.urology.2008.03.012.

30

Neonatal circumcision availability in the United States: A physician survey

Ushasi Naha[1], Hans C. Arora[2,3], Ryan F. Walton[2], Ilina Rosoklija[2], Lindsay M. Skibley[4] and Emilie K. Johnson[2,3,5*]

Abstract

Background: A significant proportion of boys present to surgical specialists later in infancy/early childhood for elective operative circumcision despite the higher procedural risks. This study aims to assess physician perspectives on access to neonatal circumcision across the United States and identify potential reasons contributing to disparities in access.

Methods: A cross-sectional survey was electronically distributed to physician members of the Societies for Pediatric Urology and the American Academy of Pediatrics Section on Hospital Medicine. Hospital characteristics and circumcision practices were assessed. Associations between NC availability and institutional characteristics were evaluated using chi-squared testing and multivariable logistic regression. Qualitative analyses of free-text comments were performed.

Results: A total of 367 physicians responded (129 urologists [41%], 188 pediatric hospitalists [59%]). Neonatal circumcision was available at 86% of hospitals represented. On univariate and multivariate analysis, the 50 hospitals that did not offer neonatal circumcision were more likely to be located in the Western region (odds ratio [OR] = 8.33; 95% confidence interval [CI] 3.1–25 vs. Midwest) and in an urban area (OR = 4.2; 95% CI 1.6–10 vs. suburban/rural) compared with hospitals that offered neonatal circumcision. Most common reasons for lack of availability included not a birth hospital (N = 22, 47%), lack of insurance coverage (N = 8, 17%), and low insurance reimbursement (N = 7, 15%). Institutional, regional, or provider availability (68%), insurance/payment (12.4%), and ethics (12.4%) were common themes in the qualitative comments.

Conclusions: Overall availability of neonatal circumcision varied based on hospital characteristics, including geography. Information from this survey will inform development of interventions designed to offer neonatal circumcision equitably and comprehensively.

Keywords: Neonatal, Circumcision, Access, Pediatrics, Pediatric urology

Introduction

Circumcisions are the most commonly performed pediatric surgical procedure [1]. For families who seek circumcision for their sons, health benefits include the decreased risk of urinary tract infections, sexually transmitted infections and penile cancer. These benefits are greatest for boys when the circumcision is performed in the neonatal period [2]. When circumcisions are done beyond the neonatal period, there are higher complication rates [3], and general anesthesia is required, leading to increased risks [4–8] and costs [9, 10].

Over time, neonatal circumcision rates in the United States (US) have modestly declined overall. However, boys with public insurance have had lower rates of circumcision compared to those with private insurance, even when controlling for demographics, geographic region, hospital and year of birth. Additionally, boys from

3
*Correspondence: ekjohnson@luriechildrens.org
Department of Urology, Northwestern University Feinberg School of Medicine, 225 E Chicago Avenue, Box 24, Chicago, IL 60611, USA

lower-income families have lower rates of circumcision in comparison to boys from families with higher income [11]. This suggests that there are barriers in access underlying the differing rates of neonatal circumcision. Indeed, a study of free-standing children's hospitals found that 28% of boys undergoing delayed surgical circumcisions were Black/African–American, and 58% of boys had public insurance [12]. After the defunding of Medicaid coverage for circumcision, state-specific rates of neonatal circumcision decreased by around 20%. In states and years without Medicaid coverage, Black infants had lower odds of undergoing neonatal circumcision [13].

Though prior data indicate differences in neonatal circumcision access by demographic factors including income, insurance type, and race, the precise reasons for these differences have not been identified. Differences in availability and efficiency of neonatal circumcision at birth hospitals may be one factor contributing to the apparent disparity in access to neonatal circumcision. The present study aims to assess physician perspectives on access to neonatal circumcision at hospitals throughout the US, and identify potential underlying reasons contributing to disparities in access to the procedure. Our hypothesis is that neonatal circumcision availability will differ based on the geographic location and by hospital characteristics.

Methods

Overview

A survey study of physicians who practice at hospitals that care for newborns was conducted. The primary outcome was neonatal circumcision availability by hospital. Survey content also aimed to describe features of hospitals that perform newborn circumcision, including those that could contribute to limited circumcision availability at certain times, or for certain patients.

Survey development

A 21-question survey was developed to ascertain hospital characteristics and circumcision practices of institutions that care for newborns across the US (Additional file 1). Hospital characteristics assessed included the teaching and metropolitan status, geographic region and whether the institution was public or private. We also assessed whether hospitals had a standard circumcision protocol used during the birth encounter. Availability of circumcision, including details of time, dates, payment options and specialties that perform circumcisions, as well as circumcision exclusion criteria, were collected. The last question was a free-text question where respondents could add any further comments about the availability of neonatal circumcisions at their institution or in their region. The study was approved by the Ann & Robert H. Lurie Children's Hospital of Chicago Institutional Review Board and the need for obtaining informed consent from subjects was waived (IRB 2020-3505).

Survey distribution

A cross-sectional, anonymous survey was electronically distributed to physician members of the Societies for Pediatric Urology (SPU) and the American Academy of Pediatrics (AAP) Section on Hospital Medicine through organizational email lists. Responses were collected starting on March 31 until May 12, 2020. One reminder email was sent to AAP members and two reminder emails were sent to the SPU email lists. Survey responses were recorded and stored without participant identifiers using REDcap [14].

Analysis

Descriptive statistics were used to summarize survey respondents and characteristics at institutions that perform circumcisions. Univariate comparisons of hospital characteristics and circumcision practices between institutions that do and do not perform circumcisions were performed using Pearson chi-square tests. Multivariable logistic regression was performed to assess adjusted associations between institutional characteristics and circumcision availability. Covariates were initially determined a priori, taking into account the statistical significance of covariates in the univariate analysis. Covariates in the regression model included geographic region, private versus public institution, metropolitan status and teaching status. Regression analyses were displayed using forest plots. All statistical analyses were performed using R 4.0.0 (R Foundation for Statistical Computing, Vienna, Austria) using 95% confidence intervals with two-sided p values < 0.05 considered significant. An inductive, qualitative analysis of free-text comments about neonatal circumcision availability was performed, and key themes were summarized.

Results

Cohort characteristics

A total of 367 physicians (165 pediatric urologists [45%], 202 pediatric hospitalists [55%]; Table 1) responded to the survey, with an estimated response rate of 9.5% (pediatric hospitalists: 6%; pediatric urologists: 23%). Response rates were estimated based on the number of clinicians on the organizational email lists. All completed surveys were included in the analysis. Most respondents (317/367 [86%]) reported neonatal circumcision availability at their institution. The geographic distribution by US region was relatively even (South: 31%, Midwest: 28%, West: 23%, Northeast: 17%). Most respondents worked

Table 1 Univariate analysis of respondents and hospital characteristics

	Total (N = 367)	Circumcisions offered (N = 317)	Circumcisions not offered (N = 50)	*p* value
Region				< 0.001*
Midwest	101 (27.5%)	95 (30.0%)	6 (12.0%)	
Northeast	62 (16.9%)	61 (19.2%)	1 (2.0%)	
South	114 (31.1%)	102 (32.2%)	12 (24.0%)	
West	85 (23.2%)	58 (18.3%)	27 (54.0%)	
Other	4 (1.1%)	1 (0.3%)	3 (6.0%)	
No response	1 (0.3%)	0 (0.0%)	1 (2.0%)	
Type of institution				0.307
Private for profit	36 (9.8%)	29 (9.1%)	7 (14.0%)	
Private non-profit	243 (66.2%)	206 (65.0%)	37 (74.0%)	
Public	69 (18.8%)	63 (19.9%)	6 (12.0%)	
Uncertain	14 (3.8%)	14 (4.4%)	0 (0.0%)	
Other	4 (1.1%)	4 (1.3%)	0 (0.0%)	
No response	1 (0.3%)	1 (0.3%)	0 (0.0%)	
Metropolitan status				0.002*
Suburban/rural	124 (33.8%)	118 (37.2%)	6 (12.0%)	
Urban	241 (65.7%)	197 (62.1%)	44 (88.0%)	
Other	2 (0.5%)	2 (0.6%)	0 (0.0%)	
Teaching status				0.885
Non-teaching	59 (16.1%)	50 (15.8%)	9 (18.0%)	
Teaching	301 (82.0%)	261 (82.3%)	40 (80.0%)	
Don't know/uncertain	5 (1.4%)	4 (1.3%)	1 (2.0%)	
No response	2 (0.5%)	2 (0.6%)	0 (0.0%)	
Respondent specialty				< 0.001*
Pediatric urology	165 (45.0%)	129 (40.7%)	36 (72.0%)	
Pediatric hospitalist	202 (55.0%)	188 (59.3%)	14 (28.0%)	

*Indicates statistical significance

at private, non-profit institutions (66%) in urban settings (66%) that were teaching hospitals (82%).

Comparison of institutions by circumcision availability

Table 1 compares characteristics of respondents and hospitals offering versus not offering neonatal circumcisions. More pediatric hospitalists than pediatric urologists were from institutions that offered circumcisions (59% vs. 41%), whereas 72% of respondents from institutions that did not offer circumcisions were pediatric urologists (vs. 28% pediatric hospitalists; $p<0.001$). A difference by geographic region was also observed: hospitals in the South were most frequently represented among hospitals that offered circumcisions whereas hospitals in the Western region were most represented among hospitals that did not offer circumcisions ($p<0.001$). Urban institutions were more highly represented among hospitals that did not offer circumcisions compared to those that do (88% vs. 62%, respectively, $p=0.002$). On multivariate analysis, the 50 hospitals that did not offer neonatal circumcision were more likely to be located in the Western region (odds ratio [OR] = 8.33; 95% confidence interval [CI] 3.1–25 vs. Midwest), and in an urban area (OR = 4.2; 95% CI 1.6–10 vs. suburban/rural), compared with hospitals that offered the procedure (Fig. 1).

Institutional factors

Table 2 displays characteristics of hospitals that offer neonatal circumcision. A standardized protocol/checklist was available at less than half of hospitals. Many specialties performed circumcisions including Pediatrics (74%), Obstetrics and Gynecology (57%), Pediatric Urology (54%), Family Medicine (31%) and Pediatric Surgery (31%), with variability depending on setting and type of anesthesia (Fig. 2). Pediatric Urology most frequently performed outpatient procedures without or under general anesthesia (56% and 80%, respectively), while Pediatrics most commonly performed circumcisions at the birth encounter without general anesthesia (70%). Hospitals offering neonatal circumcision had more availability

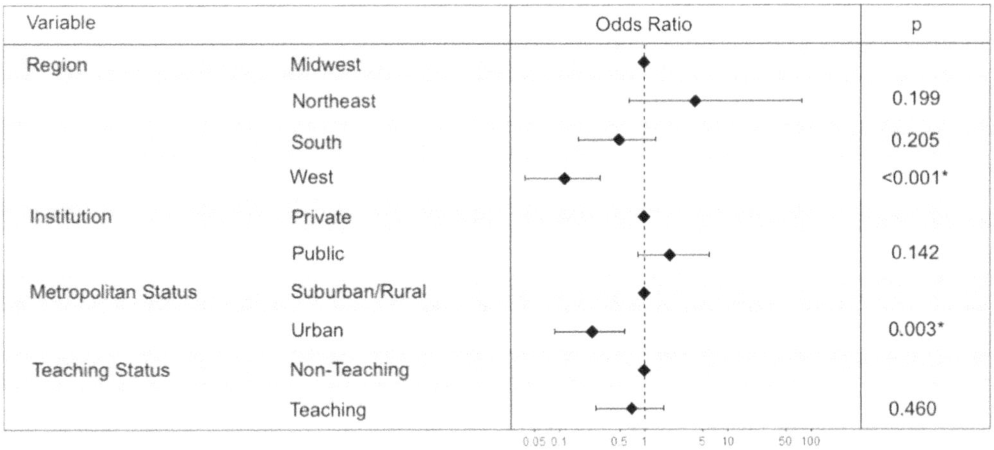

Variable	OR	2.5%	97.5%
Region (reference: Midwest)			
Northeast	4.1	0.48	35.27
South	0.51	0.18	1.44
West	0.12	0.04	0.32
Type of Institution (reference: private)			
Public	2.07	0.78	5.49
Metropolitan Status (reference: suburban/rural)			
Urban	0.24	0.1	0.63
Teaching Status (reference: non-teaching)			
Teaching	0.7	0.28	1.79

Fig. 1 Factors associated with institutions that offer circumcisions

on weekdays versus weekends, and only 21% offered the procedure 24 h per day. Most hospitals reported accepting private insurance (79%) and slightly fewer accepted Medicaid (64%) for neonatal circumcision. Over half (56%) reported that at least some patients paid cash for the procedure.

For the 50 respondents from hospitals that did not offer neonatal circumcision, the most common reasons cited for lack of availability included: not a birth hospital (N = 22, 47%), lack of insurance coverage (N = 8, 17%), and low insurance reimbursement (N = 7, 15%), (Fig. 3).

Qualitative comments

There were 105 free-text comments left by respondents (Table 3) when they were asked, "Do you have any other comments about availability of circumcision at your institution or in your region?". Institutional, regional, or provider availability (N = 71, 68%), insurance and payment (N = 13, 12.4%), and ethics (N = 13, 12.4%) were the most common themes. Within the availability and payment themes, there were varied responses that highlighted either the ease or barriers to neonatal circumcision availability. Regarding ethics, several respondents indicated that they had ethical concerns with performing circumcisions as a routine/elective procedure.

Discussion

This survey of US pediatric urologists and hospitalists indicates that neonatal circumcision availability and practices vary by hospital, region, and specialty. Approximately 1 in 6 respondents were from hospitals that do not offer neonatal circumcision. Multiple specialties performed neonatal circumcisions; pediatric urologists most frequently performed outpatient procedures with or without general anesthesia, and pediatrics most frequently performed circumcisions at the birth encounter without general anesthesia. At institutions that did offer circumcision, availability was most common during the week and during regular business hours. Almost 1 in 3 respondents added free-text comments, indicating general interest in the topic of neonatal circumcision availability. The comments provided additional insight about circumcision availability in their institution or region, provider availability or payment.

Information from the current survey study confirms findings of existing large database investigations about circumcision practice patterns and trends. Regarding

Table 2 Characteristics at institutions that perform circumcisions (N = 317)

Characteristics	N (%)
Standard protocol, checklist, or similar that is used during the birth encounter that includes offering or performing circumcision	
Yes	139 (43.4%)
No	133 (41.6%)
Don't know/unsure	44 (13.8%)
No response	1 (0.3%)
Who must initiate conversations about circumcision?	
Either hospital team or family	250 (78.9%)
Family	20 (6.3%)
Hospital team	10 (3.2%)
Don't know/uncertain	6 (1.9%)
Other	31 (9.8%)
Entity that developed this protocol, checklist, or similar	
Institution	59 (18.4%)
Department	34 (10.6%)
Group practice	21 (6.6%)
Self	6 (1.9%)
Government	1 (0.3%)
Don't know/unsure	106 (33.1%)
Other[a]	6 (1.9%)
No response	84 (26.3%)
Exclusion criteria at birth encounter for neonatal circumcision	
Penile anatomic abnormality (e.g., hypospadias, curvature, buried penis)	312 (97.5%)
Family history of bleeding disorder	233 (72.8%)
Prematurity	47 (14.7%)
Weight limit	38 (11.9%)
Older age at discharge	35 (10.9%)
Neonatal intensive care unit	25 (7.8%)
Other exclusion[b]	48 (15.0%)
Days that neonatal circumcision is available	
Monday	262 (82.6%)
Tuesday	261 (82.3%)
Wednesday	262 (82.6%)
Thursday	261 (82.3%)
Friday	261 (82.3%)
Saturday	246 (77.6%)
Sunday	242 (76.3%)
Don't know/unsure	55 (17.4%)
Times neonatal circumcision is available during birth encounter	
Regular business hours (approximately 08:00 AM–05:00 PM)	165 (51.6%)
24 h per day	67 (20.9%)
Don't know/unsure	56 (17.5%)
Other[c]	25 (7.8%)
No response	4 (1.3%)
Specialty that performs neonatal circumcisions at institution	
Pediatrics	233 (73.5%)
Obstetrics and gynecology	181 (57.1%)
Pediatric urology	170 (53.6%)
Familymedicine	98 (30.9%)
Pediatric surgery	97 (30.6%)

Table 2 (continued)

Characteristics	N (%)
Adult urology	9 (2.8%)
Other[d]	7 (2.2%)
Don't know/unsure	3 (0.9%)
Payment for neonatal circumcision	
Private insurance	251 (79.4%)
Medicaid	205 (64.9%)
Self-pay/cash	177 (56.0%)
Don't know/unsure	53 (16.8%)
Other[e]	6 (1.9%)

[a] Other entities: labor and delivery department, individual hospital unit, and pediatric urology

[b] Other exclusions: refusal of Vitamin K, heart murmurs, hyperbilirubinemia, oxygen monitoring and poor feeding

[c] Other time ranges: 8 am–9 am, 8 am–10 pm, every day at noon, only in the mornings and based on the availability of providers performing circumcisions,

[d] Other specialties: general surgery, hospitalist (adult, pediatric), midwife, neonatology, nurse practitioner

[e] Other payments: covered benefit through plan, hospital writes off the cost or covers if Medicaid, military, and Tricare

circumcision practitioner specialty, the present study findings are similar to a recent study using Pediatric Health Information Systems data by Many et al. which showed that pediatrics, obstetrics-gynecology, and perinatal medicine most commonly performed neonatal circumcisions. Beyond the neonatal period, pediatric urologists most commonly performed circumcisions in the study by Many [15], a finding also echoed in our survey. The regional and insurance coverage trends indicated by the present survey are also aligned with prior studies using national databases. While American Academy of Pediatrics recommends coverage for all desired neonatal circumcisions [2], a recent study by Navia et al. shows that male infants with private insurance had higher rates of neonatal circumcision [13]. Our study respondents indicate that private insurance is more frequently accepted as payment for neonatal circumcision, and that some families pay cash; thus financial barriers to desired circumcisions appear to exist for families with fewer financial resources.

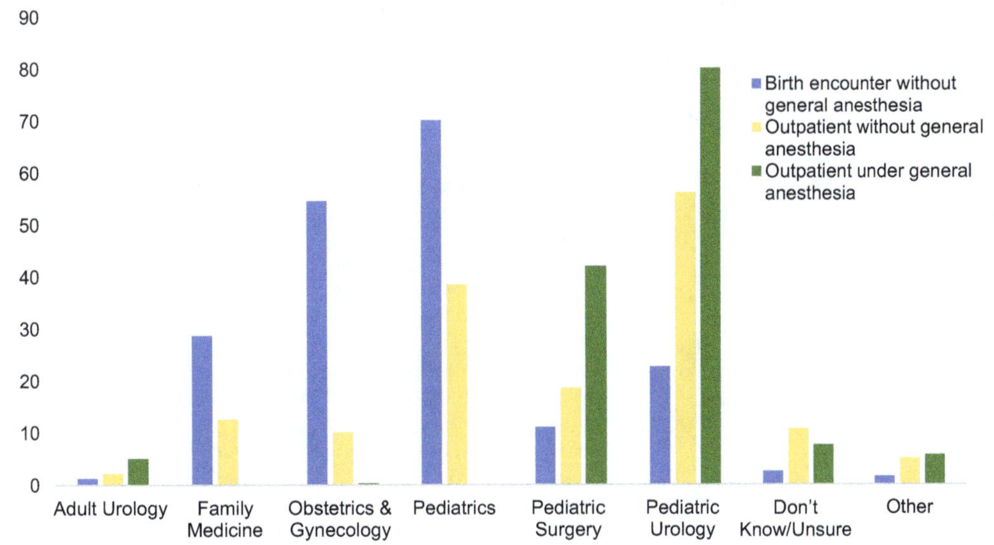

Fig. 2 Specialties that perform circumcisions (N = 317)

The present study also adds the clinician perspective to data from prior parent surveys about newborn circumcision access and reasons for delay. In the present physician survey, the most common reasons neonatal circumcision was not offered included the institution was not a birth hospital, the procedure was not covered by insurance,

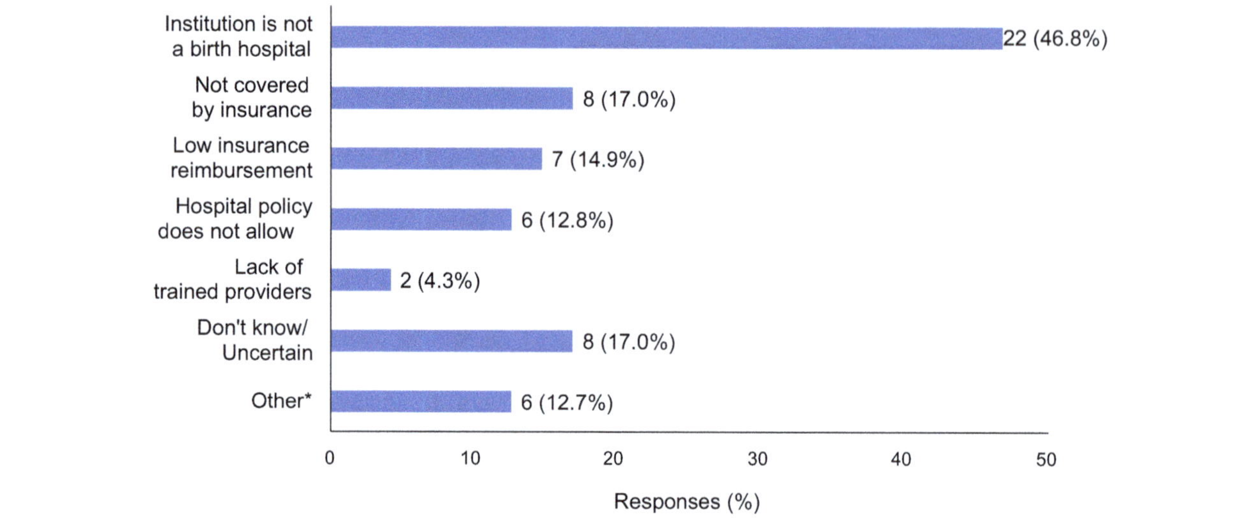

Fig. 3 Reasons institutions do not offer neonatal circumcisions. *Other reasons included high inpatient volume (1), high facility charges (1) and because providers/specialties stopped offering (2)

Table 3 Themes of respondents' free-text comments (N = 105)

Theme	Frequency	Representative auotation
Circumcision availability at institution or region	41 (39.0%)	*"If a family wants to have it done it is easy to get it performed"* *"There are no in-hospital postpartum circumcisions in the state of Nevada"*
Provider availability	30 (28.6%)	*"Providers can opt out of requested circumcision. This is increasing and parents are left to find circumcision services"* *"I get a lot of outpatient referrals because the rounding OB wasn't 'comfortable' performing circs or logistically there wasn't time to have it done before the family was discharged."*
Insurance and payment	13 (12.4%)	*"The major limitation is financial - may families can not afford to self-pay, and Medicaid and most private insurances do not cover neonatal circumcisions in our state."* *"...we accept Medicaid reimbursement so patients then don't have to pay anything. We really [don't] let it [be] known too much that we do [them] in the office and don't charge Medicaid because it would be too many coming."*
Ethics and personal opinions	13 (12.4%)	*"If this is being performed for cosmetic reasons only, it should not be permitted"* *"Just laying out my own bias that we should not do these (routine elective) procedures anymore. Sure there are indications and personal/cultural reasons but they could be outpatient."*
Circumcision eligibility	11 (10.5%)	*"Excluded if family refuses Vitamin K at birth"* *"Some OBs will not do the circumcision, for prematurity (arbitrary cutoff), if the penis is too small, or if they are NICU."*
Uncertainty about circumcision practices	6 (5.7%)	*"Unfortunately, not sure of exact weight limit at my institution"* *"Unsure what the practice is for premature infants at my institution"*

and low insurance reimbursement. Similarly, Jacobson et al. found that among patients seeking elective circumcision, one of the most common reasons for delay in desired neonatal circumcision in the Chicago area was that the hospital or physician did not perform neonatal circumcision; additional factors included prematurity, penile abnormality and low birth weight [16]. A 2016 survey of parents in San Antonio seeking delayed circumcision for boys less than 2 years old reported reasons for delay of circumcision beyond the newborn period included impaired proceduralist availability and lack of circumcision availability at the birth hospital [17].

Our study results reinforce findings in the larger body of literature that specialty/institutional availability and payment coverage are crucial factors in determining access to neonatal circumcision. To gain a more comprehensive understanding of why certain institutions experience limited circumcision availability, we are currently conducting a qualitative interview-based study of clinicians who perform circumcisions about this topic. Future studies will also focus on the development of efficient neonatal circumcision workflows for different hospital types and determine the most optimal recommendations for public and private insurance coverage of neonatal circumcision.

While the current study provides an important physician perspective on the topic of access to neonatal circumcision, there are study limitations. The survey response was relatively low, particularly amongst pediatric hospitalists, which could limit generalizability of findings. However, findings largely align with previous studies about both circumcision trends and reasons for difficulty with access, suggesting the validity of the findings. Also, percentage of survey respondents by region relatively closely align to 2019 US Census data [18]. Respondents only included pediatric urologists and pediatricians, and therefore does not represent all specialties that perform circumcisions. For some survey questions, around 15–25% of respondents were uncertain or did not respond. As such, insight about certain subtopics was suboptimal, including questions about a standardized protocol, exclusion criteria for neonatal circumcision, days of the week that circumcision were available, and reasons that institutions did not offer neonatal circumcision. Limited demographic information was ascertained for the sake of brevity and to maintain the anonymity of respondents. Therefore, some respondents could represent the same institutions, thus creating redundancy in responses.

Conclusions

The availability of neonatal circumcision varies based on hospital characteristics, including geographic location. Specialties that perform neonatal circumcision depend on setting and type of anesthesia used. Follow up research is currently focused on the institutional level to better understand potential local barriers to neonatal circumcision availability. The eventual goal is the creation of hospital-based and financial incentive structural strategies to ensure equitable access for neonatal circumcisions.

Abbreviations

AAP: American academy of pediatrics; CI: Confidence interval; OR: Odds ratio; SPU: Societies for pediatric urology; US: United States.

Acknowledgements

None.

Authors' contributions

EKJ, IR and HA conceived of the research project, with contribution from LS. EKJ supervised UN to analyze and interpret this data, and UN drafted the initial the manuscript. RFW built the survey, distributed the survey to participants via REDCap and assisted with manuscript drafting. All authors contributed to results interpretation, reviewed and edited the manuscript and approved of the final version.

Competing interests

The authors declare that they have no competing interests.

Author details

University of Illinois College of Medicine, Chicago, USA. [2]Division of Urology, Ann & Robert H. Lurie Children's Hospital of Chicago, Chicago, USA. [3]Department of Urology, Northwestern University Feinberg School of Medicine, 225 E Chicago Avenue, Box 24, Chicago, IL 60611, USA. [4]Department of Pediatrics, Northwestern University Feinberg School of Medicine, Chicago, USA. [5]Center for Health Services and Outcomes Research, Northwestern University Feinberg School of Medicine, Chicago, USA.

References

1. Pfuntner A, Wier LM, Stocks C. Most frequent conditions in U.S. Hospitals, 2010: statistical brief #148. 2006.
2. Blank S, Brady M, Buerk E, Carlo W, Diekema D, Freedman A, et al. Male circumcision. Pediatrics. 2012. https://doi.org/10.1542/peds.2012-1990.
3. El Bcheraoui C, Zhang X, Cooper CS, Rose CE, Kilmarx PH, Chen RT. Rates of adverse events associated with male circumcision in US medical settings, 2001 to 2010. JAMA Pediatr. 2014;168:625–34. https://doi.org/10.1001/jamapediatrics.2013.5414.
4. Rappaport BA, Suresh S, Hertz S, Evers AS, Orser BA. Anesthetic neurotoxicity—clinical implications of animal models. N Engl J Med. 2015;372:796–7. https://doi.org/10.1056/nejmp1414786.
5. Mellon RD, Simone AF, Rappaport BA. Use of anesthetic agents in neonates and young children. Anesth Analg. 2007;104:509–20. https://doi.org/10.1213/01.ane.0000255729.96438.b0.
6. Bhananker SM, Ramamoorthy C, Geiduschek JM, Posner KL, Domino KB, Haberkern CM, et al. Anesthesia-related cardiac arrest in children: update from the pediatric perioperative cardiac arrest registry. Anesth Analg. 2007;105:344–50. https://doi.org/10.1213/01.ane.0000268712.00756.dd.
7. Bordet F, Allaouchiche B, Lansiaux S, Combet S, Pouyau A, Taylor P, et al. Risk factors for airway complications during general anaesthesia in paediatric patients. Paediatr Anaesth 2002;12:762–9. https://doi.org/10.1046/j.1460-9592.2002.00987.x.
8. Cronjé L. A review of paediatric anaesthetic-related mortality, serious adverse events and critical incidents. S Afr J Anaesth Analg. 2015;21:147–53. https://doi.org/10.1080/22201181.2015.1119503.
9. Schoen EJ, Colby CJ, To TT. Cost analysis of neonatal circumcision in a large health maintenance organization. J Urol 2006;175:1111–5. https://doi.org/10.1016/S0022-5347(05)00399-X.
10. Hart-Cooper GD, Tao G, Stock JA, Hoover KW. Circumcision of privately insured males aged 0 to 18 years in the United States. Pediatrics 2014;134:950–6. https://doi.org/10.1542/peds.2014-1007.
11. Jacobson DL, Balmert LC, Holl JL, Rosoklija I, Davis MM, Johnson EK. Nationwide circumcision trends: 2003 to 2016. J Urol. 2021;205:257–63. https://doi.org/10.1097/JU.0000000000001316.
12. Roth JD, Keenan AC, Carroll AE, Rink RC, Cain MP, Whittam BM, et al. Readmission characteristics of elective pediatric circumcisions using large-scale administrative data. J Pediatr Urol. 2016;12:27.e1-27.e6. https://doi.org/10.1016/j.jpurol.2015.10.006.
13. Navia MZ, Jacobson DL, Balmert LC, Rosoklija I, Holl JL, Davis MM, et al. State-level public insurance coverage and neonatal circumcision rates. Pediatrics. 2020. https://doi.org/10.1542/peds.2020-1475.
14. Harris PA, Taylor R, Thielke R, Payne J, Gonzalez N, Conde JG. Research electronic data capture (REDCap)-a metadata-driven methodology and workflow process for providing translational research informatics support. J Biomed Inform. 2009;42:377–81. https://doi.org/10.1016/j.jbi.2008.08.010.
15. Many BT, Rizeq YK, Vacek J, Cheon EC, Johnson E, Hu YY, et al. A contemporary snapshot of circumcision in US children's hospitals. J Pediatr Surg 2020;55:1134–8. https://doi.org/10.1016/j.jpedsurg.2020.02.031

16. Jacobson DL, D'Oro A, Abdullah F, Barsness KA, Liu DB, Maizels M, et al. Caregiver reported reasons for delay of neonatal circumcision. Urology. 2020;140:143–9. https://doi.org/10.1016/j.urology.2020.01.043.
17. Otto R, Evans G, Boniquit C, Peppas D, Leslie J. Why desired newborn circumcisions are not performed: a survey. Urology. 2016;97:188–93. https://doi.org/10.1016/j.urology.2016.06.054.
18. United States Population Growth by Region [cited 2021 October 1]. Available from: https://www.census.gov/popclock/data_tables.php?component=growth.

Permissions

All chapters in this book were first published by BioMed Central; hereby published with permission under the Creative Commons Attribution License or equivalent. Every chapter published in this book has been scrutinized by our experts. Their significance has been extensively debated. The topics covered herein carry significant findings which will fuel the growth of the discipline. They may even be implemented as practical applications or may be referred to as a beginning point for another development.

The contributors of this book come from diverse backgrounds, making this book a truly international effort. This book will bring forth new frontiers with its revolutionizing research information and detailed analysis of the nascent developments around the world.

We would like to thank all the contributing authors for lending their expertise to make the book truly unique. They have played a crucial role in the development of this book. Without their invaluable contributions this book wouldn't have been possible. They have made vital efforts to compile up to date information on the varied aspects of this subject to make this book a valuable addition to the collection of many professionals and students.

This book was conceptualized with the vision of imparting up-to-date information and advanced data in this field. To ensure the same, a matchless editorial board was set up. Every individual on the board went through rigorous rounds of assessment to prove their worth. After which they invested a large part of their time researching and compiling the most relevant data for our readers.

The editorial board has been involved in producing this book since its inception. They have spent rigorous hours researching and exploring the diverse topics which have resulted in the successful publishing of this book. They have passed on their knowledge of decades through this book. To expedite this challenging task, the publisher supported the team at every step. A small team of assistant editors was also appointed to further simplify the editing procedure and attain best results for the readers.

Apart from the editorial board, the designing team has also invested a significant amount of their time in understanding the subject and creating the most relevant covers. They scrutinized every image to scout for the most suitable representation of the subject and create an appropriate cover for the book.

The publishing team has been an ardent support to the editorial, designing and production team. Their endless efforts to recruit the best for this project, has resulted in the accomplishment of this book. They are a veteran in the field of academics and their pool of knowledge is as vast as their experience in printing. Their expertise and guidance has proved useful at every step. Their uncompromising quality standards have made this book an exceptional effort. Their encouragement from time to time has been an inspiration for everyone.

The publisher and the editorial board hope that this book will prove to be a valuable piece of knowledge for researchers, students, practitioners and scholars across the globe.

List of Contributors

Li Wan, Shucheng Liu, Mingyong Li, Libo Chen, Zhengwu Hou and Wang Zhang
Department of Urology, The First Affiliated Hospital of University of South China, Hengyang 421001, China

Qing Li
Department of Urology, The Fifth Affiliated Hospital of Southern Medical University, Guangzhou 510900, China

Ken Batai, Aye Lwin and Joel T. Funk
Department of Urology, The University of Arizona, 1501 N Campbell Ave, Tucson, AZ 85724-5077, USA

Michael Phung
Department of Urology, University of California Los Angeles, 10833 Le Conte Avenue, Los Angeles, CA 90095-1738, USA

Robert Bell
Department of Pathology and Immunology, Washington University in St. Louis, 660 S Euclid Ave, Campus, St. Louis, MO 63110, USA

Kieran A. Hynes
Department of Surgery, University of Mississippi Medical Center, 2500 N State St, Jackson, MS 39216, USA

Elinora Price
Department of Surgery, University of Arizona, 1501 N. Campbell Ave., Tucson, AZ 85724, USA

Karleen M. Meiklejohn and Erika R. Bracamonte
Department of Pathology, University of Arizona, 1501 N. Campbell Ave., Tucson, AZ 85724, USA

Zoë G. Baker, Arthi Hannallah and Melissa Trabold
Division of Urology, Children's Hospital Los Angeles, Los Angeles, CA, USA

Andy Y. Chang, S. Scott Sparks, Roger De Filippo and Evalynn Vasquez
Division of Urology, Children's Hospital Los Angeles, Los Angeles, CA, USA
Keck School of Medicine of Medicine of USC, University of Southern California, Los Angeles, CA, USA

Danielle Estell
Keck School of Medicine of Medicine of USC, University of Southern California, Los Angeles, CA, USA

Cherry Deng
Thomas J. Long School of Pharmacy, University of the Pacific, Stockton, CA, USA

Adam Cole, Jaya Telang, Tae-Kyung Kim, Kavya Swarna, Ji Qi, Casey Dauw, William Roberts, John Hollingsworth and Khurshid R. Ghani
Department of Urology, University of Michigan, Ann Arbor, MI 48103, USA

Brian Seifman
Michigan Institute of Urology, West Bloomfield, MI 48322, USA

Mazen Abdelhady
Detroit Medical Center, Department of Urology, Detroit, MI 48201, USA

Xiang Ren
Graduate School, Shanxi Medical University, Taiyuan 030000, China

Jiwen Shang
Graduate School, Shanxi Medical University, Taiyuan 030000, China
Department of Urology, Shanxi Bethune Hospital, No. 99 Longcheng Street, Taiyuan 030032, Shanxi, China

Ruimin Ren, Huajun Zhang and Xue Yao
Department of Urology, Shanxi Bethune Hospital, No. 99 Longcheng Street, Taiyuan 030032, Shanxi, China

Katsuya Hikita, Masashi Honda, Shogo Teraoka, Ryoma Nishikawa, Yuske Kimura, Panagiota Tsounapi, Hideto Iwamoto, Shuichi Morizane and Atsushi Takenaka
Division of Urology, Department of Surgery, Faculty of Medicine, Tottori University, 36-1 Nishicho, Yonago, Japan

K. Sisa and S. Huoponen
Perioperative Services, Intensive Care and Pain Medicine, Turku University Hospital, Turku, Finland

H. Antila, T. I. Saari and P. Uusalo
Perioperative Services, Intensive Care and Pain Medicine, Turku University Hospital, Turku, Finland
Department of Anaesthesiology and Intensive Care, University of Turku, Kiinamyllynkatu 4-8, Turku, Finland

O. Ettala
Department of Urology, University of Turku, Turku, Finland

Yi-Zhong Chen
Department of Urology, MacKay Memorial Hospital, No. 92, Sec. 2, Zhongshan N. Rd., Zhongshan Dist., Taipei 104, Taiwan

Wun-Rong Lin, Yung-Chiong Chow and Wei-Kung Tsai
Department of Urology, MacKay Memorial Hospital, No. 92, Sec. 2, Zhongshan N. Rd., Zhongshan Dist., Taipei 104, Taiwan
School of Medicine, MacKay Medical College, New Taipei City, Taiwan

Marcelo Chen
Department of Urology, MacKay Memorial Hospital, No. 92, Sec. 2, Zhongshan N. Rd., Zhongshan Dist., Taipei 104, Taiwan
School of Medicine, MacKay Medical College, New Taipei City, Taiwan
Department of Cosmetic Applications and Management, MacKay Junior College of Medicine, Nursing and Management, Taipei, Taiwan

Allen W. Chiu
Department of Urology, MacKay Memorial Hospital, No. 92, Sec. 2, Zhongshan N. Rd., Zhongshan Dist., Taipei 104, Taiwan
School of Medicine, MacKay Medical College, New Taipei City, Taiwan
School of Medicine, National Yang-Ming University, Taipei, Taiwan

Qi Wang, Liang Tang, Liangkuan Bi, Jie Min, Lu Fang, Wei Sun and Dexin Yu
Department of Urology, The Second Affiliated Hospital of Anhui Medical University, Hefei, China

Jing Shen and Luke Vale
Population Health Sciences Institute, Newcastle University, Newcastle upon Tyne, UK

Beatriz Goulao
Health Services Research Unit, University of Aberdeen, Aberdeen, UK

Paul Whybrow
Hull York Medical School, University of Hull, Hull, UK

Stephen Payne
Central Manchester Hospitals NHS Foundation Trust, Manchester, UK

Nick Watkin
Department of Urology, St George's University of London, London, UK

Shigenori Kakutani
Department of Urology, Chiba Tokushukai Hospital, Chiba, Japan
Department of Urology, Graduate School of Medicine, The University of Tokyo, 7-3-1 Hongo, Bunkyo-Ku, Tokyo 113-8655, Japan

Yuta Yamada, Yuji Hakozaki, Naoki Kimura, Taro Teshima, Yoshiyuki Akiyama, Yusuke Sato, Taketo Kawai, Daisuke Yamada and Haruki Kume
Department of Urology, Graduate School of Medicine, The University of Tokyo, 7-3-1 Hongo, Bunkyo-Ku, Tokyo 113-8655, Japan

Yuta Takeshima
Division of Innovative Cancer Therapy, Advanced Research Center, The Institute of Medical Science, The University of Tokyo, Minato-Ku, Tokyo, Japan

Tetsuya Fujimura
Department of Urology, Jichi Medical University, Tochigi, Japan

Shoichi Nagamoto and Yutaka Enomoto
Department of Urology, Mitsui Memorial Hospital, Tokyo, Japan

Weinan Chen, Liulin Xiong and Xiongjun Ye
Urology and Lithotripsy Center, Peking University People's Hospital, Peking University, 133 Fuchengmen Inner Street, Xicheng District, Beijing 100034, People's Republic of China
Peking University Applied Lithotripsy Institute, Peking University, Beijing 100034, China

Jingjun Zhang
Department of Urology, Peking University BinHai Hospital (Fifth Tianjin Central Hospital), Tianjin 300450, China

Won Tae Kim, Ho Won Kang, Yong-June Kim, Sang Cheol Lee, Wun-Jae Kim and Seok Joong Yun
Department of Urology, College of Medicine, Chungbuk National University, 62, Kaeshin-dong, Heungduk-ku, Cheongju, Chungbuk 361-711, South Korea
Department of Urology, Chungbuk National University Hospital, Cheongju, South Korea

Sung Pil Seo
Department of Urology, Chungbuk National University Hospital, Cheongju, South Korea

Bum Sang Cho
Department of Radiology, College of Medicine, Chungbuk National University, Cheongju, South Korea

Yun Sok Ha and Tae Gyun Kwon
Department of Urology, College of Medicine, Kyungpook National University, Daegu, South Korea

Jinsung Park
Department of Urology, College of Medicine, Eulji University, Daejeon, South Korea

Seung Chol Park
Department of Urology, College of Medicine, Won Kang University, Iksan, South Korea

Young Beom Jeong
Department of Urology, College of Medicine, Jeonbuk National University, Jeonju, South Korea

Taek Won Kang
Department of Urology, College of Medicine, Jeonnam National University, Kwangju, South Korea

Sung-Woo Park
Department of Urology, College of Medicine, Pusan National University, Pusan, South Korea

Xue Dong, Dongnv Wang, Huangqi Zhang, Shuzong You, Wenting Pan and Wenbin Ji
Department of Radiology, Taizhou Hospital, Zhejiang University, Taizhou 318000, Zhejiang, China

Chaoqian Chen
Department of Urology, Taizhou Hospital of Zhejiang Province, Taizhou 318000, Zhejiang, China

Hongjie Hu
Department of Radiology, School of Medicine, Sir Run Run Shaw Hospital, Zhejiang University, Hangzhou 310023, Zhejiang, China

Peipei Pang
Department of Pharmaceuticals Diagnosis, GE Healthcare, Hangzhou, China

Qinxin Zhao, Feiya Yang, Sujun Han and Nianzeng Xing
Department of Urology, National Cancer Center/ National Clinical Research Center for Cancer/Cancer Hospital, Chinese Academy of Medical Sciences and Peking Union Medical College, Beijing, People's Republic of China

Dongdong Han
Department of Urology, National Cancer Center/ National Clinical Research Center for Cancer/Cancer Hospital, Chinese Academy of Medical Sciences and Peking Union Medical College, Beijing, People's Republic of China
Department of Urology, Beijing Chaoyang Hospital, Capital Medical University, Beijing, People's Republic of China

John Culhane and Johar Raza Syed
Department of Trauma, Saint Louis University, 1008 Spring Ave, Saint Louis, MO 63110, USA

Sameer Siddiqui
Department of Urology, Saint Louis University, 1008 Spring Ave, Saint Louis, MO 63110, USA

Wei Wang, Xiaoshuai Gao, Jixiang Chen, Zhenghuan Liu, Liao Peng and Xin Wei
Department of Urology, Institute of Urology, West China Hospital, Sichuan University, No. 37 Guo Xue Xiang, Chengdu, Sichuan 610041, People's Republic of China

Ling Zhu and Yan Huang
Health Management Center, West China Hospital, Sichuan University, Chengdu, China

Zhenghao Wang, Ye Zhou, Liping Gou and Xiaofeng Zheng
Department of Endocrinology and Metabolism, Center for Diabetes and Metabolism Research, West China Hospital, Sichuan University, Chengdu, China

Xiaoqian Ying and Limin Liao
Department of Urology, Beijing Boai Hospital, China Rehabilitation Research Centre; School of Rehabilitation of Capital Medical University, No 10. Jiaomen Beilu, Fengtai District, Beijing 100068, China

Jianpo Zhai, Guanglin Huang and Libo Man
Department of Urology, Beijing Jishuitan Hospital, No. 68, Huinanbei Road, Changping District, Beijing 100096, China

Danhui Zhao, Guoqiang Yan and Chengai Wu
Beijing Research Institute of Traumatology and Orthopaedics, No. 31 Xinjiekou East Street, Xicheng District, Beijing 100035, China

Jun Liu, Jiayi Lan, Yang Hong, Xiaobo Huang and Bo Yang
Urology and Lithotripsy Center, Peking University People's Hospital, 133 Fuchengmen Inner Street, Xicheng District, Beijing 100034, People's Republic of China
Peking University Applied Lithotripsy Institute, Peking University, Beijing 100034, People's Republic of China

Qingya Yang
Department of Urology, Qilu Hospital (Qingdao), Cheeloo College of Medicine, Shandong University, Qingdao 266035, People's Republic of China

Xuwei Lu
Department of Urology, Minhang Hospital, Fudan University, Shanghai 201199, China
Department of Urology, Zhongshan Hospital, Fudan University, Fenglin Rd 130, Shanghai 200032, China

Chang He, Fan Yang, Zhuifeng Guo, Jiaqi Huang, Minke He and Jiawen Wu
Department of Urology, Minhang Hospital, Fudan University, Shanghai 201199, China

Sihong Zhang, Jianming Guo and Hang Wang
Department of Urology, Zhongshan Hospital, Fudan University, Fenglin Rd 130, Shanghai 200032, China

Xia Sheng
Department of Pathology, Minhang Hospital, Fudan University, Shanghai 201199, China

Wenyao Lin and Jie Cheng
Department of Urology, Xuhui Hospital, Fudan University, Shanghai 200031, China

Xiaochuan Wang, Yu Zhang, Fengbo Zhang, Zhengguo Ji, Peiqian Yang and Ye Tian
Department of Urology, Capital Medical University Affiliated Beijing Friendship Hospital, No. 95, Yongan Road, Xicheng District, Beijing, People's Republic of China

Stephan Buse
Department of Urology, Alfried Krupp Krankenhaus, Hellweg 100, 45276 Essen, Germany
Department of Urology and Paediatric Urology, University Medical Center, Johannes-Gutenberg-University, Mainz, Germany

Axel Haferkamp
Department of Urology and Paediatric Urology, University Medical Center, Johannes-Gutenberg-University, Mainz, Germany

Assen Alexandrov
Landesklinikum Wiener Neustadt, Vienna, Austria

Elio Mazzone
Division of Oncology/Unit of Urology, URI, IRCCS Ospedale San Raffaele, Milan, Italy
Vita-Salute San Raffaele University, Milan, Italy

Alexandre Mottrie
Department of Urology, OLV Aalst, Aalst, Belgium
ORSI Academy, Melle, Belgium

Mohammed El Imam M. Ahmed and Sami Mahjoub Taha Awad
Department of Surgery, Faculty of Medicine, University of Gezira, Wad Medani, Gezira State, Sudan
Department of Urology, Gezira Hospital for Kidney Disease and Surgery, Wad Medani, Gezira State, Sudan

Mohamed Daffalla-Awadalla Gismalla
Department of Surgery, Faculty of Medicine, University of Gezira, Wad Medani, Gezira State, Sudan

Yassin Mohamed Osman Abdalla
Department of Urology, Gezira Hospital for Kidney Disease and Surgery, Wad Medani, Gezira State, Sudan

Musab Abdalla M. Ahmed
Department of Urology, Gezira Hospital for Kidney Disease and Surgery, Wad Medani, Gezira State, Sudan
Sudan Medical Specialization Board, Khartoum, Sudan

Hai Lin, Yu-Yun Wang, Shi-Bing Li, Ze-Ting Chen and Liang-Ju Su
Department of Pediatric Surgery, Hainan General Hospital (Hainan Affiliated Hospital of Hainan Medical University), Xiuying District, Haikou 570311, Hainan, People's Republic of China

Federico Soria
Endoscopy-Endourology Department, Jesús Usón Minimally Invasive Surgery Centre Foundation, Carretera N-521, Km. 41.8, C.P.10071 Cáceres, Spain

Julia E. de La Cruz
Endoscopy-Endourology Department, Jesús Usón Minimally Invasive Surgery Centre Foundation, Cáceres, Spain

Juan Pablo Caballero-Romeu
Urology Department, Alicante University General Hospital, Alicante Institute for Health and Biomedical Research (ISABIAL Foundation), Alicante, Spain

Manuel Pamplona
Urology Department, 12 de Octubre University Hospital, Madrid, Spain

Daniel Pérez-Fentes
University Hospital Santiago de Compostela, Santiago de Compostela, Spain

Luis Resel-Folskerma
Urology Department, University Hospital Clínico San Carlos, Madrid, Spain

Francisco M. Sanchez-Margallo
Jesús Usón Minimally Invasive Surgery Centre Foundation, Cáceres, Spain

Hannah Botkin, Brian Barnes and Amy Pearlman
University of Iowa Hospitals and Clinics, 200 Hawkins Drive, Iowa City, IA 52242, USA

Jacopo Durante, Francesca Manassero, Tiziana Fidecicchi, Alessio Tognarelli, Tommaso Di Vico and Cesare Selli
Department of Translational Research and New Technologies in Medicine and Surgery, Section of Urology, University of Pisa, via Paradisa 2, 56126 Pisa, Italy

Pinuccia Faviana
Department of Surgical, Medical, Molecular Pathology and Critical Area, Section of Pathology, University of Pisa, via Roma 67, 56124 Pisa, Italy

Ushasi Naha
University of Illinois College of Medicine, Chicago, USA

Ryan F. Walton and Ilina Rosoklija
Division of Urology, Ann & Robert H. Lurie Children's Hospital of Chicago, Chicago, USA

Hans C. Arora
Division of Urology, Ann & Robert H. Lurie Children's Hospital of Chicago, Chicago, USA
Department of Urology, Northwestern University Feinberg School of Medicine, 225 E Chicago Avenue, Chicago, IL 60611, USA

Lindsay M. Skibley
Department of Pediatrics, Northwestern University Feinberg School of Medicine, Chicago, USA

Emilie K. Johnson
Division of Urology, Ann & Robert H. Lurie Children's Hospital of Chicago, Chicago, USA
Department of Urology, Northwestern University Feinberg School of Medicine, 225 E Chicago Avenue, Chicago, IL 60611, USA
Center for Health Services and Outcomes Research, Northwestern University Feinberg School of Medicine, Chicago, USA

Index

www.ingramcontent.com/pod-product-compliance
Lightning Source LLC
LaVergne TN
LVHW082217200926
848484LV00008B/2268